Child Refugee and Migrant Health

Christian Harkensee · Karen Olness
B. Emily Esmaili
Editors

Child Refugee and Migrant Health

A Manual for Health Professionals

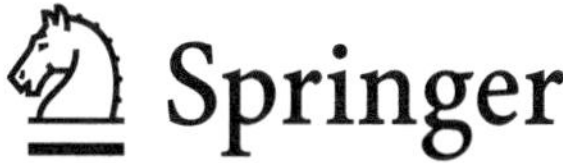
Springer

Editors
Christian Harkensee
Queen Elizabeth Hospital
Gateshead
UK

Karen Olness
Department of Pediatrics
Case Western Reserve University
Cleveland, OH
USA

B. Emily Esmaili
Duke Global Health Institute
Duke University
Durham, NC
USA

Lincoln Community Health Center,
Durham, NC
USA

ISBN 978-3-030-74908-8   ISBN 978-3-030-74906-4   (eBook)
https://doi.org/10.1007/978-3-030-74906-4

This Springer imprint is published by the registered company Springer Nature Switzerland AG
The registered company address is: Gewerbestrasse 11, 6330 Cham, Switzerland

Foreword

I met Dr. Christian Harkensee in one of the medical missions that were organized by my organization MedGlobal to help Syrian refugee children in Bekaa Valley in Lebanon. We were close to the epicenter of the worst humanitarian crisis in recent decades. Half of the Syrian population have been displaced because of the ongoing civil war. More than 6.5 million remained as refugees.

A group of Pediatricians and medical volunteers traveled from different countries to provide basic healthcare services to children in Arsal camp at the Lebanon Syrian border. More than 50% of the 1 million Syrian refugees in Lebanon are children.

We are living through a global refugee crisis that is the worst since WWII. Children represent at least half of the 28 million refugees and 78 million displaced people in the world. It is imperative for medical or global health professionals to understand the psychological, developmental, physical, and medical aspects of caring for child refugees before embarking on such work.

This book is intended to be read from cover to cover by anyone who is new to the topic. It serves as an introduction before getting involved in working with refugees. As this book offers a more longitudinal, "life-cycle" approach to child health, even experienced humanitarians will find it useful. It was written by field workers with decades of experience as a guide to finding answers and inspiration. It is not intended to be a textbook, academic text, or exhaustive handbook, but a practical guide for anyone working with children and families in a humanitarian context.

The style of this book is intended to be interactive, focusing on practical "on-the-ground experience," providing tips, and tricks that are not normally found in books, but giving the reader a realistic impression of the challenges working with refugees.

The gist of this book is to stimulate readers to make the best of the often extremely limited resources; often contrasting or contradicting options available in high-income countries; or evidence-based practice.

There is a strong emphasis on children and families, a focus on preventative measures rather than only curative in all settings, a perspective on the effects of what we do in the future and the next generations, recognizing the necessity of cultural acceptability of the aid we offer, recognizing that refugees have a human right to health as anyone else, and striving for health equality of refugees within the population where they are settled.

I invite you to read the book and embark on a life mission of compassion and care to the refugees among us.

Zaher Sahloul
University in Illinois of Chicago,
Chicago, IL, USA
December 2020

Acknowledgments

The editors and the authors thank their partners and families for their support and patience writing this book—the time should have been theirs.

Contents

Part III   A Lifetime Perspective on Child Refugee and Migrant Health

Part IV   Editor's Introduction: Field Guide

Contributors

Saleh M. Al Salehi Princes Nourah bint Abdulrahman University, Riyadh, Saudi Arabia

Ramin Asgary, MD, MPH, FASTMH Department of Global Health, Milken Institute School of Public Health and Elliott School of International Affairs, George Washington University, Washington, DC, USA

Department of Medicine, Weill Cornell Medical College, Cornell University, New York, NY, USA

Zoë Bell, BSc, MSc Newcastle University, Baddiley Clark Building, Population Health Sciences Institute, Newcastle, UK

Martha C. Carlough, MD, MPH Department of Family Medicine, University of North Carolina—Chapel Hill, Chapel Hill, NC, USA

Office of Global Health Education, University of North Carolina—Chapel Hill, Chapel Hill, NC, USA

Ayesha Cheema-Hasan, MD Cleveland Clinic Abu Dhabi, Abu Dhabi, UAE

Children's Neurodevelopment Center, Warren Alpert Medical School of Brown University, Providence, RI, USA

Johnny Mahippathorn Chinnapha, MB, BCh, MRCPCH Ambulatory Pediatric and Adolescent Medicine Division (APAM), Pediatric Department, Ramathibodi Hospital, Mahidol University, Bangkok, Thailand

Megan Doherty, MD, FRCPC Program Director, Pediatric Palliative Care, Two Worlds Cancer Collaboration Foundation, Kelowna, BC, Canada

Children's Palliative Care Initiative in Bangladesh, World Child Cancer, Dhaka, Bangladesh

Pediatric Palliative Care, Children's Hospital of Eastern Ontario and Roger Neilson House, Ottawa, ON, Canada

University of Ottawa, Ottawa, ON, Canada

Naomi N. Duke, MD, PhD, MPH Duke University School of Medicine, Durham, NC, USA

B. Emily Esmaili, DO, MA, FAAP Duke Global Health Institute, Duke University, Durham, NC, USA

Lincoln Community Health Center, Durham, NC, USA

Christine Fernandes, MSc Save the Children, Amman, Jordan

Aurora Teresa Gadsden-Hevia Doctors Without Borders/Médecins Sans Frontières (MSF), Toronto, ON, Canada

Daniel Martinez Garcia, MD, MPH Médecins Sans Frontières (MSF), Geneva, Switzerland

EveryWhereSchools (EWS), Geneva, Switzerland

Marlene Goodfriend, MD Medecins Sans Frontieres, Jacksonville, FL, USA

Christian Harkensee, MD, PhD, MSc, DLSHTM, FRCPCH Queen Elizabeth Hospital, Gateshead, UK

Maria Isabel Herran, MD MetroHealth Medical Center, Cleveland, OH, USA

Eva Holsinger, MD Liaoning International General Health Trainers, Shenyang, China

H'Image Doctor International Clinic, DeJi Hospital, Shenyang, China

Farzana Khan, MA, MPH, MBBS Fasiuddin Khan Research Foundation (FKRF), Dhaka, Bangladesh

Minh Tram Le UNICEF Regional Office for South Asia (ROSA), Kathmandu, Nepal

Siyana Mahroof-Shaffi, MBBS, MRCGP, DRCOG Kitrinos Healthcare, London, UK

Philip Bruce Murray, MD, DTM&H Josephine County Public Health Department, Grants Pass, OR, USA

Medical Teams International, Portland, OR, USA

Ramzi Nasir, MD, MPH Royal Free London NHS Foundation Trust, London, UK

The Portland Hospital, London, UK

Karen Olness, MD, FAAP Department of Pediatrics, Case Western Reserve University, Cleveland, OH, USA

Maria Filipa Pereira, PharmD, MBA, CEFA Faculty of Pharmacy, University of Coimbra, Coimbra, Portugal

University of Aberdeen, Aberdeen, UK

Porto Business School, Porto, Portugal

Venkateswaran Ramesh, MBBS, DCH, MRCP King's College Hospital, London, UK

David J. Schonfeld, MD National Center for School Crisis and Bereavement, Children's Hospital Los Angeles, and USC Keck School of Medicine, Los Angeles, CA, USA

M. Leila Srour, MD, FAAP, MPH, DTM&H Health Frontiers, Vientiane, Laos

Sarah Walpole, MBChB, MSc, Med Educ, MRCP Health Education England North East, Newcastle, UK

Newcastle University, Newcastle, UK

Infectious Diseases Department, Newcastle Hospitals, RVI, Newcastle, UK

Newcastle Hospitals/Health Education England North East/Newcastle University, Newcastle upon Tyne, UK

Ante Wind, MD Unity Health Care, Washington, DC, USA

Part I

Introduction

Refugee Children and their Families: The Bigger Picture

1

Christian Harkensee and Sarah Walpole

Introduction

Humanitarian workers can begin to appreciate the situation of refugee children and their families by trying to understand the context of their current situation. The purpose of this book is to offer a perspective to humanitarian work that moves away from programs that are designed as short-term crisis-fighting or narrow-scoped, towards a life-cycle view that considers a broader context of refugee health. This book is not intended to be a comprehensive textbook of all topics and conditions, but a practical guide and toolkit on child and family health for humanitarian workers from all backgrounds, with any level of experience.

This book is about children. While doing humanitarian work and making decisions in the field, we often ask ourselves the question often, "Is this what's best for these children?"

Migration is not a new phenomenon. Virtually all human populations have some history of migration or ancestors who have migrated, whether to find better land or livelihoods, or to escape adverse conditions. Anyone who has migrated has experienced at least three phases: the setting that they lived in predeparture, a journey, and a place of arrival or settlement, be that temporary or permanent. Journeys may last anywhere from a few hours to decades, and most involve stops en route. Every refugee's experience is different.

Refugee health settings are hugely diverse, and each refugee's perception of their particular setting will be unique. Working in this field you may engage with refugees who still consider themselves to be in the journey phase, whether they are

C. Harkensee (✉)
Queen Elizabeth Hospital, Gateshead, UK

S. Walpole
Newcastle Hospitals/Health Education England North East/Newcastle University,
Newcastle, UK
e-mail: sarah.walpole@doctors.org.uk

© Springer Nature Switzerland AG 2021
C. Harkensee et al. (eds.), *Child Refugee and Migrant Health*,
https://doi.org/10.1007/978-3-030-74906-4_1

temporarily settled or they are making a short stop during travel. Some refugees may consider that they have arrived at their destination, whether or not they have a secure home, family contacts, legal status, or income. Some may have settled in a new place for decades, but still regard this as temporary, hoping to return home one day.

The term "migrant" is an umbrella term for people who leave their usual residence to live in another place, for any reason. Categorizing individuals according to their "nation," "race" or other cultural or political definition risks racism, political abuse, or discrimination. Similarly, attempting to categorize people according to their reasons for migration, e.g., as an "economic" migrant, could be both artificial, because migration is rarely caused by one factor alone, and unhelpful, because it risks implying that some reasons for migration are more valid than others. Similarly, it is important to recognize that forced and voluntary migration are two ends of a spectrum and in most cases both choice and necessity influence the decision to migrate [1].

Recognizing this, the narrative in this book advocates for understanding individual children according to their unique experiences, vulnerabilities, and health needs. Barriers to living a healthy lifestyle and accessing appropriate and effective health care are not only determined by different personal factors, but also how their community and society recognize and respond to their health and social needs.

The decision to leave home is not one that is taken lightly. A person may decide to migrate in order to find a livelihood and a standard of living for him/her/themself and family that he/she/they deem acceptable, or in order to avoid the threat of death from a natural or human-made disaster. Regardless of the cause or multiple causes, humanitarian workers should focus on migrants' vulnerabilities, health needs, and wider advocacy needs.

As humanitarian workers, we will meet refugee children and their families at some point along their journey, in different settings. Such settings are aligned along the trajectory of the journey but may overlap. Settings include:

- Within the immediate humanitarian post-disaster setting—which can be man-made (e.g., war) or natural (e.g., earthquake).
- Along the journey (displacement inside/outside own country, while moving on foot, by car, boat, or plane).
- During initial or preliminary settlement (such as makeshift, evolving camps).
- Living in more established settlements (which may persist over decades).
- In permanent resettlement in host countries, or permanent return/repatriation.

Each of these settings comes with different risks and vulnerabilities, health needs, and barriers to accessing health care that humanitarian workers need to consider (Table 1.1).

This chapter briefly examines how drivers of good and ill health in individual people, local communities, and wider society affect the health of children over their lifetimes, in particular refugee children who may be in more unfortunate circumstances. This may be a somewhat fluid framework—all levels of each of these drivers extensively interact with other drivers, at every level. Figure 1.1 describes these interactions.

Table 1.1 Overview of different settings in which you may work with refugees and some of the health needs, vulnerabilities, and barriers to accessing healthcare that may be experienced in such a setting

Setting	Detail	Exposures/vulnerabilities	Specific health needs	Barriers to accessing care
Humanitarian disaster setting	An event or a series of events causes societal breakdown and a humanitarian disaster. People may migrate from, through, or to zones affected by humanitarian disasters.	Threat of violence may be ongoing Access to resources including water, food, sanitation, and shelter, may be restricted Instability and fear of violence, e.g., nearby shelling	Violence and unsafe living conditions may lead to traumatic injuries Mental health problems Vulnerability to malnutrition, dehydration Vaccine preventable diseases may occur locally	Breakdown of local health infrastructure Insecurity limiting freedom of movement
During flight (land, sea, or air)	Rescue boats are the most well-known example of healthcare provision during flight, e.g., MSF boats rescuing migrants from the sea or unsafe vessels in the Mediterranean Sea	Unsafe Sea crossings Unsafe travel in vehicles for extended time periods, e.g., excess exposure to fumes, dehydration, or musculoskeletal pain/injuries Risk physical, sexual, and psychological abuse, including from traffickers	Dehydration Malnutrition Communicable diseases due to extended close proximity and lack of hygieneconsequences of physical, sexual, and psychological abusemental health problems	Few health services available Lack of continuity of care between providers Access to secondary care particularly limited Translation services less likely to have been established

(continued)

Table 1.1 (continued)

Setting	Detail	Exposures/vulnerabilities	Specific health needs	Barriers to accessing care
Newly established/ evolving camps/ informal settlements	New camps may be set up when there is a developing crisis causing mass migration, or where influx of refugees is ongoing and existing camps no longer have space for new arrivals. In some locations, informal camps exist for many years without recognition or support from authorities	Often lack basic facilities, including shelter, safe drinking water, cooking equipment, and sanitation. Physical access routes and arranging nearby accommodation for NGO workers may be difficult. Newer camps may have few or no NGOs supporting their work	Communicable disease Malnutrition Dehydration	Health services less likely to be established in newer camps/informal settlementshealth promotion and sexual and reproductive health services in particular may be lacking. Lack of access to previous healthcare records. Access to secondary care may be limited. Language barriers may be a problem, especially if addressing mental health, stigmatized or intimate problems
Established refugee camps	Established camps have varying levels of support from government and nonstate actors	Close living conditions, lack of accessibility or acceptability of WASH facilities, adequate shelter, and cooking facilities may be ongoing	Mental health problems may be compounded by uncertainty about the future and lack of occupation/educational opportunities. Substance misuse. Domestic violence	Language and knowledge barriers to accessing health care. Formal and informal restrictions imposed in host country to access health care

Dispersed in a rural or urban setting	Relocation programs may send refugees to homes in urban or rural settings. This may be part of "permanent resettlement" or may be temporary. Experiences of refugees there may vary greatly depending on the number of refugees sent, local community attitudes, employment or education opportunities, etc.	Living conditions and shelter may vary in quality—Risk of extremes of heat, cold and damp Discrimination, re-traumatization Integration is a challenge, and lack of occupation or other means of community engagement is a risk to mental and physical health	Mental health problems, particularly where refugees are isolated, and/or receive negative reactions from the local community Malnutrition Mental health Usual risks of urban locations— Inactivity, air pollution, poor diet cardiovascular problems	Lack of knowledge of local health systems Language barriers Financial barriers

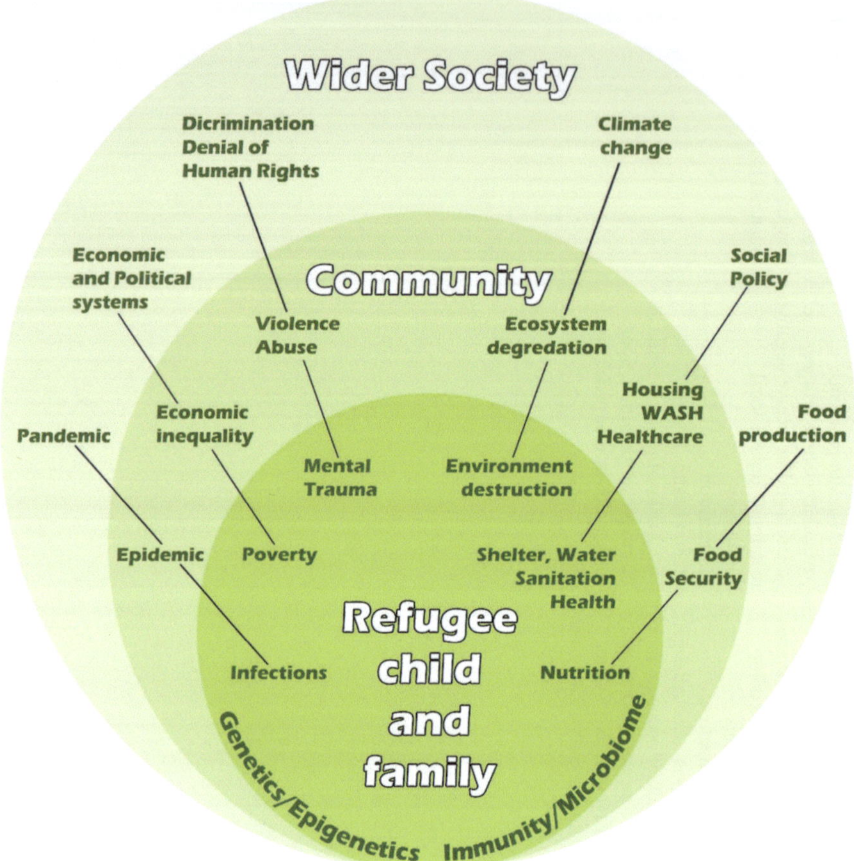

Fig. 1.1 Wider determinants of health for refugee children and their families (graph courtesy of Robert Cooper)

What Are the Drivers of Good and Ill Health in Refugee Children and their Families?

Figure 1.1 provides a framework for understanding the factors that influence health in refugee children and families. This framework aims to put determinants of health in a wider context, illustrating that holistic (i.e., considering physical, emotional, mental, environmental, social, political, economic drivers) and long-term (i.e., over a lifetime and intergenerational) perspectives are needed to best serve the health and well-being of refugee families. This involves alleviating acute suffering, practicing preventative medicine, and strongly advocating for social, political, and economic changes that benefit refugees, or obviates the factors that result in forced displacement. This book will explore these aspects in more detail. Here we outline some of the important aspects that determine child refugee health at an individual, family, and community level, and in the wider global context.

The Child, their Family, and Community

Child development can be described as the sequence of physical, emotional, and psychological changes that occur between conception and completion of adolescence [2–4]. The nutritional status, physical, mental, and emotional health of a woman preconception and during pregnancy is crucial for the lifelong health of her child. Development can be described as a continuum where the largest leaps are made early in life, with further development building on and determined by early developmental progress. Missing out on early developmental opportunities, or exposure to detrimental events at an early stage may have a lifelong impact on physical health, cognitive abilities, social status and quality of life, and may also affect the next generation.

The degree to which young people grow up to become physically, mentally, and emotionally strong depends on complex, interacting intrinsic and extrinsic factors experienced during childhood. Intrinsic factors include those that a child is born with, such as their physical health at birth and their genetics, which may predispose them to illness, but also the way their brain works, their character, and even experiences in utero. The speed and scope of a child's development are controlled by genetic (the structure of the DNA) and epigenetic (the way genes are switched on and off) factors. Environmental factors can also influence child development in a promoting as well as an inhibitory way.

Environmental factors are key to promoting healthy development and allowing children to excel, feel fulfilled and happy, feel part of their family and society, and achieve in education in childhood and employment in adult life. Examples of supportive environmental factors include:

- Care and love from parents or caregivers.
- Predictable routines for meals, sleep, play, and personal hygiene.
- Rules and discipline without harshness, and caregivers responding predictably.
- Adequate housing, nutrition, sanitation, health care, and security.
- Access to education and facilitation of socialization.

On the other hand, individual factors as well as environmental conditions can hinder the full attainment of a child's genetic potential. This includes poor antenatal health and inadequate care of the mother, adverse events in pregnancy and childhood, or sustained adverse environmental conditions such as poverty, discrimination, poor physical and mental health, and malnutrition of children or their caregivers.

Family, community, and society's perspectives on health greatly influence the treatment of childhood diseases, developmental disability, and chronic illness, and can vary widely in different societies—which can be difficult to grasp for humanitarian workers with a "Western" perspective on health. As an example, in some societies developmental delay, incurable chronic diseases or genetic syndromes may not be regarded as a health problem—merely as individual needs that require extra help, care, compassion, and love from the family and the community. There are countries where families hide children who have disabilities such as hydrocephalus. There are others where communities blame parents for congenital conditions such as Down syndrome. Regardless of the particular country of origin, in the refugee situation, family and community networks often break down, making these children more vulnerable.

The health of the mother has a major influence on the future health and life prospects of her children. During pregnancy, maternal malnutrition, iron deficiency anemia and vitamin deficiencies, smoking, alcohol, and drug use all affect the growth, health, and long-term quality of life of her child. After birth, lack of food for the mother or the child, feeding problems, recurrent infections, postnatal depression, and problems with bonding and attachment can result in adverse physical and mental health outcomes, manifesting throughout a child's lifetime. The Developmental Origins of Health and Disease hypothesis [5] has emphasized the particular importance of the first 1000 days of life (from the point of conception) for life expectancy and chronic disease risk. Providing optimal nutrition, health care, and disease prevention (e.g., vaccination) during this time period offers a child the best start in life. Studies have shown that not meeting these basic needs may predispose to problems such as early heart disease and death. Stable families and communities can mitigate some of these effects even in the face of poverty. Displacement, however, often disrupts family and community structures, making families and their children more vulnerable.

Infections early in life can also result in malnutrition and thus negatively impact a child's cognitive, mental, emotional, and physical development. Early weaning from breastfeeding, breastfeeding failure, or bottle feeding in living conditions where good hygiene could not be maintained can result in recurrent gastrointestinal infections, malnutrition, stunting, and impaired cognitive abilities [6, 7]. These children may grow up to become undernourished parents, trapped in the same cycle with their own children. The right amount of macronutrients (e.g., protein, fats, and carbohydrates) and micronutrients (e.g., iron, vitamins) during pregnancy, breastfeeding, and early childhood is critical for normal and optimal brain development. If a mother is undernourished or has iron or vitamin deficiency, babies can be born small and their brain development can already be impaired in utero. Infections such as gastroenteritis in the first year of life result in higher energy consumption, but also malabsorption of macro- and micronutrients, promoting malnutrition. Nutrients are also essential for a healthy immune system development; malnutrition weakens the immune system resulting in a vicious cycle of infection/malnutrition, and impaired cognitive and physical development. This is why the promotion of breastfeeding and vaccination against infections (e.g., rotavirus, measles) are so critical in early childhood to move health provision from emergency care to care with a more preventative and long-term perspective.

The microbiome is the community of microorganisms that naturally colonizes our skin, respiratory, and intestinal tracts. Recent research highlights the importance of the microbiome not only for the digestion of nutrients but also the health of the immune system [8–11]. Introducing "healthy" bacteria early, e.g., through early and sustained breastfeeding, shapes both the microbiome and the immune system in a way that it becomes more resistant to intestinal infections, hence preventing malnutrition from recurrent gastroenteritis. Early disruption (in the first year of life) of microbiome development, e.g., by early bottle feeding, recurrent gastrointestinal infections, or unnecessary use of antibiotics is associated with adverse long-term health outcomes.

As for extrinsic factors, disaster and flight are hugely disruptive to a child's emotional well-being, and in this situation stabilizing factors such as an intact family or community are also often disrupted. Prolonged hardships such as flight, displacement, loss, poverty, and discrimination can result in progressive erosion of resilience. The concept of Adverse Childhood Experiences (ACEs) can be used to describe such events, experiences, and their long-term effects on health and well-being. ACEs are defined as traumatic experiences that occur in childhood; these can be acute events or "toxic stress" sustained over a long period of time. The hypothesis of ACEs is that early trauma has neurobiological effects on the developing brain, predisposing the child to adverse physical and mental health outcomes later in life in a dose-response pattern (e.g., the more ACEs, the worse health is affected) [12]. Research studies have linked the presence of ACEs to many physical (e.g., diabetes, heart disease, obesity, cancer) and mental health problems (anxiety, depression, low life satisfaction, low mental health self-rating, delinquency, violent behavior, suicide risk) in later life [13]. ACEs are presumed to affect genetic expression and epigenetics through physical stress signals via the hypothalmo-pituitary-adrenal axis, effects that can be long-lasting and even passed on through generations [14], which demonstrates how vital it is to prevent exposure to ACEs where possible.

The effect of ACEs on refugee and asylum-seeking children and adults are less well studied, but results from various countries, including non-Western and low-income regions, replicate the findings of large ACEs studies [15–18]. Refugee children are not only exposed to the same stressors as non-displaced populations but often have additional ACEs related to their situation, such as direct exposure (seeing or being a victim of or forced perpetrator of violence, loss of close family members and friends, loss of home, loss of education). Many have florid PTSD. These exposures are strongly related to adverse physical outcomes (i.e., heart disease, respiratory disease) and mental health outcomes (i.e., depression, suicidal ideations, PTSD, antisocial and aggressive behavior) as well as risk-taking lifestyle choices (e.g., alcohol and drug use).

A Wider Perspective on Health: Globalization and Refugee Health

No human being lives in total isolation. To a large degree, our thinking, behavior, health, and well-being are determined by the societal context we are living in. Early humans were shaped by their local community and immediate fight for survival; currently, an economy that is increasingly globalized shapes societies around the globe. The last 200 years have brought enormous technological advances. In recent decades, the digital revolution and an economy dominated by free trade ideology have resulted in the removal of trade barriers and increased communication, which impact individuals' and societies' health.

Global Change and Health

It is important to have a closer look at how globalization shapes health and healthcare. International borders exist to limit the flows of goods and people between regions under different jurisdictions, but not all transborder crossings can be regulated. Globalization is the process of borders becoming more porous, be that through the flow of materials, financial capital, information, people, or animals.

Globalization brings increasing interdependence and complexity as our everyday activities are affected by and have an increasing effect on a wider scope of factors and actors [19]. This comes with a sense of responsibility for communities and people far away. Awareness of this responsibility may motivate some to work in global health or refugee health.

How does the global change we are experiencing result in increased migration? While there remains controversy over the benefits and disadvantages of globalization, on one hand, increased international trade and advances in transport capacity and information technology have brought unprecedented economic growth in both developed and developing countries. The economy of many poor countries has substantially improved, allowing them to invest more in infrastructure and health. The Internet allows rapid exchange of information and ideas, breaking down cultural barriers. Transportation has gained capacity and speed while becoming cheaper, thus bringing the world closer together. In general, access to healthcare has improved in many low-income countries, in particular in urban areas, as has food security through trade and increased productivity.

Critics of globalization, however, argue that it reinforces inequality and strengthens the already powerful large global companies, which can force open and control the economy of poorer countries, resulting in an increasing gap between poor and rich. These greater inequalities may lead to a weakened democracy, political entanglements in worker's rights, and undermining of social welfare and access to healthcare. Healthcare in many low-income countries has become privatized and unaffordable, and removal of trade barriers has resulted in the weakening of vital local food production, dependence on food imports from large multinational companies, and promotion of an unhealthy lifestyle (e.g., increased access to processed food, tobacco, and alcohol). Poverty is the strongest predictor of ill health and mortality in any society. The increasing gap between the rich and poor can be observed in all countries, even the wealthiest. Breakdown of these social safeguards lead to conflict, both within and between societies; and conflict becoming one of the strongest drivers for migration. People always have moved, and always will move to find resources, work, safety, education, food, and freedom.

Climate Change and Environmental Degradation

While disasters such as earthquakes and volcanic eruptions are genuinely natural, many of the floods and storms that have led to the displacement of people in recent years are the result of climate change, a man-made disaster. Climate change, the result of the increasing concentration of greenhouse gases in the Earth's atmosphere, is intrinsically linked to globalization. The destruction of natural habitats and biodiversity, and increased use of fossil fuels have accelerated in line with the increase in free trade, travel and transport, and deregulation of markets particularly in developing countries. This has resulted in increased exploitation of the natural resources that form the basis of all life on Earth.

Environments and ecosystems exist in a constant state of flux, however, particularly consequential for human societies and human migration are variations outside of the normal range, which overwhelm usual homeostatic systems and cause extreme, irreversible changes, with effects on resource availability and/or the safety of environments. The loss of biodiversity, for example, can lead to the collapse of ecosystems and resultant food insecurity, such as through loss of insects which pollinate 35% of crops that we consume [20, 21]. Another domain is atmospheric greenhouse gas concentrations, where we have already breached safe limits.

All of these environmental issues are highly relevant to migration because loss of lands and livelihoods and social, economic, and political upheaval all affect decisions to migrate, as well as experiences during migration and after resettlement. The UN estimated that one aspect of climate change alone, climate disasters, caused around 17 million people to be displaced in 2018.

In 2001, for the first time, the number of refugees displaced due to environmental issues was higher than the number displaced due to war and conflict [22]. Environmental changes are causing migration both by directly destroying homes and livelihoods, and through impacts on and interaction with other social, economic, political, and cultural factors. Direct impacts of climate change which cause migration include natural disasters such as flooding, hurricanes, and bush fires causing loss of homes and livelihoods, sea-level rise causing loss of homes or salination of freshwater causing loss of livelihoods for people who depend on freshwater fishing, and changes to environmental conditions affecting crop survival and yields causing loss of livelihood or starvation. Pathways through which environmental change causes migration indirectly may involve conflict over resource scarcity, unemployment, or famine. The World Bank estimated that climate change would push over 100 million people into poverty over 15 years [23].

The interactions between environmental change and migration are multiple and multidirectional. Migration itself has significant environmental impacts, related to the breakdown of social structures and governmental systems, resource use, and waste production. In mass displacement of populations, their journey and relocation may be through and to locations where systems are not in place to manage large and concentrated human impacts. Areas may need to be cleared to make space for dwellings. Even basic sanitation and waste disposal systems are usually lacking at the point of arrival of a large refugee population and may take some time to establish, which can result in local environmental degradation. It is important to ensure that blame is avoided and that the environmental impacts of refugee settlements are seen in context. Refugees themselves often do not have resources and choices to avoid negative environmental impacts, and this problem is solvable or avoidable with planning and resources from governments and/or local or international NGOs. While local environmental impacts can be significant, the environmental footprint of a refugee living with very few resources is a tiny fraction of the footprint of the average person living in a high- or middle-income country setting. Humanitarian actors are beginning to recognize this and actions to mitigate this effect are emerging [24].

Summary

Returning to the child in front of us in a refugee camp clinic, what can we bring to this setting from having looked at the wider context? Firstly, we need to consider the lifetime perspective of the refugee child and their family. Humanitarian settings are often focused on relieving immediate health needs, which is important and the right thing to do. However, we best serve children's physical and mental health if we promote healthy living conditions, supportive relationships, healthy nutrition, development and play, education, and regular healthcare including vaccinations. Children can only grow up healthy if their caregivers are healthy—ensuring they are in the best state to look after their children well is one of the strongest interventions.

Secondly, and equally important, as humanitarian workers we need to be advocates for a healthier and more just world. On a global scale, children are among the most vulnerable and neglected groups of people, and yet many humanitarian settings focus primarily on adults. We have a duty to prioritize children's needs to ensure that they develop to their best capabilities, and one day take on this challenging world.

You will find these two lessons throughout every chapter of this book.

Acknowledgments The authors thank Mr. Robert Cooper, Fishburn, UK for the graphic design of Fig. 1.1.

Appendix 1: Refugee Children and their Families: The Bigger Picture

See Table 1.1

References

1. Schütte S, Gemenne F, Zaman M, Flahault A, Depoux A. Connecting planetary health, climate change, and migration. Lancet Planet Health. 2018;2(2):e58–9.
2. Shute RH, Slee PT. Child development: theories and critical perspectives. 2nd ed. Hove, UK: Routledge; 2015.

3. May P. Child development in practice. 1st ed. Oxon: Routledge; 2011.
4. Ertem IO, Dogan DG, Gok CG, Kizilates SU, Caliskan A, Atay G, et al. A guide for monitoring child development in low- and middle-income countries. Pediatrics. 2008;121(3):e581–9.
5. Barouki R, Gluckman PD, Grandjean P, Hanson M, Heindel JJ. Developmental origins of non-communicable disease: implications for research and public health. Environ Health. 2012;11:42.
6. Dawson-Hahn E, Pak-Gorstein S, Matheson J, Zhou C, Yun K, Scott K, et al. Growth trajectories of refugee and nonrefugee children in the United States. Pediatrics. 2016;138:6.
7. Lozoff B, Beard J, Connor J, Barbara F, Georgieff M, Schallert T. Long-lasting neural and behavioral effects of iron deficiency in infancy. Nutr Rev. 2006;64(5 Pt 2):S34–43. discussion S72-91
8. Olszak T, An D, Zeissig S, Vera MP, Richter J, Franke A, et al. Microbial exposure during early life has persistent effects on natural killer T cell function. Science. 2012;336(6080):489–93.
9. Hooper LV, Littman DR, Macpherson AJ. Interactions between the microbiota and the immune system. Science. 2012;336(6086):1268–73.
10. Rautava S, Luoto R, Salminen S, Isolauri E. Microbial contact during pregnancy, intestinal colonization and human disease. Nat Rev Gastroenterol Hepatol. 2012;9(10):565–76.
11. Robertson RC, Manges AR, Finlay BB, Prendergast AJ. The human microbiome and child growth—first 1000 days and beyond. Trends Microbiol. 2019;27(2):131–47.
12. Dube SR, Felitti VJ, Dong M, Giles WH, Anda RF. The impact of adverse childhood experiences on health problems: evidence from four birth cohorts dating back to 1900. Prev Med. 2003;37(3):268–77.
13. Hughes K, Bellis MA, Hardcastle KA, Sethi D, Butchart A, Mikton C, et al. The effect of multiple adverse childhood experiences on health: a systematic review and meta-analysis. Lancet Public Health. 2017;2(8):e356–66.
14. Jiang S, Postovit L, Cattaneo A, Binder EB, Aitchison KJ. Epigenetic modifications in stress response genes associated with childhood trauma. Front Psych. 2019;10:808.
15. Opaas M, Varvin S. Relationships of childhood adverse experiences with mental health and quality of life at treatment start for adult refugees traumatized by pre-flight experiences of war and human rights violations. J Nerv Ment Dis. 2015;203(9):684–95.
16. Hanes G, Sung L, Mutch R, Cherian S. Adversity and resilience amongst resettling Western Australian paediatric refugees. J Paediatr Child Health. 2017;53(9):882–8.
17. Calam R. Public health implications and risks for children and families resettled after exposure to armed conflict and displacement. Scand J Public Health. 2017;45(3):209–11.
18. Dong M, Anda RF, Felitti VJ, Williamson DF, Dube SR, Brown DW, et al. Childhood residential mobility and multiple health risks during adolescence and adulthood: the hidden role of adverse childhood experiences. Arch Pediatr Adolesc Med. 2005;159(12):1104–10.
19. Lee K, Collin J. Global change and health. 1st ed. London: Open University Press; 2005. (Understanding Public Health)
20. Rockstrom J, Steffen W, Noone K, Persson A, Chapin FS, Lambin EF, et al. A safe operating space for humanity. Nature. 2009;461(7263):472–5.
21. Whitmee S, Haines A, Beyrer C, Boltz F, Capon AG, de Souza Dias BF, et al. Safeguarding human health in the Anthropocene epoch: report of the Rockefeller Foundation–lancet commission on planetary health. Lancet. 2015;386(10007):1973–2028.
22. Durkova P, Gromilova A, Kiss B, Plaku M. Climate refugees in the 21st century. 2012. United Nations.
23. Shock waves: managing the impacts of climate change on poverty—background papers [internet]. World Bank. [cited 2020 Nov 13]. https://www.worldbank.org/en/topic/climatechange/brief/shock-waves-managing-the-impacts-of-climate-change-on-poverty-background-papers
24. Environmental Impact Toolkit—MSF transformational investment capacity [internet]. [cited 2020 Nov 27]. https://msf-transformation.org/news/environmentalimpacttoolkit/

Christian Harkensee, MD, PhD, MSc, DLSHTM, DiMM, MAcadMEd, MFPHC (RCSEd), FHEA, FRCPCH Made his first humanitarian experience in Central America in 1987. Since, became a doctor (Humboldt University Berlin, Germany, 1997), pediatrician and pediatric infectious diseases and immunology specialist (UK, 2012), researcher (PhD in immunogenetics, UK, 2012), medical educator (2003), and mountain and expedition doctor (2017). Humanitarian disaster relief, development and capacity building work in many countries ever since; and currently leading a health service for refugee children and families in the North East of England.

Sarah Walpole, BSc Int Health, MBChB, Med, MSc(Res), Med Educ, MRCP is an Infectious Diseases registrar in Newcastle, UK. She has worked in various medical and pediatric specialties, completed an Academic Clinical Fellowship in medical education with cardiology, and worked as a Medical Activities Manager and Medical Educator for MSF in DRC, SAMS in Greece, Doctors Worldwide in Bangladesh, and Health in Harmony in Indonesia. She continues to provide telemedicine consultations to junior doctors in Bangladesh. She champions planetary health, including the Association of Medical Education in Europe and the Centre for Sustainable Healthcare. She cofounded the UK's Climate and Health Council and IFMSA's "Healthy Planet" during her studies of International Health at University College London and medicine at Leeds University. She is committed to protecting access to healthcare, including by maintaining the UK's NHS as a publicly funded and publicly provided service, and has undertaken research on privatization with the Centre for Health in the Public Interest.

Part II

Introduction: Psychosocial Section Helping Children in Humanitarian Emergencies

Karen Olness

The editors of this manual have all had hands-on experience working in humanitarian emergencies. They all know how important it is to provide the basic necessities of life to displaced children, to do medical triage, to provide acute medical care, and to assess the nutritional status of displaced children. They have also witnessed the psychosocial issues of these children and their families, important issues that need to be addressed by relief workers in humanitarian emergencies. There are hundreds of articles and books that provide information about the long-term effects of disasters on children. They document the negative long-term psychological effects on children, especially when their mental health issues are not recognized or are ignored during the early period after a disaster. These range from problems such as life-long weather phobia in children who have lived through a hurricane to chronic depression and/or PTSD in children who have experienced a manmade disaster [1–6]. There are also many articles describing successful early interventions for children who have experienced humanitarian emergencies [7, 8].

We now know enough about the psychosocial issues to be able to list risk factors, to perform psy triage, and to suggest early interventions to prevent or mitigate life-long psychological suffering for these children. The overall purpose of this manual is to provide practical information for relief workers whom we know are often overwhelmed and exhausted. In this psychosocial section, we intend to provide practical information on how to identify children who are suffering and who need psychological help, how schools can help, how to help children who have lost close family members, how to help parents, and how to provide palliative care for children who are very ill. The experience of resettlement in a different country leads to additional mental health trauma for some children. So we provide a section on how to assess and help children in hospital and clinic settings after resettlement.

We also emphasize the innate resilience of children and their families; we include some ways to facilitate or enhance that resilience.

K. Olness
Case Western Reserve University, Cleveland, OH, USA

References

1. Pfefferbaum B, Jacobs A, Van Horn R, Houston J. Effects of displacement in children exposed to disaster. Curr Psychiatry Rep. 2016;18:71–5.
2. Mclaughlin KA, Fairbank JA, Gruber MJ, et al. Serious emotional disturbance among youths exposed to hurricane Katrina 2 Years post disaster. J Am Acad Child Adolesc Psychiatry. 2009;48:1069–78.
3. Feldman R, Vengrober A. Posttraumatic stress disorder in infants and young children exposed to war-related trauma. J Am Acad Child Adolesc Psychiatry. 2011;50:645–58.
4. Iwadare Y, Usami M, Suzuki Y, et al. Posttraumatic symptoms in elementary and junior high school children after the 2011 Japan earthquake and tsunami: symptom severity and recovery vary by age and sex. J Pediatr. 2014;164:917–21.
5. School S, Elbert T. Ten years after the genocide: trauma confrontation and post-traumatic stress in Rwandan adolescents. J Trauma Stress. 2006;19:95–105.
6. Coleman JSM, Newby KD, Multon KD, Taylor CL. Weathering the storm: revisiting severe weather phobia. Bull Am Meteor Soc. 2014;95:1179–83.
7. Pairojkul S. Psychosocial First Aid: support for the child survivors of the Asian tsunami. J Dev Behav Pediatr. 2010;31:723–27.
8. Weine SM, Ware N, Hakizimana L, Tugenberg T, Currie M, Dahnweih G, Wulu J. Fostering resilience: protective agents, resources, and mechanisms for adolescent refugees' psychosocial well-being. Adolescent Psychiatry. 2014;4:164–76.

Karen Olness is board certified in Developmental and Behavioral Pediatrics and Professor Emerita of Pediatrics, Global Health, and Diseases at Case Western Reserve University (CWRU) in Ohio. She has been a field worker, helping children in humanitarian emergencies in many countries. In 1996, she initiated programs at CWRU to train relief workers about the special needs of children in disasters. These workshops have been replicated in many resource-poor settings. She is past chair of the Global Child Health Section of the American Academy of Pediatrics (AAP) and the Technical Advisory Group on Children in Humanitarian Emergencies of the IPA. She is past President of the Society for Developmental and Behavioral Pediatrics. She has more than 150 publications and has received many awards from universities and professional organizations.

Psychosocial Assessment and Early Intervention

2

Ayesha Cheema-Hasan

Introduction

It is important to keep in mind that regardless of what type of crisis is occurring; manmade or natural, the immediate effects will be physical and psychological in nature. While the physical effects will be the same across nations, the psychological effects and the response to the stress will be different across cultures [1, 2]. Manmade events are associated with higher levels of stress as compared to climate-related disasters [3]. War, religious persecution or any conflict related event causes children to experience death, loss of possessions, home, and relocation. This also happens in climate-related events but the children are more likely to encounter a loving adult and immediate assistance after these than in conflict-related events.

Children experience and express symptoms based on their developmental age. Though many impacts seem to subside in the short to medium term, larger effects that occur at critical points in a child's development can persist for their lifetime and even be passed to the next generation.

The other thing to keep in mind is that the parents and immediate family are also experiencing stress, fear, grief, and loss. Children sense these feelings and feel even more vulnerable.

Describing symptoms and assessment by age group is a pragmatic way to approach mental health and trauma experience in children.

A. Cheema-Hasan (✉)
Cleveland Clinic Abu Dhabi, Abu Dhabi, UAE

Children's Neurodevelopment Center, Warren Alpert Medical School of Brown University, Providence, RI, USA
e-mail: cheemaa@clevelandclinicabudhabi.ae

Infancy: (0–1 Years)

Issues with the quality of attachment; be it secure or insecure; can occur in infants particularly 6 months and older. Parents play a central role in this developmental period. Any disruption can cause them to have changes in eating patterns and/or sleeping. They can appear cranky or irritable, hard to soothe or can appear listless and appear as a "good baby." Younger infants can exhibit an exaggerated startle response.

Toddlerhood (1–3 Years)

This is the time of autonomy and exploration. They are testing limits; physical and relational. Temperament affects behavior at an individual level. So, a slow to warm up child will exhibit clinginess and separation distress. A child with a difficult temperament might externalize, have tantrums and be difficult to console. At this age, they might regress, stop talking, refuse to do or have difficulty with previously learned self-help tasks. They might have regression in toileting/bowel bladder control. It is important to remember that overly good behavior or acting like "adults" is a sign of stress.

Young Children (Preschool Age 3–6 Years)

Around this age, children develop a vivid imagination and use magical thinking to solve problems or explain things. Many are not logical thinkers and are egocentric meaning that they are unable to distinguish between their point of view and the point of view of others. They have misunderstandings of death and believe it is reversible or just means that the person has gone somewhere. Children at this age may exhibit disrupted and or repetitive play, nightmares, acting out, being aggressive, or oppositional.

School Age (6–12 Years)

They now begin to see themselves as individuals capable of basic problem-solving. Peer acceptance and conformity start taking precedence and they start understanding peer hierarchy. Many still prefer structured activities over open-ended ones. Children may show symptoms of poor academic performance, withdrawal from normal activities, or decreased interest in peers. They may be anxious or depressed or may show externalizing behaviors like aggression or hyperactivity. The responses may vary based on gender. Boys show more antisocial and aggressive behaviors and girls display more emotions and or ask more questions.

Adolescence (12–18 Years)

During this age, children change in how they interact with family, friends, and peers. They are searching for their identity and this can be influenced by gender, peers, cultural background, media, and family expectations. They seek to be independent and responsible and look for new experiences and can engage in risk-taking behaviors. They start to develop a sexual identity and may start to explore or question it. In times of crisis, adolescents may go through an identity crisis, have feelings of despair, hopelessness, and loss of direction. They may experience disillusionment with their faith, become radicalized, or cling to a new idea. They might become parentified, engage in risk-taking behaviors, have difficulty concentrating, and have difficulty feeling pleasure.

How to Support Children and Teenagers

Those who are working with vulnerable children after a life-altering event or in a camp/detention center, first and foremost should remain calm. Children look to adults for support and care. Most children and adolescents will regain normal functioning provided that basic survival needs are met, safety and security are reestablished and developmental opportunities are restored as much as possible based on the resources available. Preexisting risk factors like preexisting mental health problems, reactive temperament, parental maladaptation, and social isolation can affect the response to emotional trauma and long-term well-being. On the other hand, intelligence, physical health, beliefs/religion, and supportive social frameworks, which include immediate and extended family, friends, and institutions, all promote resilience.

Meet Basic Requirements

A safe and loving home is a basic need for any child. Reunification and keeping families together is very important and should be encouraged and implemented as soon as possible. Make sure basic requirements that include food, clothing, shelter, and sanitation are being met. Children of different ages have specific dietary needs. For example, an infant requires breast milk and/or formula. Supply for breast milk is affected by whether the mother is present or not, maternal stress, and nutrition.

Make sure that children have appropriate clothing, including shoes. Clothing can be overlooked especially in poor countries. Shelters protect against the elements and also against exploitation. Efforts should be made to ensure safe water and good sanitation. Otherwise, children will likely become ill with infectious diseases and also infect their caretakers and other household members sick as well.

Establish Routines

The most important thing is to establish routines. Resilience in children who experience a disaster is facilitated by establishing routines. Routines provide predictability and regularity which is comforting to kids. Therefore, it is important to encourage parents to be consistent in establishing routines for meals, naps, and bedtime and to set appropriate limits. Incorporate holidays and festivals that are important to the family into these routines. Set up a time to read together or to children daily [4]. Relief workers should speak with parents about their important role in helping children feel secure and should be encouraged to spend time with their children.

For toddlers, help parents to teach limit settings without excessive punishment. Expect temporary regression at all ages. Young children, especially toddlers, may test limits and caregivers should accept them as a learning opportunity and redirect them rather than taking it personally. Teach parents that the "bad" behavior is possibly a sign of distress or a cry for help as children do not know how to express themselves verbally like adults.

For older youth giving them chores and responsibilities will give them an opportunity to influence what is happening to them. Keeping them involved in the day-to-day management can decrease opportunities for risky behaviors. It also facilitates a connection with other peers who may be going through something similar. Fostering a sense of hope is important for their recovery. Explain to them that their feelings are normal, respect their emotions and do not minimize or dismiss their reactions.

Education/Learning

Reestablish schools when safe to do so. This helps in providing routines and a sense of normalcy to the day, provides safety, allows opportunities for children to meet with peers in a group environment where possible and, most importantly, gives hope for a future. Education is rarely a core focus after a disaster. But the impact it can have on children and young adolescents can be profound and long-lasting. Schools and school teachers can be integral in helping children and their families recover after a disaster has struck the community. It is important to also keep in mind that the teachers will also be struggling with stress-related symptoms and personal losses and it is important they also care for themselves. Please see Chap. 4 on schools for detailed information.

Reunification where Possible

It should be a priority to reunite children with parent/caregivers as soon as possible. Relief workers should assess parental/caregiver supports. It is important to remember that parental emotional and physical well-being will impact how they will interact and take care of their children. For infants that are being breastfed, monitoring maternal nutrition and hydration will be important. Make sure you focus on parental/caregiver care along with the children. Be culturally sensitive to the needs of families. For unaccompanied minors, it is preferable to place them with kind and experienced foster mothers instead of having them in orphanage-type settings. Caring interactions between adults and children even if they are not related helps develop resiliency in children. It improves self-esteem in children and can also impact negative trajectories in teens and can prevent exposure to risky situations. These supports can be added at any developmental stage in a child's life and can compensate for missing familial support [5].

Allow Play

Make time for play. Play is critical for children and adolescent's development. It provides opportunities for them to learn critical social skills [6, 7].

Allocate safe areas where children can explore and play. Allow opportunities for imaginative and expressive play. Try to organize group sporting activities like soccer. Having a connection with others through play, particularly with peers, and the involvement of an older adult or older youth from the community can give a sense of belonging for the involved children and the teaching adult or youth. It helps them develop a sense of community.

Be aware of gender norms, in many cultures girls after a certain age cannot participate in sporting activities with boys or play sports in the presence of men. Try to find ways to get the girls involved in play or sports activities by either finding a time that does not take them away from chores or a place which can meet societal and cultural norms of segregation.

Disaster and Media

Avoid overexposure to disasters or events through media as they may contain graphic images or details that can be upsetting for children and adolescents. This can cause them to incessant worry about what is happening incessantly. For younger children, it can be more frightening than for older youth. Restricting media exposure for younger children is a good strategy. However, expect that children can hear frightening messages from neighbors or friends. In this day and age for older children, given the prevalence of media devices and social media access, the chances of them hearing or watching it are very likely. So, it is best to be prepared to answer questions and monitor for any changes in behavior. Parents should be encouraged to listen to their children and, taking their cues, to explain the context and provide reassurance [8].

Some parents might prefer that their children hear about an event from them. The recommendation is to provide information that is truthful and age appropriate. Keep it simple and brief and provide reassurance in a calm manner.

Tools Available for Health Professionals for Rapid Assessment after a Catastrophic Event (Disaster)

PsySTART

PsySTART is a rapid mental health triage system that can be used immediately after a disaster by health, mental health or first responders that are nonmental health workers. It can help ascertain how severe the disaster exposure is and how urgent are the mental health needs of an individual that has arrived at a hospital, healthcare facility, or any other setting after a disaster. It helps streamline and allows for targeted response by mental health providers based on the urgency of the mental health needs of individuals [9].

The Strength and Difficulties Questionnaire

The SDQ is another useful tool. It is an emotional and behavioral screening questionnaire that can be completed by children and youth as a self-report or by parents and teachers. It can take between 5 and 10 min to complete and comprises 25 questions divided between five subscales. These are

  (i). emotional symptoms,
 (ii). conduct problems,
(iii). hyperactivity/inattention,
 (iv). peer relationship problems,
  (v). prosocial problems.

An impact supplement and follow-up section are also available. The impact supplement asks questions about the chronicity of the problem, social impairment, and its impact on the child's life. The follow-up section asks two questions to detect change after an intervention. The SDQ is free and available in 20 languages. It can be printed or completed online [10].

Considerations for Health Relief Responders Working in Refugee Camps and Health Professionals in Resettlement Clinics

Refugee children have unique needs including catch-up immunizations, nutritional deficiencies, mental health, and trauma concerns. It is important to remember that these children may have experienced specific infections, specific nutrient deficiencies, and/or traumatic experiences during important developmental stages of their lives. These can impact their development and future learning significantly and being aware and assessing development can greatly impact their lives. It is also important to note that caregivers might not be aware of any delays in their child's development. They might not have the word "development" in their language and have limited awareness of developmental milestones, poor health care knowledge, or have strong beliefs in traditional healing practices [11].

Therefore, it is important to obtain a detailed birth history and maternal gestational history focusing on toxic exposures, nutritional status, prematurity, anemia, lead exposure, specific infections like cerebral malaria, parasitic infestations/intestinal worms, etc.

Parental mental health/trauma can also greatly impact their relationship with their children. These can manifest as atypical bonding relationships in younger children or contentious relationships with teenaged children.

The following are some structured developmental tools that can help identify developmental issues.

- Ages and Stages Questionnaires (ASQ).

    The ASQ is a screening tool that looks at five developmental areas; communication, fine motor, gross motor, problem-solving, and personal social. It helps identify concerns in these domains in children from 2–60 months of age. Parents can complete this in 12–18 min independently or with assistance by professionals. It is available in English, Spanish, Somali, Hmong, French, Arabic, Dutch, Norwegian, Vietnamese, Turkish, Chinese, Hindi, and Persian [12].
- Survey of Well-being of Young Children (SWYC).

    The SWYC is a short free developmental screening tool for parents to complete for their children between 2 and 60 months. It screens for motor, cognitive, social emotional, language delays as well as autism and family risk factors like domestic violence, substance use, food insecurity, and parental mental health concerns. The SWYC has been translated into Spanish, Burmese, Nepali, Portuguese, Haitian-Creole, Vietnamese, Somali, and Arabic [13].
- Parents' Evaluation of Developmental Status (PEDS).

    PEDS is an evidence-based screening tool that can detect and also address developmental and behavioral problems in children from birth to 7 years 11 months of age. It is available in many languages and can be administered as an interview with the parents or can be completed at home or prior to the visit by the parents/caregivers.
- PEDS: Developmental Milestones (PEDS:DM).

    This is a tool that can be used with PEDS or on its own targeting the same age group. This measure includes 6–8 items for each age/encounter. The questions elicit responses that cover the following developmental domains. Gross motor, fine motor, expressive language, receptive language, self-help and for older children; math and reading. These responses can give information and help monitor development. There are additional supplemental measures that assess psychosocial risk, resilience, an autism-specific screening (M-CHAT-R), and the Vanderbilt ADHD scale (for older children). There is also an assessment level version for children at risk that are already in early intervention or in a NICU graduate.

PEDS is printed in English and Spanish. There are translations in Albanian, Amharic, Arabic, Armenian, Bengali, Bulgarian, Burmese, Cambodian, Chinese (Traditional and Simplified characters), Congolese Swahili, Danish, Dutch, Dzongkha, Farsi, Filipino Tagalog, French, Galician, German, Greek, Gujarati, Haitian-Creole, Hebrew, Hindi, Hmong, Icelandic, Indonesian, Karen, Korean, Laotian, Malay, Nepali, Polish, Portuguese and Cape Verdean, Punjabi, Quechua, Russian, Serbian (Cyrillic and Latin), Samoan, Somali, Sotho, Swahili, Swedish, Tagalog available as well [14].

Advocating for an integrated health care model with collaboration between health care professionals, social workers, and schools could help facilitate appropriate supports for refugee children in schools [15]. One needs to be aware of the differences in access to assistance in refugee camps versus organized settlements and self-settlements. Increased use of detention centers in developed countries is also impacting the development and mental well-being of children. Studies have shown that increased parental employment, improved language proficiency, and integration into the resettled host country are strong predictors of improved overall outcome in the long term [16].

References

1. Fazel M, Reed RV, et al. Mental health of displaced and refugee children resettled in high-income countries: risk and protective factors. Lancet. 2012;379:266–82.
2. Perreira K, et al. Painful passages: traumatic experiences and post-traumatic stress among immigrant Latino adolescents and their primary caregivers. Int Migr Rev. 2013;47:4. https://doi.org/10.1111/imre.12050. https://www.ncbi.nlm.nih.gov/pmc/articles/PMC3875301/
3. Makwana N. Disaster and its impact on mental health: a narrative review. 2019;8(10):3090–5. https://doi.org/10.4103/jfmpc.jfmpc_893_19. https://www.ncbi.nlm.nih.gov/pmc/articles/PMC6857396/
4. San Agustin M, Ramos-Bonoan C, Lorenzana R, Klass P, Needlman R. Picture books and Reading aloud to support children after a natural disaster: an exploratory study. Int J Emergency Mental Health Human Resilience. 2018;21:1–6.
5. Robert Henley, PhD. Swiss Academy for development; helping children overcome disaster trauma through post-emergency psychosocial sports programs. Jan 2005.
6. Erickson E. Identity, youth and crisis. New York: Norton; 1968.
7. Richmond PG. Introduction to Piaget. Boca Ratan, FL: Taylor and Francis; 1970.
8. Ahern J, Galea S, Gold J, et al. Television images and psychological symptoms after September 11 terrorist attacks. Psychiatry. 2002;65:289–300.
9. J Emerg Manag 10(5):349–358. https://doi.org/10.5055/jem.2012.0112.
10. SDQ, https://www.sdqinfo.org/a0.html).
11. Kroening ALH, et al. Developmental screening of refugees. A qualitative study. Pediatrics. 2016;138(3):e20160234. https://doi.org/10.1542/peds.2016-0234.
12. http://www.agesandstages.com/.
13. https://www.floatinghospital.org/the-survey-of-wellbeing-of-young-children/overview.
14. http://www.pedstest.com/online.

15. Zwi K, et al. J Paediatr Child Health. 2017;53(9):841–849. https://doi.org/10.1111/jpc.13551. Epub 2017 May 29.
16. Zwi K, Woodland L, Mares S, et al. Arch Dis Child. 2018;103:529–32.

Ayesha Cheema-Hasan, MD is a Staff Physician in the Neurological Institute at Cleveland Clinic Abu Dhabi. Previously she was the Chief Developmental and Behavioral Pediatrician at LIH-Olivia's Place, Shenzhen, China, and also worked as a Consultant at the American Center for Psychiatry and Neurology, Abu Dhabi. She is an Assistant Professor of Pediatrics (Adjunct) at the Warren Alpert Medical School of Brown University. Dr. Cheema-Hasan is a member of the steering committee for Society for Developmental and Behavioral Pediatrics International Interprofessional Collaborative office rounds and a technical advisor on the American Academy of Pediatrics first Global Early Childhood Development Project Advisory Committee (AAP-GECD PAC). Dr. Cheema-Hasan served as the Co-Chair of the International Special Interest Group for SDBP from 2016 until 2020. She has participated, facilitated, and organized workshops on Emergency Preparedness and Disaster Management with a focus on children and families in several countries.

The Return to Happiness Program

Maria Isabel Herran

Introduction

We all have witnessed how children and families are affected by disasters. Family disruptions, forced displacements, refugees, unaccompanied minors, orphans, child soldiers, child trafficking, malnutrition, child neglect and abuse, school closings, gender discrimination, and Gender-Based Violence (GBV) are some of the issues impacting children affected by disasters. Professionals working with children affected by disasters, such as pediatricians, behavioral and developmental pediatricians, child psychiatrists, child psychologists, counselors, teachers, therapists, nurses, realize children need special programs for their psychosocial recovery. As the twenty-first Century dawned on us, child health professionals, especially those working with the psychosocial and developmental needs of children, realized the need for implementing programs for the psychosocial recovery of children affected by disasters. Institutions and universities train professionals to carry out individual clinical, therapeutic, and educational assessments but do not generally train professionals to provide mass treatment for children affected by disasters. The Return to Happiness Program (RTH) is such a program. This chapter provides the history of RTH, how it works, and some specific examples of its implementation. The author encourages the reader to consider how this program might be adapted and implemented for the displaced children with whom he/she is working.

History

RTH is a project created and implemented by UNICEF for the psychosocial recovery of children affected by wars and conflict, human-made, and natural disasters. It was first implemented in Mozambique in 1992 as part of the psychosocial

M. I. Herran (✉)
MetroHealth Medical Center, Cleveland, OH, USA

© Springer Nature Switzerland AG 2021
C. Harkensee et al. (eds.), *Child Refugee and Migrant Health*,
https://doi.org/10.1007/978-3-030-74906-4_3

rehabilitation of children affected by drought and the civil war that lasted from 1977 to 1992 [1].

In the early 90s, the RTH program was translated from Portuguese to Spanish and implemented in Colombia for children affected by armed conflicts and natural disasters. By 1996 more than 20,000 children benefited from this project, helping to repair the damage caused by decades of conflicts and violence [2].

In 1998 Hurricane Mitch devastated Central America, causing more than 10,000 deaths, more than three million displaced people, and more than 9 billion dollars in damage. UNICEF Nicaragua implemented the RTH program for the psychosocial recovery of children affected by Hurricane Mitch [3].

Many countries have implemented the RTH program after experiencing natural or human-made disasters. In 1999, after the end of the conflict in Timor Leste, UNICEF in the region collaborated with local professionals and executed the RTH for affected children. The RTH program was performed in Venezuela in 1999 after massive floods. On August 1, 2004, a devastating fire in a supermarket in Asuncion, Paraguay, left more than 400 deaths, 200 of them were children, 138 were orphans after the event, and many children suffered physical and emotional trauma after the event. UNICEF Paraguay implemented the RTC for the affected population [4].

The 2004 Indian Ocean Tsunami devastated coastal communities on the western coast of Thailand. A group of pediatricians, behavioral, and developmental pediatricians at Case Western Reserve University School of Medicine in Cleveland worked as liaisons between Nicaragua and Thailand, translated the RTH program from Spanish to English, and sent it to Thailand. A group of pediatricians, developmental and behavioral pediatricians, nurses, and counselors from Khon Kaen University in Thailand, translated the RTH from English to Thai and implemented an RTH modified program tailored to the needs of the Thai children [5].

In 2005, after the Pakistan earthquake, the World Health Organization (WHO) created the cluster approach to improve logistics and adequate coordination of humanitarian response in disasters [1]. Until then, UNICEF had been mostly responsible, among other priorities, for mental health and psychosocial recovery programs for children such as the RTH. After the implementation of the clusters, the WHO became responsible for all physical and mental health evaluations and recovery programs. With this new approach, UNICEF switched priorities. Since then, UNICEF serves as Global Cluster Lead Agency (CLA) for three clusters: Nutrition, Water, Sanitation, and Hygiene (WASH) and serves as co-CLA with Save the Children in charge of Education. UNICEF is also responsible as the Focal Point Agency for Child Protection area of responsibility (AOR) and co-Focal Point Agency with the United Nations Population Fund (UNFPA) for the Gender-based Violence (GBV) AOR. UNICEF is the organization with the most cluster and AORs under its responsibility [1]. (Evaluation Office, 2013) With these changes, the work performed by UNICEF changed and projects such as the RTH program moved to a lesser priority. Nevertheless, UNICEF trained professionals have implemented RTH in some places such as Colombia, the Dominican Republic, Haiti after the 2010 earthquake, and the Caribbean islands after several devastating hurricanes [6].

Methodology: The Nicaragua and Colombia Experiences

Mental health professionals usually perform classic mental health interventions in hospitals and offices. Methods used include interviews, diagnostic tests, and psychological tests.

However, interventions in disasters need to be nonconventional.

Ideally, mental health professionals should work in disasters, but they are in short supply. So other professionals, such as public health, general health, social sciences professionals, teachers, and volunteers, must help. The location for RTH, rather than individual offices, could be open parks, churches, schools, or sports centers. Methods used are required to be flexible, interactive, multigenerational, involving the community and families. It is essential to be sensitive and observant of local traditions and cultures. Local materials are critical to the success of the intervention, including the use of well-known games, songs, toys, stories, plays, dolls and puppets, and pets, and known characters [2].

Mental health interventions are essential soon after a disaster, or the number of survivors with long-term problems can increase. Psychosocial rehabilitation, as soon as possible, is vital.

UNICEF Nicaragua [7]

Hurricane Mitch devastated Nicaragua in 1998. A mudslide at Las Casitas Volcano caused close to 3000 deaths. Soon after the hurricane, UNICEF Nicaragua moved into action and looked for options to help children recover from the catastrophe and trauma they lived through. UNICEF professionals, including pediatricians with public health backgrounds and allied professionals who had training in the RTH program, joined efforts to implement the RTH program among affected communities. They agreed upon and defined the goals of the RTH program, including a psychosocial rehabilitation program focused in the community with attention to the unique needs of children. UNICEF Nicaragua designed the program in a way that required community and school participation, and it was essential to build educational bridges between the schools and the community to support the psychosocial recovery of children. These professionals realized that the mental health interventions needed to be fast and straightforward, using knowledge acquired in the clinical setting to prevent adverse mental health outcomes and to promote psychosocial rehabilitation of children. The general objectives were to implement a program to help the psychosocial rehabilitation of children affected by Hurricane Mitch through intervention with a global strategy, including the Ministry of Health, the Ministry of Education, Culture and Sports, and the civil society.

The specific objectives included the need to implement a program for the community's social recovery and focus on children in areas affected by Hurricane Mitch, develop activities to support adults' participation in children's rehabilitation, and establish "educational bridges" to support the program through the education system.

The methodology and strategy included two interventions: a health component coordinated through the Ministry of Health and its health workers and an educational component implemented through the Ministry of Education, Culture and Sports, including its teachers and schools in the affected area. These two components complemented each other: the schools provided places for socialization and psychosocial recovery, and the Ministry of Health took care of cases requiring specialized care. The health strategies included activities coordinated by the Ministry of Health, paying attention to physical and mental health needs, providing necessary assistance, and promoting prevention with mental health programs and integrated well-childcare.

An essential component of the RTH program implemented in Nicaragua was the Carousel activities. The Carousel was the first step in the process of recovery. It was a community activity and included the use of "Psycho-affective Backpacks." The second health strategy was the Mobile Health Brigades after the Carousel identified children at risk of developing post-traumatic issues. These brigades required trained professionals and trained community members to follow-up cases identified through Carousel until remission.

What was the Carousel? It was 4–6 h of community activities developed in circles. These activities ran simultaneously, and children went through different stations involving psychosocial care.

The different stations or circles of activities included the first circle to gather the group and exit at the end of the activity, a circle of games/recreation, another circle for drawing or catharsis, the fourth circle for orientation, and the fifth circle for physical activities and detection of affected cases. Each station lasted 45 min.

Each carousel activity targeted 300–800 children of all ages. National workshops trained 467 people, including physicians, nurses, teachers, psychologists, health promoters, brigade participants, volunteers, and adolescents. The whole community got involved in the planned activity performed in open spaces, fields, community areas, and schoolyards. Mental health workers and previously trained community members coordinated the efforts. It involved the use of "Psycho-affective or Psychosocial Backpacks," which included toys and supportive material for children's recovery. The RTH Carousel provided support services to 7126 children and adolescents and 855 adults.

The lessons learned showed that the Carousel activities promoted an increase in community participation and integration among different groups. Each community was responsible for decisions regarding their planning and goals. The community realized the positive results and significant benefits to different communities immediately after the Carousel activity. Among the positive outcomes were low cost, identification of local resources, creation of local meeting places, extensive coverage in a short time, reinforcement of the importance of community education, detection of previously missed cases, creation of local capability, the rescue of local values and culture, and follow-up with reasonable expectations.

Based on the screening and results found through Carousels in affected communities, groups of professionals provided coverage for affected children and families at the community level. These professionals assisted emotionally and physically all the cases identified at risk. The mental health workers and community-trained members required intensive training for mental health before follow-up interventions.

The Ministry of Education, Culture and Sports were responsible for organizing and training the teams of educators and selecting content of training workshops for the Educational Bridges. The workshops' content included the Rights of the Child, community organization, commitment to Earth, disaster prevention, preparation and mitigation, anti-personal mines, and helping children under adverse circumstances.

The education strategies included Educational Bridges to facilitate the reopening of schools. Instructors from the National Emergency system, including the Red Cross and Civil Defense, trained the Educational Brigades. Another component was the School Brigades organized by groups of young people and teenagers after each Educational Bridge.

Each Educational Brigade organized groups of young people and teenagers to promote self-heal and grass-root organizations to prevent similar events. These groups formed the School Brigades.

UNICEF Colombia Experience Evaluation in 2009 [8]

Colombia had been the second country in the world to implement the RTH program, first in 1996 and second in the years 2006–2009. The RTH program's second implementation by UNICEF Colombia took place from November 25, 2008, to March 31, 2009. Evaluation of this program focused on four agreements signed between UNICEF and counterpart organizations in the departments of Cauca, Chocó, and Córdoba.

The evaluation included the criteria of relevance, efficacy, efficiency, sustainability, and impact. It also incorporated qualitative evaluations based on the methodology used in critical ethnography. The most common method used were focal groups, semi-structured interviews, conversation groups, and observation. The RTH's essential program was to promote the psychosocial recovery and rehabilitation of children and adolescents in areas of wars and conflicts and to prevent the recruitment of children and adolescents as illegal soldiers.

The RTH programs benefited 1500 children and 1000 adolescents from black and indigenous communities in the Middle San Juan, Istmina, and Upper, Middle, and Lower Baudó. 7956 indigenous children and 1200 adolescents from alto Andagüeda, Highway Zone and Murindó; 7000 Afro-descendant's children and 700 Afro-descendant adolescents and youths in 21 rural communities and urban areas in the municipalities of Atrato, Quibdó, Lloró, Bagadó, and Carmen de Atrato. 4210 children and adolescents participated in the municipalities of Montería, Tierralta, Valencia, and Canalete.

In conclusion, RTH methodology had many strengths. It was dedicated to community needs when there were psycho-affective needs to be addressed. It helped to create conscience to avoid the recruitment of children and adolescents by armed groups and to protect children and adolescents. The methodology and agenda improved and transformed teachers' way of communicating with children, improved their way of doing their job, and increased their motivation. RTH program became not an end, but a means for community building.

Lessons learned included improving attitudes towards psycho-affective recovery and prevention of children and adolescents' participation in illegal armed groups. It was useful to use the RTH methodology with indigenous groups because it allowed respect for the cultural needs of groups that wanted to preserve identity, without imposing its interest over those found in the community. The adolescent volunteers were the essence of the activities of the RTH program. Promoting this kind of participation helped youth promotion and protection of the rights of children and adolescents. In the RTH programs, the recreational learning activities associated with the preparation of foods emphasized cultural traditions and provided valuable support for healthier and newer nutritional behaviors in the community respecting culture and traditions.

The experiences in Colombia with the RTH program showed that in a short time, the program helped thousands of children through in-service peer training of young people and adolescents. Through recreation and play, these young people were able to help children express their feelings and analyze the events that made them feel guilty. Enabling adolescents and children to participate in humanitarian action removes them from the danger of the spiral of violence [9].

Latest Implementations

On September 6, 2017, Hurricane Irma roared across the Atlantic and brought destruction to Anguilla, Barbuda, the British Virgin Islands, Turks and Caicos, the Dominican Republic, Haiti, and Cuba. Two weeks later, Maria devastated Dominica, Guadalupe, and Puerto Rico. With so much devastation UNICEF responded quickly with water, food, medicine, and other emergency supplies. UNICEF also provided educational supplies, temporary learning spaces, and launched the "Return to Happiness" program in Anguilla and other islands to provide psychosocial support to traumatized children. The RTH workshops focused primarily on helping young children cope with the traumatic memories of the devastating storms. From Monday, November 20 through Wednesday, November 22, 2017, UNICEF organized a 3-day training workshop at the Community College in Anguilla. This workshop was a "training the trainers" exercise for 3 days, and on the fourth day, they moved into the classroom to deliver the program to affected children and to receive a Return to Happiness certificate [10].

Future

As catastrophic disasters and conflicts continue affecting children worldwide, the need for psychosocial recovery programs increases. WHO and PAHO work with clusters related to mental health and psychosocial recovery. However, there are no programs similar or equivalent to RTH currently run by WHO or PAHO. UNICEF professionals, especially in Latin America and the Caribbean, are motivated to update the RTH program and evaluate and implement programs in the region. Among the most active professionals are UNICEF professionals from the Dominican Republic. Some of them are presently working with the Ministry of Education, reviewing and adapting the RTH program to the present COVID-19 emergency. UNICEF's commitment includes working for the psycho-affective recovery of children affected by disasters. UNICEF in the Dominican Republic is planning to create an educational plan adapted to the local circumstances and to provide psychosocial and emotional support to children and adolescents confronting the COVID-19 emergency. The global objective is to review and adopt the "Return to Happiness" program of psycho-affective recovery together with the socio-emotional support in disaster situations prepared by UNESCO aimed at children and adolescents so that the program resulting from interagency collaboration responds to the current situation generated by the COVID-19 pandemic and its psycho-affective effects on the staff, students, and families in the Dominican Republic [11].

Summary

Since the 90s, when the UNICEF RTH program started in Mozambique, thousands of children worldwide benefited from this strategy for the rehabilitation and recovery of children affected by disasters. Through psychosocial interventions utilizing local resources, health workers, mental health professionals, teachers, volunteers, and people from the community, this program helped communities affected by disasters to help themselves to a new future full of hope. The implementation of the RTH programs helps communities, its people, and especially their children to return to a sense of normalcy and happiness. Nowadays, the professionals working most actively with the RTH program are UNICEF workers from the Dominican Republic, the Caribbean, and some countries in Latin America.

References

1. UNICEF website. Updated May 25, 2012, accessed online May 1, 2020, https://www.unicef.org/infobycountry/grenada_23364.html
2. *Psychoaffective recovery of children affected by armed conflict and natural disasters* by Nidya Quiroz 1999 ©United Nations Emergency Fond for Children UNICEF, Regional Office for Colombia and Venezuela.
3. *"Huracán Mitch: Una mirada a algunas tendencias tematicas para la reducción del riesgo."*. San José, Costa Rica Noviembre 2000 p11 (254 pp), accessed May 1, 2020, https://www.preventionweb.net/files/4095_Mitch.pdf
4. UNICEF backs emotional recovery plan for child survivors of Paraguayan fire https://news.un.org/en/story/2004/08/112362-unicef-backs-emotional-recovery-plan-child-survivors-paraguayan-fire August 16 2004, accessed May 5 2020.
5. Pairojkul S, et al. Psychosocial first aid: support for the child survivors of the Asian tsunami. J Dev Behav Pediatr. 2010;31(9):723–7. https://doi.org/10.1097/DBP.0b013e3181f46de2.

https://pubmed.ncbi.nlm.nih.gov/21057257/?from_single_result=srivieng+thailand+tsunami &expanded_search_query=srivieng+thailand+tsunami accessed May 21 2020

6. Evaluation of UNICEF's cluster lead agency role in humanitarian action final report. ©United Nations Children's Fund, New York, 2013. 97 pp. Accessed online May 2020 https://www.unicef.org/evaldatabase/files/UNICEF_CLARE_Final_Report_FINAL.pdf

7. El Retorno a la Alegría: "Volver a reír es…como Volver a empezar." Rehabilitación psicosocial de la población infantile afectada por el Huracán Mitch. Publication by Ministry of Education, Culture, and Sports, Ministry of Health and UNICEF. 48 pp. EMCOR, Managua 1999.

8. Evaluation Report: Project: "Evaluation of the 'Return to Happiness' methodology as a strategy for psychosocial recovery and as a component of the strategy for preventing the recruitment of children and adolescents by illegal armed groups." Evaluator Oscar Solano Forero, Consultancy hired directly by UNICEF April 2009. 32 pp https://www.unicef.org/evaldatabase/files/Colombia_2009-002_-_Return_to_happiness_evaluation_report_final_English.pdf Accessed May 8 2020.

9. Children first…organization and recovery in Latin America by Nidya Quiroz 2 pp https://www.fmreview.org/displaced-children-and-adolescents/quiroz accessed online May 2 2020.

10. UNICEF Eastern Caribbean's responses in emergencies. UNICEF supporting the return to normality after devastating crises. https://www.unicef.org/easterncaribbean/unicef-eastern-caribbeans-responses-emergencies Accessed online May 23, 2020.

11. https://www.unicef.org/about/employ/?job=531635 Accessed online May 10, 2020.

Maria Isabel Herran, MD, FAAP was born in Cuba, lived in Spain, and grew up in Puerto Rico where she graduated from the Puerto Rico School of Medicine and then completed her pediatric residency there. She has been on the faculty of Case Western Reserve University since 1999. She was a child refugee and that experience shaped her life. She has worked in the field to help displaced children in Kosovo, Sudan, El Salvador, Haiti, Nepal, Puerto Rico, and Laos. She has served as faculty in the CWRU workshop, "How to help children in humanitarian emergencies" in Nicaragua, India, Syria, Thailand, Pakistan, El Salvador, Sudan, Lebanon, Saudi Arabia, Cuba, Nepal, Panama, and Nigeria.

How Can Schools and Teachers Help Displaced Children?

4

Johnny Mahippathorn Chinnapha

Introduction

Relief workers or those who see refugee children once resettled ought to be aware of the importance of continued education. Resumption of schooling should be a high priority. All displaced children benefit from the regular schedules, teacher guidance, and peer interaction associated with the recommencement of their education. Relief workers can assist by asking children about school and by establishing communication with teachers and other school workers, and by assisting to find resources for schools.

The following pages, with a series of examples, provide a narrative of how different schools or groups in diverse locations have resumed and functioned after disasters and tragic events.

The Everywhere Classroom—Schools Conducted without a Formal School Building

The photograph below illustrates an alternative classroom structure, created after the tsunami that wrecked through Asia in 2004, out of a teacher's garage (Fig. 4.1). The original school building in the south of Thailand was completely destroyed by the tsunami. Relocation of the school into a teacher's garage allowed for a safe, temporary classroom space. The flexibility and quick thinking of local educators made possible the recommencement of "school" within weeks after the natural disaster struck, allowing for resumption of normal routines for children and augmenting their recovery. The children had their teachers and most of their friends

J. M. Chinnapha (✉)
Ambulatory Pediatric and Adolescent Medicine Division (APAM), Pediatric Department, Ramathibodi Hospital, Mahidol University, Bangkok, Thailand
e-mail: johnny@stjohn.ac.th

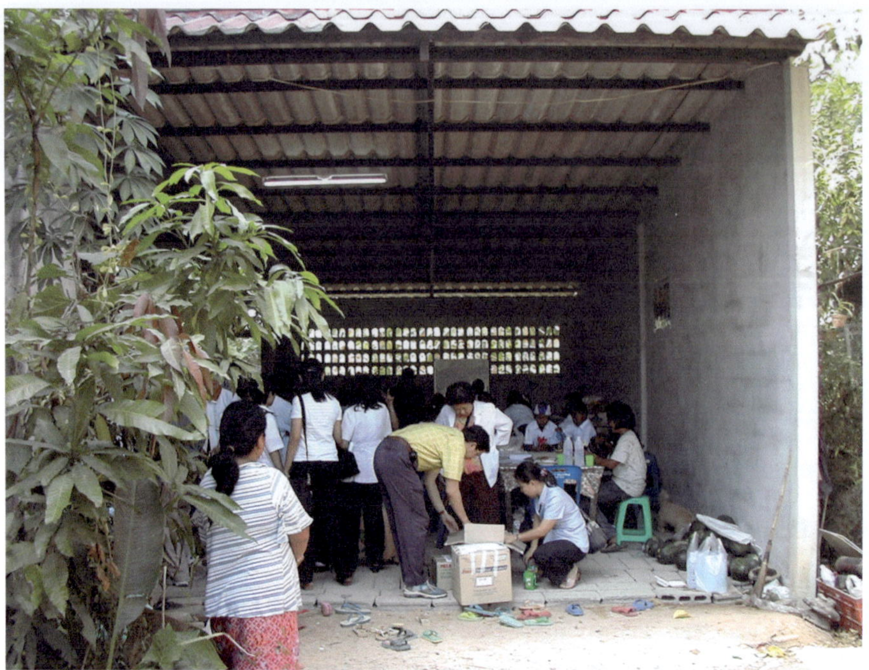

Fig. 4.1 Alternative classroom in Asia tsunami 2004. (J.M.Chinnapha)

with them and were in a safe environment, despite being in a different location. The temporary school shelter not only protected them from the elements, but also served as a barrier from exploitation, abuse, and other negative influences [1]. The children and families could also access healthcare providers in this one location, rather than scattered places.

In the subsequent Uttaradit Province landslide in 2006, in the north of Thailand, the school itself became a shelter and a place of safety. This concept of a "school-centered community building" was in line with the suggestion from previous work by Shiwaku and Shaw [2]. Some of the rooms were taken up by affected families, while others continued to be used as classrooms. In many parts of Japan as well, school buildings themselves are designated safe evacuation zones.

In the year 2011, extensive flooding occurred in the north and central parts of Thailand, including Bangkok and the surrounding provinces. A public university and one government facility were used to house a large displaced population. The indoor sports complex of Thammasat University's Rangsit Campus was turned into a shelter, a school, and play spaces. The children, their carers, teachers, and relief workers were actively engaged in a safe and pleasant environment. Here, both the government and non-governmental organizations effectively worked hand-in-hand, though the latter involved less bureaucracy [3].

After the Nepal 2015 earthquake, one school building was deemed unsafe, so an outdoor area was put to use. An overhead cover was erected using two poles and a part of a classroom wall. Three sides were open to the natural elements. The students and their teacher enjoyed learning together amid the gentle seasonal breeze. As the school was in the vicinity of a forest, there was minimal human activity or noise to distract the students.

UNICEFs concept of "A lifeline" points out that for children in emergencies, education is more than just the right to learn. UNICEF encourages safe learning spaces, and often supplies learning materials and supports governments to reduce the risks from disaster experiences. When children can continue to learn, the whole community benefits [4]. The recommencement of education paves way for the young minds to grow while propelling adults to envisage hope.

Volunteerism to Help Displaced Children

Education comes in many forms. During the recovery period of the Asian tsunami of 2004 in the south of Thailand, when a group of volunteers from Japan was not busy helping inside the hospital building, they went around in pairs to collect rubbish around the hospital (Fig. 4.2). They were a role model for local hospital staff, community, and the children. Children learned first-hand and onsite.

The second Saturday of January is Children's Day in Thailand. Many events for children took place on Children's Day in 2005. The military band provided music

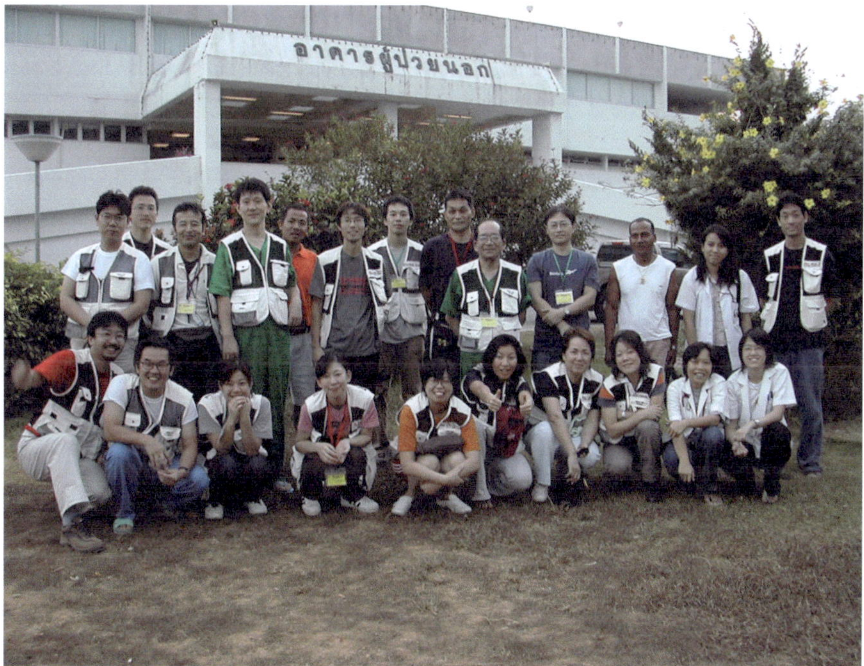

Fig. 4.2 Japanese volunteers in Thailand south, 2004 tsunami. (J.M. Chinnapha)

"therapy" within the camp, bringing joy to both adults and children. When parents are happy, so are the children. Teachers and schools permitted pediatricians to be part of psychosocial rehabilitation wherever possible, such as through outreach programs where pediatricians visited the children in their schools. A significant proportion of displaced children lived in makeshift tents and could not access school. Visitors and teachers went around to ensure their welfare and handed out food, toys, and books. The idea of homeschooling evolved into tent classrooms.

Another example of medical relief workers reaching out to children is demonstrated in this photo in Pakistan. A team of Thai child health professionals went to visit these children who were displaced by an earthquake in their tent homes. They discussed their favorite sport, cricket. These sorts of social interactions are critical to a child's post-disaster recovery (Fig. 4.3).

In yet another example, in 2006 following a landslide in the north of Thailand, Buddhist monks played an important part in education, keeping the community close and cohesive. They were regarded as teachers as they went around to visit people in the affected areas. Teachers who live in disaster-affected areas also need psychosocial support. During this particular natural disaster, the Thai government and universities held joint workshops to support local teachers, giving them time to unwind and express their fears, frustrations, and fraternity.

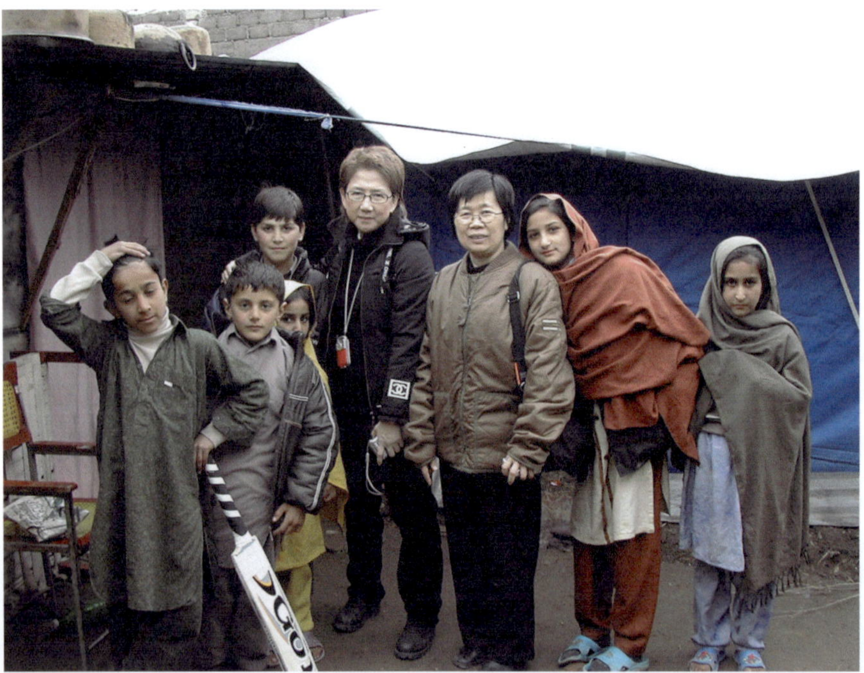

Fig. 4.3 Khon Kaen Faculty with children in Pakistan earthquake 2006. (J.M. Chinnapha)

Grassroots Initiatives

In 2010, the plight of a group of young people in the southern provinces of Thailand came to light. Chompoo, pictured in the yellow-white dress below, had to leave her village due to violence caused by a combination of politics, religion, and self-protection (Fig. 4.4). She and a group of friends together started their own home, looked after each other, and taught themselves while attending schools whenever possible. Eventually, this group became known as the Luuk Rieang Group, and now, every year holds a "Family Camp" for about 100 children and teenagers. They cook together and enjoy many activities together, including constructing a "Graph of Life" where the children take a supported journey through the ups and downs in their lives over the last 1 year. Examples of ups were: school was good, had friends, and they visited different places. Downs included hearing loud noises, such as fireworks, which reminded the children of gunfire and caused some children to remain very still while others cried, before coming to understand that it was only fireworks. Ten years on, the Luuk Rieang Group has flourished in leaps and bounds, benefiting many children from different backgrounds.

A few months after the earthquake in Nepal in 2015, letters written by American children from a small community were brought to the children in the school pictured below (Fig. 4.5). Nepali teachers helped their students to reply to these letters

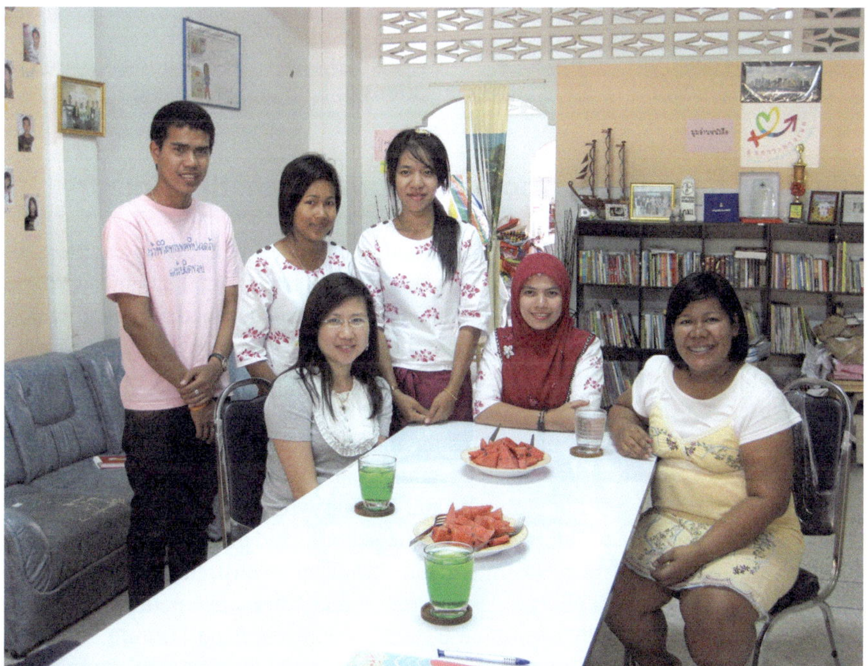

Fig. 4.4 Luuk Rieang Group in 2010. (J.M. Chinnapha)

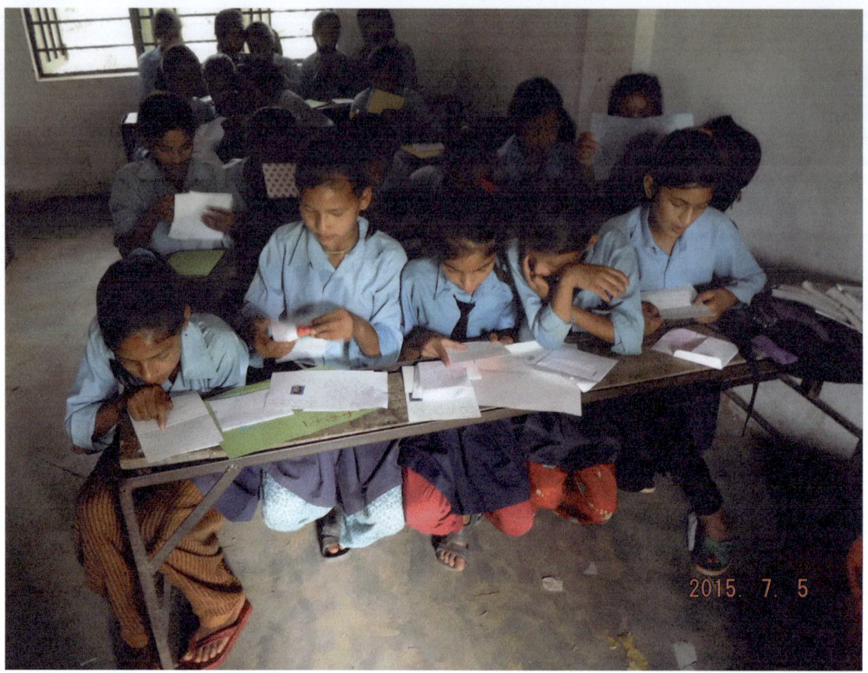

Fig. 4.5 Nepal 2015 earthquake and writing penpals. (J.M. Chinnapha)

and to include their drawings. Relief workers in refugee camps can make arrangements for similar child-to-child communications to help in healing and recovery.

Education for Children Who Are Resettled in another Country

Providing ongoing education for children and adolescents who await resettlement can take many forms. One example is a program in Bangkok, Thailand where a combined effort involving several organizations established a day-center which cares for approximately 100 children aged 4–18 years from Asia and the Middle East. Teaching is in Thai language, with three main subjects being mathematics, Thai culture, and English language. If the student needs additional learning assistance there is a nearby government resource center for children and adolescents with learning difficulties or who need additional psychological support. Social workers are responsible for home visits and link up with local religious groups to provide extra assistance to families. When the school, student, and family feel that children are ready, then they are integrated into Thai mainstream school, where education is mostly free of charge. At the same center, alternative pathways of education are provided through vocational training, mainly in hand knitting and craft making. Local community members also help to provide additional support to female students thereby providing community-based learning and vocational training support.

Unfortunately, child bullying is a common occurrence when resettled children integrate into local schools. In one government school near Bangkok where many pupils are non-Thai, bullying is mitigated by frequent reminders of the equal rights of all the children. Everyone joins in school activities equally and collaboratively.

To help ease integration into local schools, some locations emphasize language acquisition. For example, the Turkish Ministry of Education mandated all temporary education centers to hold 15 h minimum per week of Turkish language for Syrian refugee children, in order to prepare them for transition to mainstream school [5]. Another organization, Syria Bright Future, offers individual education and mental health support services for Syrian refugee children and their families, through the help of professionals and volunteers [6]. Finally, as another protective factor for immigrant children, a unified ethnic identity can buffer children from discrimination [7].

From the work offered to refugee children in Norway, the following points were learned: Firstly, parental figures, as persons providing care, support, and guidance, are paramount. Also, relief workers should focus on helping the child understand and integrate into the new environment. Active participation and self-expression should be encouraged as part of settling into the larger community. Meeting peers through sports and other activities promotes integration and can raise future aspirations. Finally, teachers of refugee children must serve both academic and psychosocial roles. There is currently no effective structure within Norwegian schools to identify, monitor, and refer refugee students. It is mainly up to the individual teachers to take action [8].

In the United Kingdom, noteworthy programs are "Welcoming Refugee Children To Your School" [9] and the anti-bullying "KiVa" programme [10]. Generally, the task faced by teachers is the same with regard to all newcomers. In these programs, teachers obtain support from interpreters, cultural centers, and other organizations. Creating a climate where new pupils feel welcome and valued is emphasized, including arrangements for religious observances and dietary needs. Local children can be taught to say hello and goodbye in many languages and to approach refugee children as learning opportunities. When everyone in the school can appreciate different cultures, then bullying is less likely to occur. The KiVa strategy, originally from Finland, has been applied in Welsh schools and has shown positive results. Keys to the success of KiVa are the following elements: certain teachers and students are designated to support refugee children; continual cultural awareness teaching; individual case management; and involvement of the parents and community members.

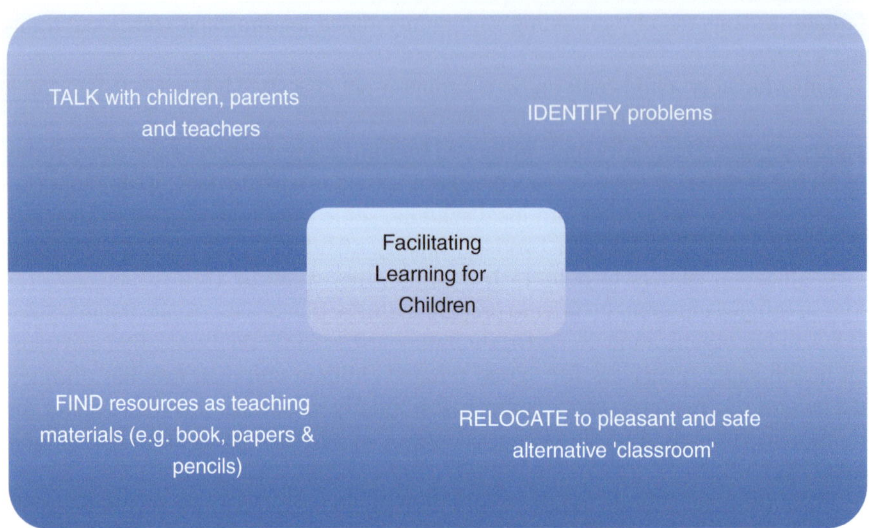

Chart 4.1 Action plan examples for relief workers

Conclusion

Children who are displaced by disasters and untoward events benefit from the resumption of their education as soon as possible. Temporary shelters can serve as a space for schools. Organizations such as UNICEF can provide guidelines and materials on education support for refugee and displaced children. Teachers may need additional support, especially if they are themselves from the disaster area. Relief workers should communicate with children and with teachers about their educational programs and needs (Chart 4.1). Once children are resettled, schools should plan tailored programs for them, including psychosocial support.

References

1. Mandalakas A, Torjesen K, Olness K. Priorities for children: shelter and protection. How to help the children in disasters. 4th ed. Health Frontiers; 2015. p. 34.
2. Shiwaku K, Shaw R. Introduction: disaster risk reduction and education system. In: Shisaku K, Sakurai A, Shaw R, editors. Disaster resilience of education systems: experiences from Japan. Springer; 2016. p. 2–3.
3. Mondel D, Chowdhury S, Dasu D. Role of non governmental organization in disaster management. Res J Agric Sci. 2015;6:1489. http://www.researchgate.net. Accessed 16 Mar 2020
4. UNICEF: Education in Emergencies. https://www.unicef.org/education/emergencies. Accessed 11 Mar 2020.
5. Refugee Education 2030. A strategy for refugee inclusion. 2019 edition. UNHCR. 2019. p. 19. https://www.unhcr.org/5d651da88d7.pdf Accessed 27 Jun 2020.
6. Sirin SR, Rogers-Sirin L. The educational and mental health needs of Syrian refugee children. Migration Policy Institute. 2015. p. 16–17. https://www.migrationpolicy.org/research/educational-and-mental-health-needs-syrian-refugee-children Accessed 27 Jun 2020.

7. Spears BC. The educational, psychological, and social impact of discrimination on the immigrant child. Migration Policy Institute. 2015. p. 12 https://www.migrationpolicy.org/research/educational-psychological-and-social-impact-discrimination-immigrant-child . Accessed 27 Jun 2020.
8. de Wal Pastoor L. The meditational role of schools in supporting psychosocial transitions among unaccompanied young refugees upon resettlement in Norway. Int J Educ Dev. 2015;41:252.
9. Welcome Refugee Children To Your School. A National Education Union Teaching Resource. National Education Union. https://neu.org.uk/refugee Accessed 27 Jun 2020.
10. Hutchings J, Clarkson S. KiVa anti-bullying programme. Centre of Evidence Based Early Intervention. 2017 https://www.bangor.ac.uk/psychology/cebei/documents/KiVaInfoBookletFeb2017pdf.pdf Accessed 27 Jun 2020.

Johnny Mahippathorn Chinnapha: During the Asia tsunami 2004 the author offered help to a colleague in one local hospital in the south of Thailand. The following year an opportunity arose to join the workshop of Professor Karen Olness on helping children during disaster in Khon Kaen, north-east of Thailand. Since then, the author has gained insight into the overall management in this field, particularly for school children. Professor Srivieng of Khon Kaen Univeristy and Professor Olness have allowed the author to join them on numerous international workshops, from which first-hands experiences has been gained and remain to this day.

Trauma and PTSD in Children Who Are Refugees or Immigrants

5

Karen Olness

Introduction

Children in humanitarian emergencies are at risk of experiencing further trauma of several types, including physical or mental abuse. Studies have shown that a majority of children will have experienced at least one significant trauma by age 18, regardless of whether or not they are in a humanitarian emergency [1, 2]. An estimated 10–15% of these will develop PTSD [3]. If children experience repeated traumatic events, they are more likely to develop PTSD. A systematic review of psychological distress of refugee children found prevalence rates of PTSD between 19% and 54% [4]. The higher rates could reflect multiple or complex trauma.

The PTSD prevalence figure varies significantly with the type of trauma, age, and sex of the child. PTSD may evolve from the horrifying experiences leading to family displacement, from the abuse experienced in a refugee setting or in transit, from traumas experienced during resettlement, and even from medical or surgical procedures experienced in clinics or hospitals. Whether or not a child manifests PTSD after a traumatic event will depend on the child's innate personality, the adult support received immediately after the event, and whether or not the child receives appropriate psychological assistance. The traumatic events that are most likely to lead to PTSD include the death of a parent, loss of a home, repetition of displacements or physical and mental abuse. The children at greatest risk for both abuse and PTSD are unaccompanied minors [5]. If relief workers fail to recognize or intervene early, the negative impacts on displaced children may lead to lifelong psychiatric illness.

K. Olness (✉)
Department of Pediatrics, Case Western Reserve University, Cleveland, OH, USA
e-mail: karen.olness@case.edu

© Springer Nature Switzerland AG 2021
C. Harkensee et al. (eds.), *Child Refugee and Migrant Health*,
https://doi.org/10.1007/978-3-030-74906-4_5

How to Recognize the Trauma from Child Abuse

Children who are displaced may experience several types of abuse after the initial trauma of leaving a home and being part of family uncertainty. Even in a well-organized refugee camp children may experience mental or physical (including sexual) abuse sometimes perpetrated by family members or teachers, traffickers, or even relief workers. Young children may have left home carrying precious toys that are stolen by other children. This can be significant trauma to a child who has already lost nearly everything. Child bullies may inflict both physical and mental abuse. Parents who are stressed by many aspects of a disaster may be more likely to beat their children or criticize them. The loss of supportive connections with relatives, friends, religious leaders, and teachers may lead to increased abuse by parents or caretakers [6]. Childhood maltreatment, including neglect and physical, emotional, and sexual abuse, is the leading risk factor for mood disorders and psychiatric disorders, according to a review by Lippard and colleagues [7].

Relief workers should be alert for signs of abuse such as unexplained bruises, strange descriptions for injuries, evidence of fear, the child clinging to a relative stranger, hyperventilation, frequent frightening nightmares, recurrent abdominal pain without a clear diagnosis, anxiety about attending school, or violent or graphic drawings. Some children will have elevated blood pressure for prolonged periods after experiencing abuse.

If physical abuse is suspected, a thorough skin examination should be done. A mnemonic for remembering when to suspect that bruises were caused by physical abuse is TEN-4-FACESp. TEN refers to bruising on the torso, ears, or neck. 4 refers to bruising in a child less than 4 years or ANY bruising in a child 4 months or younger. FACES refers to physical injury to the frenulum of the tongue, angle of the jaw, cheek, eyelid, or sclera. P refers to a pattern of injury, e.g., bruise that is in the shape of a hand or a belt.

Abusive head trauma may manifest as the shaken baby syndrome. If severe, the infant may be unconscious, have seizures or apnea. If less severe, the infant may manifest vomiting, poor feeding, or rapid increase of head circumference. Such infants should have head imaging and a skeletal survey if available.

The Child Protection App developed by Children's Mercy Hospital, Kansas City, and the University of Texas Health Sciences Center is available for free download from Apple or Google Play stores. It provides realistic animations of how childhood injuries may happen, photos of various injuries, history-taking tools, descriptions of medical findings, decision trees for use in determining the likelihood of abuse, appropriate medical evaluations, and further investigative needs [8].

How to Recognize PTSD

The term PTSD is in general casual usage today, and it is probable that there are children and adults who are incorrectly labeled as having PTSD. It is best to make the diagnosis of PTSD based on the rather complex diagnostic requirements as described in the DSM V that were published in 2013, by the American Psychiatric Association [9]. Keep in mind that the listed criteria must be present for more than 1 month in order to qualify for a PTSD diagnosis.

Diagnostic Criteria for PTSD

The following are the specific criteria for the diagnosis of PTSD for adults, adolescents, and children *6 years of age or older.*
Criterion *A*: Stressor (one required)

- Direct exposure.
- Witnessing the trauma.
- Learning that a relative or close friend was exposed to trauma.
- Indirect exposure to aversive details of the trauma.

Criterion *B*: Intrusion Symptoms (one required)

- Unwanted or upsetting memories.
- Nightmares.
- Flashbacks.
- Emotional distress after exposure to traumatic reminders.
- Physical reactivity after exposure to traumatic reminders.

Criterion *C*: Avoidance of trauma-related stimuli after the trauma in the following way (one required)

- Trauma-related thoughts or feelings.
- Trauma-related external reminders.

Criterion *D*: Negative alterations in cognitions and mood (two required)

- Inability to recall key features of the trauma.
- Overly negative thoughts and assumptions about oneself or the world.
- Exaggerated blame of self or others for causing the trauma.
- Negative affect.
- Decreased interest in activities.
- Feeling isolated.
- Difficulty experiencing positive affect.

Criterion *E*: Alterations in arousal and reactivity. (These symptoms began or worsened after the trauma) (one required)

- Irritability or aggression.
- Risky or destructive behavior.

- Hypervigilance.
- Heightened startle reaction.
- Difficulty concentrating.
- Difficulty sleeping.

Criterion F: Duration (required)

– Symptoms have lasted for more than 1 month.

Criterion G: Functional significance (required)

– Symptoms create distress or functional impairment in social interactions or in work.

Criterion H: Exclusion (required)

– Symptoms are not due to medication, substance use, or other illness.

Two Additional Specifications for PTSD Diagnosis

Dissociative Specification. In addition to meeting the criteria for diagnosis, an individual experiences high levels of either of the following in reaction to trauma-related stimuli:

- Depersonalization. Experience of being an outside observer or detached from oneself (e.g., feeling as if one is in a dream or "this is not happening to me").
- Derealization. Experience of unreality, distance, or distortion (e.g., "things are not real").

Delayed Specification. Full diagnostic criteria are not met until at least *6 months* after the trauma, although onset of symptoms may occur immediately after the trauma.

Diagnostic Criteria of the DSM V that Apply Specifically to Children *Younger than Age Six* Include the Following

Exposure to actual or threatened death, serious injury, or sexual violation:

- Direct experience.
- Witnessing the events as they occurred to others, especially primary caregivers *(Note: Does not include events witnessed only in electronic media, television, movies, or pictures.)*
- Learning that the traumatic events occurred to a parent or caregiver.

The presence of one or more of the following:

- Spontaneous or cued recurrent, involuntary, and intrusive distressing memories of the traumatic events *(Note: Spontaneous and intrusive memories may not necessarily appear distressing and may be expressed as play reenactment.)*
- Recurrent distressing dreams related to the content and/or feeling of the traumatic events *(Note: It may not be possible to ascertain that the frightening content is related to the traumatic event.)*
- Reactions as if the traumatic events are recurring; the most extreme being a complete loss of awareness of present surroundings. *(Note: Such trauma-specific reenactment may occur in play.)*
- Intense or prolonged psychological distress at exposure to internal or external cues.
- Marked physiological reactions to reminders of the traumatic events.

One of the following related to traumatic events:

- Persistent avoidance of activities, places, or physical reminders.
- People, conversations, or interpersonal situations that arouse recollections.
- Diminished interest or participation in significant activities such as play.
- Socially withdrawn behavior.
- Persistent reduction in the expression of positive emotions.

Two or more of the following:

- Irritable, angry, or aggressive behavior, including extreme temper tantrums.
- Hypervigilance.
- Exaggerated startle response.
- Problems with concentration.
- Difficulty falling or staying asleep or restless sleep.

Clinically significant distress or impairment in relationships with parents, siblings, peers, or other caregivers, or with school behavior not attributable to another medical condition.

PsySTART Rapid Mental Health Triage System

In many settings where families are displaced by man-made or natural disasters, symptom-based screening tools have been used to identify those with disorders. However, in the immediate aftermath of traumatic events, these screeners are problematic because they do not differentiate children with transitory distress from those with more permanent distress. During the first weeks after displacement, we recommend the use of the PsySTART rapid mental health triage system which was developed to address the limitations of early screeners [10].

As opposed to symptom-based PTSD screening tools, PsySTART is an evidence-based rapid mental health triage system that can be completed by non-mental health workers. It relies on evidence-based, objective risk factors such as deaths of family members, displacement from home, and exposure to mutilated bodies. Relief workers can apply PsySTART in a matter of seconds (see Appendix). Those identified with high scores in the aftermath of a disaster should be monitored closely and referred for mental health evaluation and treatment if they meet the criteria for PTSD or have other psychological symptoms of concern.

After more than a month following a disaster, relief workers can consider using a PTSD screening tool such as the UCLA PTSD Reaction Index for Children and Adolescents (PTSD-R). This widely used assessment tool can be administered to children and adolescents or to parents [11]. It is available in many languages including Spanish, Japanese, Simplified Chinese, Korean, German, and Arabic.

Appropriate Interventions for a Traumatized Child

We do not recommend that relief workers ask specific questions about the trauma. However, if a child wishes to talk about the specifics, the relief worker should listen and express empathy to the child [12]. Some children will reflect fear and anxiety in their play or in their drawings. For example, a 5-year-old child who had lost a parent in the Asian tsunami of 2004 kept playing with a toy boat and tipping the boat. The father had been a fisherman who was lost in the tsunami. Relief workers should make efforts to provide paper, crayons, pencils, and markers for children. They should also identify coaches and teachers who can guide adolescents to organize games and activities for younger children.

Treatment for Physical Abuse of Young Children

Children are often reluctant or unable to describe abuse from family members. If relief workers believe that physical abuse has occurred they should explain the significance of symptoms to parents or caretakers. Depending on the culture or language issues, it may be necessary to engage assistance from the medical staff of the same culture or from leaders in the refugee community. The perpetrator should be directly confronted if he/she is an older sibling or a classmate. Direct confrontation of parents or caretakers may be more complicated if, for example, the culture permits child-beating. International child protection laws should be explained as well as local child protection laws if they exist.

Treatment for Physical Abuse of Adolescents

Adolescents also may be reluctant to describe abuse or identify a perpetrator. Refugee camp leaders should assign persons to organize advocacy programs that include safe shelters for abused women, adolescent females, and adolescent males. The program should include a system for notifying all persons about the safe shelters or names of persons whom they may contact about abuse.

Facilitating Resilience

Although the literature on refugee youth contains many examples of risk for mental health and educational challenges, researchers are increasingly documenting the importance of viewing the experiences of refugee children through a lens of recovery and resilience [13, 14].

It is helpful to remember that the majority of people, including children, are inherently resilient. Resilience can be facilitated by providing basic needs such as food, clothing, and shelter. For children, it is important to provide routines including reestablishment of schools as soon as possible following a disaster and to arrange for children to attend school wherever they are resettled. In refugee settings play tents or playgrounds that are closely monitored for safety are helpful and often therapeutic to children. The Nubader program [15] includes a variety of interventions, such as play therapy, parenting courses, and mindfulness, and has been used in a dozen countries.

When disasters happen children often cannot see the wider perspective. They see the world they once knew as coming to a standstill. Ideally, parents should lead by example and stay calm as the changed life circumstances evolve. Children who feel cared for and safe may find it easier to bounce back during challenging situations. Children reflect the mental health of their parents. If possible, mothers with several children should have access to a respite center. In some refugee camps, volunteers have organized "daycare" for children so that parents can get a break for at least a few hours [16]. This need may be even greater when the family is resettled in a new country and less likely to have close neighbors of the same ethnic group and experience.

There are a number of programs and activities that have helped displaced children to regain resilience. These include the Return to Happiness program originally developed by UNICEF and used in many countries (see Chapter on Return to Happiness). The Child to Child Programme [17] provides programs for teaching displaced older children how to help younger siblings. Culbert designed Comfort Kits with items appealing to children that have specific therapeutic benefit. Items include finger puppets, crayons, stress squeeze balls, bubbles or pinwheels, biodots, and small toys. He included instructions for parents or caretakers on how these benefit children in disasters. These have been translated into many languages and used extensively in disasters such as the tsunami of 2006, the Haiti earthquake of 2010, and the severe floods in Laos in 2018. Instructions for making comfort kits can be downloaded from the website of the International Pediatric Association [18]. Providing children with picture books is also comforting as demonstrated after a typhoon in the Philippines [19].

If there is access to the Internet or to a smartphone there are a number of apps designed to promote a sense of control and self-regulation in the children who use them. Examples include the following:

The Meg Foundation for Pain — www.themegfoundationforpain.org. This website provides excellent, free videos for young children about non-pharmacologic pain management. The videos have been translated into Spanish, Arabic, Chinese, and Thai.

Healing Buddies Comfort Kit — www.healingbuddiescomfort.org. This free app provides appealing guidance to help children who are anxious, afraid, or having sleep problems.

Heart Math — www.heartmath.com. This biofeedback system measures heart rate variability and has several formats including an app for smartphones (Inner Balance), a hand-held portable monitor (EmWave), and a computer program. The latter provides feedback for children as appealing games.

Promoting Resilience after Resettlement

In order to facilitate resilience children should be regarded as children, not as refugees. Factors that seem most important for children include meaningful involvement in school, social connections including some with people from the home culture, and family connectedness. If children develop an area of success in academics, music, art or sports, this facilitates feelings of belonging and adaptation to the new culture. However, it is also helpful for children to maintain contact with relatives or friends from the same ethnic or cultural group.

Conclusion

There is substantial data to validate the recommendation that relief workers should assess the trauma experiences of children. This should happen soon after a disaster. Those children at risk for PTSD or who manifest other psychological disorders should be treated as soon as possible to avoid lifelong mental illness. Programs in refugee camps should be alert to the possibility of continuing or recurrent trauma. Resettlement may occur years after a trauma. Once resettled, children should also be evaluated for mental illness and provided treatment if needed. And the remarkable resilience of humans should be respected and fostered.

References

1. Lewis SJ, Arseneault L, Caspi A, et al. The epidemiology of trauma and post-traumatic stress disorder in a representative cohort of young people in England and Wales. Lancet Psychiatry. 2019;6:247.

2. Orozco R, Borges G, Benjet C, et al. Traumatic life events and posttraumatic stress disorder among Mexican adolescents: results from a survey. Salud Publica Mex. 2008;50(Suppl 1):S29.

3. McLaughlin KA, Koenen KC, Hill ED, et al. Trauma exposure and posttraumatic stress disorder in a national sample of adolescents. J Am Acad Child Adolesc Psychiatry. 2013;5:815.

4. Bronstein I, Montgomery P. Psychological distress in refugee children: a systematic review. Clin Child Fam Psychol Rev. 2011;14:44–56.

5. Gartland MG, Hidalgo JA, Danaher FS. A girl with severe psychological distress after family separation. NEJM. 2020;382:2557 66.

6. Rosenthal CM and Thompson LA. Child abuse awareness month during the Coronavirus Disease 2019 pandemic. Published online. April 24, 2020. doi:https://doi.org/10.1001/jamapediatrics.2020.1459.

7. Lippard ET, Nemeroff CB. The devastating clinical consequences of child abuse and neglect: increased disease vulnerability and poor treatment response in mood disorders. Am J Psychiatry. 2020;177:20–36.

8. https://www.cdc.gov/violenceprevention/childabuseandneglect/resources.html

9. American Psychiatric Association. Diagnostic and statistical manual of mental disorders, fifth edition (DSM-5). Arlington: American Psychiatric Association; 2013.

10. Schreiber M, Gurwitch R, Wong M. Listen, protect, connect, model & teach: psychological first aid (PFA) for students and teachers 2006. https://www.ready.gov/sites/default/files/documents/files/PFA. Accessed on September 29, 2020.

11. Steinberg AM, Brymer MJ, Decker KB, Pynoos RS. The University of California at Los Angeles post-traumatic stress disorder reaction index. Psychiatry Rep. 2004;6:96–100.

12. World Health Organization, War Trauma Foundation and World Vision International. Psychological first aid: guide for field workers. Geneva: WHO; 2011.

13. Weine SM, Ware N, Hakizimana L, Tugenberg T, Currie M, Dahnweih G, Wulu J. Fostering resilience: protective agents, resources, and mechanisms for adolescent refugees' psychosocial Well-being. Adolesc Psychiatry. 2014;4:164–76.

14. Pieloch KA, McCullough MB, Marks AK. Resilience of children with refugee statuses: a research review. Can Psychol. 2016;57:330–9.

15. Underwood E. Lessons in resilience. Science. 2018;359(6379):976–9.

16. Torjesen H, Olness K, Torjesen E. The gift of the refugees. Eden Prairie MN: Health Frontiers; 1980.

17. www.childtochild.org.uk/about Accessed on September 29, 2020.

18. https://ipa-world.org/uploadedbyfck/Comfort-Kits-for-IPA-website.pdf   Accessed   on September 20, 2020.

19. San Agustin M, Ramos-Bonoan C, Lorenzana R, Klass P, Needleman R. Picture books and reading aloud to support children after a natural disaster: an exploratory study. Int J Emerg Ment Health Human Resilience. 2018;21:1–6.

Karen Olness, MD is board certified in Developmental and Behavioral Pediatrics and Professor Emerita of Pediatrics, Global Health and Diseases at Case Western Reserve University (CWRU) in Ohio. She has been a field worker, helping children in humanitarian emergencies in many countries. In 1996 she initiated programs at CWRU to train relief workers about the special needs of children in disasters. These workshops have been replicated in many resource-poor settings. She is past chair of the Global Child Health Section of the American Academy of Pediatrics (AAP) and the Technical Advisory Group on Children in Humanitarian Emergencies of the IPA. She is past President of the Society for Developmental and Behavioral Pediatrics. She has more than 150 publications and has received many awards from universities and professional organizations.

Children's Understanding of and Adjustment to Death in the Aftermath of a Crisis

6

David J. Schonfeld

Introduction

The vast majority of all children experience the death of a close family member or friend at some point during their childhood. Although common, such loss can have a profound and lasting impact on children's emotional adjustment, psychological functioning, academic achievement, physical health, developmental trajectory, and social and behavioral adaptation. When bereavement occurs among migrant or refugee children, the impact can be even more dramatic.

Unique Aspects of Grief in Migrant and Refugee Populations

After a significant death, children not only grieve the absence of the loved one (i.e., the primary loss), but also everything that person did, could have done or might have done on their behalf (i.e., the secondary losses). The death of a parent/guardian generally results in a large number of secondary losses, such as loss of income, stability, and emotional support. Among migrant or refugee children, these secondary losses, by themselves, can be overwhelming and threaten the safety, health, and overall well-being of children.

The circumstances of the death may also complicate adjustment. Migrants and refugee populations may have experienced crises that are related to war, genocide, large-scale natural disasters, or other mass casualty events. Family/community members may be missing without the ability to verify the deaths, which can prolong and complicate the grieving process. In such situations where there is a persistent uncertainty about whether people have died or are missing, authorities should make

D. J. Schonfeld (✉)
National Center for School Crisis and Bereavement, Children's Hospital Los Angeles, and USC Keck School of Medicine, Los Angeles, CA, USA
e-mail: schonfel@usc.edu

© Springer Nature Switzerland AG 2021
C. Harkensee et al. (eds.), *Child Refugee and Migrant Health*,
https://doi.org/10.1007/978-3-030-74906-4_6

all reasonable efforts to determine their status. Adults who are close and trusted by the children can share information about the steps being taken and their conclusions about the most likely status, updating them as significant new information becomes available. Support then should focus on coping with the unavoidable uncertainty, acknowledging that this is a tremendous challenge even for adults.

Those that are known to have died may not have received an appropriate burial; surviving family members may not have been able to engage in other rituals or traditions. Efforts to follow to the extent possible the cultural practices associated with the death of members of the family/community are important considerations. Survivors may also be concerned about ongoing dangers, whether additional violence or the continuing natural disaster. Such stressors may intensify and/or prolong the grieving process. Efforts to ensure that all children have a trusted, consistent, and nurturing caregiver, and are in an environment that is safe from additional harm, can help mitigate some of this distress and should be an initial focus. In contrast, placement with caregivers or in settings that place children at risk of sexual or physical abuse or neglect will dramatically increase challenges with adaptation. It is vital to recognize basic needs, such as safety and reunification and communication with family and other loved ones, as a top priority.

Refugee and migrant children often come from communities that have experienced preexisting chronic violence and/or cumulative loss. It is often assumed, incorrectly, that such children have become accustomed to these circumstances. In reality, children never get used to the death of someone very close to them. They may, though, come to realize that the adults in their lives are unable to ensure their safety and unable or unwilling to provide emotional support after a death has occurred. As a result, they may withhold their outward expressions of distress or requests for support if feel that they are futile. In some situations, they turn to peers for support that they find lacking among adults; this is one reason why youth in these communities join gangs. Migrant and refugee children are generally separated from the preexisting supports in their communities of origin, often with limited capacity for ongoing communication. When communication can be arranged (e.g., through phone calls or web- or Internet-based messages), preexisting supports may assist children in adjusting to their loss.

Deaths experienced as a result of war, genocide, large-scale natural disasters, and other mass casualty events may expose children to trauma as well as grief, especially if they felt their life in jeopardy at the time. Children experiencing both grief and trauma may experience traumatic grief, which may benefit from trauma treatment before children are able to process their grief. In some situations where both trauma and grief occur, grief may be the predominant issue even in the immediate aftermath. Overall, it is important to look for and address both when they are both present.

Children's Understanding of Death

Infants and toddlers will react to the death of close family members but will likely have a limited understanding of what has occurred. Since understanding the concepts of death (outlined in Table 6.1) assists children in coping after a significant loss, parents should inquire about what children of any age understand and provide explanations and information that is appropriate to their developmental level. For example, toddlers generally understand "all gone" which can be used to convey the irreversibility of the loss. Children with intellectual disabilities or other neurodevelopmental disabilities are likely to understand these concepts at a level consistent with their developmental, rather than chronologic, age. In order to assess children's understanding of these concepts, it is often best to ask children about their understanding of the key concepts. Children with very limited cognitive and/or communicative abilities may demonstrate their grief in other ways, such as through withdrawn or disruptive behavior, crying, head-banging, and loss of appetite. These behaviors may also be seen in refugee and migrant children due to the distress of displacement even in the absence of bereavement.

Table 6.1 Component Death Concepts and Implications of Incomplete Understanding for Adjustment to Loss

Irreversibility: Death is a permanent phenomenon from which there is no recovery or return
• Example of incomplete understanding: The child expects the deceased to return, as if from a trip
• Implication of incomplete understanding: Failure to comprehend this concept prevents the child from detaching personal ties to the deceased, a necessary first step in successful mourning
Finality (nonfunctionality): Death is a state in which *all* life functions cease *completely*
• Example of incomplete understanding: The child worries about a buried relative being cold or in pain; the child wishes to bury food with the deceased
• Implication of incomplete understanding: May lead to preoccupation with physical suffering of the deceased and impair readjustment
Inevitability (universality): Death is a natural phenomenon that no living being can escape indefinitely
• Example of incomplete understanding: The child views significant individuals (e.g., self, parents) as immortal
• Implication of incomplete understanding: If the child does not view death as inevitable, he/she is likely to view death as punishment (either for actions or thoughts of the deceased or the child), leading to excessive guilt and shame
Causality: The child develops a realistic understanding of the causes of death
• Example of incomplete understanding: The child who relies on magical thinking is apt to assume responsibility for the death of a loved one by assuming that bad thoughts or unrelated actions were causative
• Implication of incomplete understanding: Tends to lead to excessive guilt that is difficult for the child to resolve

Reproduced with permission from Schonfeld D. Crisis intervention for bereavement support: a model of intervention in the children's school. *Clin Pediatr (Phila).* 1989;28(1):29, © Copyright Sage Publications 1989

Many adults feel uncomfortable talking about death with children, even though they unwittingly engage in games that focus on death with very young children. Once they develop object permanence (beginning in the second half of the first year of life), children of all cultures will engage in a game about death, which is called "peek-a-boo" in the United States. During the game, children fix their gaze on another, and experience heightened concern when separated and joy at reunion—and then are compelled to keep repeating. It has been suggested that this is one of the first games children play about death; of note, the literal translation of "peek-a-boo" from Old English is "alive-or-dead." After a traumatic loss impacting a community, children may also demonstrate post-traumatic play involving a reenactment of the specific trauma. Such play has an infective quality and may spread quickly through resettlement or refugee camps and be quite persistent. For example, Ring Around the Rosie started after the Great Plague of London and is still played by many children. The words relate to the experience of the plague (e.g., ringed red lesions were seen in victims; flowers were used to cover the smell of decaying flesh; cremation was implemented to decrease the spread of the illness; and "we all fall down" represented the many people dropping dead).

Adults may worry that raising questions about the death may unnecessarily upset grieving children. In reality, asking children how they feel after a significant loss does not cause upset, but rather gives them permission to share their feelings so that they do not have to grieve alone. It provides an opportunity to provide support and promote adjustment. Adults may also be concerned that they do not know the "right" thing to say. Table 6.2 outlines some considerations about what not to say and what to say to grieving children.

Literal misinterpretations are commonly seen among grieving children and may undermine both comprehension and adjustment. A young child told that a deceased parent has gone to sleep may become afraid to fall asleep him- or herself and may expect the deceased to awaken and return. It is therefore best to avoid euphemisms and use direct and simple language, including the words "dead" or "died." Religious concepts tend to be abstract and therefore should be accompanied by explanations that address the physical reality. Discussions that are conducted in a language that is not native to children are prone to introduce misunderstandings and miss-interpretations, underscoring the need for qualified interpreters. Given the discomfort adults have in talking about death, especially to children with whom they have a close relationship or when they too are grieving the individual's death, this is an important reminder to avoid the use of family members as translators, especially the use of other children in the family.

Notifying children about the death of a loved one in the setting of a disaster or crisis requires attention to a number of key principles and practices. A practical step-by-step guide to death notification in this setting can be found at https://downloads.aap.org/DOCHW/Topical-Collection-Chapter-4.pdf [1].

Table 6.2 What Not to Say to a Grieving Child

Do not Say This: "I know just what you're going through." you cannot know this. Everyone's experience of grief is unique.
Say this Instead: "Can you tell me more about what this has been like for you?"
Do not Say This: "You must be incredibly angry." It is not helpful to tell people how they are feeling or ought to feel. It is better to ask. People in grief often feel many different things at different times.
Say this Instead: "Most people have strong feelings when something like this happens to them. What has this been like for you?"
Do not Say This: "This is hard. But it's important to remember the good things in life, too." This kind of statement is likely to quiet down true expressions of grief. When people are grieving, it is important they be allowed to experience and express whatever feelings, memories, or wishes they are having.
Say this Instead: "What kinds of memories do you have about the person who died?"
Do not Say This: "At least he's no longer in pain." Efforts to "focus on the good things" are more likely to minimize the student or family's experience (see above). Any statement that begins with the words "at least" should probably be reconsidered.
Say this Instead: "What sorts of things have you been thinking about since your loved one died?"
Do not Say This: "I lost both my parents when I was your age." Avoid comparing your losses with those of students or their families. These types of statements may leave children feeling that their loss is not as profound or important.
Say this Instead: "Tell me more about what this has been like for you."
Do not Say This: "You'll need to be strong now for your family. It's important to get a grip on your feelings." Grieving children are often told they should not express their feelings. This holds children back from expressing their grief and learning to cope with these difficult feelings.
Say this Instead: "How is your family doing? What kinds of concerns do you have about them?"
Do not Say This: "My dog died last week. I know how you must be feeling." It is not useful to compare losses. Keep the focus on grieving children and their families.
Say this Instead: "I know how I've felt when someone I loved died, but I don't really know how you're feeling. Can you tell me something about what this has been like for you?"

Reprinted from Schonfeld D, Quackenbush M, and the Coalition to Support Grieving Children: What Not to Say. Accessed July 6, 2019 http://grievingstudents.org/wp-content/uploads/2016/05/NYL-1B-What-to-Say.pdf

Talking with Grieving Children

Adults who are concerned about upsetting grieving children or saying the wrong thing and making the situation worse may conclude, falsely, that it is better to say nothing at all. But saying nothing says a lot to grieving children—it communicates that adults are uninformed, uninterested, or unwilling or unable to be of assistance. It leaves children confused about what has happened or what it means for them and their family and requires them to grieve alone.

Instead, adults should initiate the conversation, following the practical steps outlined in Table 6.3. Adults can also use expressive techniques, such as drawing pictures, to encourage children to express their feelings. Ask children to share a story

Table 6.3 Initiating a conversation about death

1. Express concern. Let children know you are aware of their loss and are available to listen and offer support.
2. Be genuine. Children can tell when adults are authentic in their communications. For example, do not tell a child you will miss her uncle if you did not know the man. Do tell the child you are sad she has experienced this loss.
3. Invite the conversation. Use simple, direct, open-ended questions. For example, ask, "how are you and your family doing?"
4. Listen and observe. Listen more and talk less. Share observations about children's behavior or responses in a nonjudgmental manner.
5. Limit personal sharing. You can draw on personal experiences to help you better understand children, but do not need to share this with them. Keep the focus on the student.
6. Offer practical advice. For example, discuss ways to respond to questions from peers or adults about the death.
7. Offer reassurance. Without minimizing their concerns, let grieving children know that over time they will be better able to cope with their distress and that you will be there to help them.
8. Maintain contact. At first, children may not accept your invitation to talk or offers of support. Their questions will evolve over time. Remain accessible, concerned, and connected.

(adapted from Schonfeld D, Quackenbush M, and the Coalition to Support Grieving Children: Talking with Children. Accessed July 6, 2019 http://grievingstudents.org/wp-content/uploads/2016/05/NYL-1A-Talking-With-Children.pdf)

about what the picture or other artwork communicates and use that as an opportunity to assess their understanding of the concepts of death, which may not be apparent in the picture or art project.

Guilt and Other Common Reactions

The magical thinking and egocentrism of young children make them vulnerable to feeling guilty after a crisis. They will often wonder what they did, did not do, or should have done that would have changed the outcome, even if an outside observer might see no logical reason for this guilt. Older children, and to a great extent adults as well, often feel this way. At some level, this assumption of personal responsibility can provide the grieving individual with an illusion of control. If they accept responsibility for something they did or did not do, then they can reassure themselves if they do not make the same mistake again, then they will be spared further tragedy. This results in strong feelings of guilt that complicate the adjustment process. It is often helpful to explain to children (and adults) that after a significant death, people often feel bad and wonder what they did bad. Many children may question if there was something that they did, did not do, or should have done that may have prevented the death. But thoughts and feelings do not cause deaths. When possible, reassure children that you know that there was nothing they did to contribute to the death but wonder if they feel responsible as many other children do after the death of someone they love.

When children do not understand the reason for a death, especially if they do not appreciate that everyone eventually dies, they may question if the person who died did something to cause the death and/or God chose to have the person die for something the deceased had done. This may result in shame about the death and the deceased, which will discourage the child from talking about the individual, the death, and the child's feelings about the death. After any crisis, victims may feel embarrassed or even ashamed and reluctant to share their experience with others. Migrant and refugee populations are too often treated in ways that make them feel marginalized and unwanted, that can only further exacerbate these perceptions.

As would be anticipated, migrant and refugee children have many reasons to be worried and fearful. They may worry about additional losses or trauma, become concerned that any surviving adults caring for them may also die and leave them alone, worry about the financial stability of the family, become concerned that they will not be able to attend or succeed in school, etc.

Despite the wide range of significant concerns and reactions that grieving children may experience, they are often reluctant to share these feelings with parents or other guardians. They may worry that such feelings are abnormal or inappropriate or hesitate to add further burden to the adults around them who seem overwhelmed or upset themselves. Children may instead attempt to support their parents and other caregivers and deny any difficulties. It is important that parents and other caregivers try to access other adults for their own support and encourage children to share their feelings. They should be cautious about requesting, or allowing, children to take on too much adult responsibilities (such as care of younger children or for adolescents, contributing to the financial well-being of the family) after the death of a family member. While some of this may be a necessity in some situations for migrant and refugee families, it should be minimized to the extent possible.

Cultural Considerations and Children's Participation in Funerals and Other Rituals

Bereavement is in many ways both a universal and personal experience. While there are differences in the rituals and practices associated with death among people of different cultures, the basic needs of grieving children are still similar. Adults should therefore not hesitate to reach out to grieving children of different backgrounds to offer support—keep an open heart and open mind and inquire about what might be helpful to the child and family. Refugees and migrants are likely to want to follow the rituals and practices typical of their home communities and culture, although in some situations they may prefer to adopt other practices—communities are not homogenous and increasingly individuals are part of families that have members from different cultures and communities.

Ask families what rituals and practices are important and/or likely to bring comfort and make a concerted effort to honor those wishes. When it is not possible to follow a particular ritual (e.g., the deceased's body has not been recovered and therefore a proper burial of the remains is impossible), work with the family to identify an alternative ritual (e.g., burying a coffin containing a possession of the deceased). In some situations, the usual rituals or practices may be seen as possible by the family but prohibited, such as having the family bathe the deceased's body after a death due to Ebola. In these situations, it is important to work with the family to identify compromises that preserve to the extent possible the intention of the cultural practice while conforming to the necessities of the situation.

Children should be invited to participate in funerals and other rituals after the death of someone close to them. Begin by explaining to children what they are likely to see and experience, including that some people may be crying or telling pleasant or even funny stories about their memories of the person that died. Invite them to ask questions and to participate to the extent they wish in the rituals. Ask them if they have any suggestions or preferences about how they wish to be engaged; do not force or coerce them to do something that is very uncomfortable to them. It is often helpful to ask an adult who is not personally grieving to mentor the child through the experience so that the grieving child's needs can be met, and the level of participation adjusted based on the child's reactions.

Reactions over Time

Grief after the death of someone close is not limited to a particular time period, such as a number of months or even a number of years. As children get older and they accumulate a better understanding of death in general, as well as the particular circumstances surrounding the death of someone they love, they will have new questions or seek more satisfying answers to questions they may have asked in the past. Secondary losses they had not anticipated prior may now become apparent—a child whose mother died when she was 5 years of age may miss her acutely at the time she has her own child and realizes her mother is unavailable to provide important advice and support.

Children may experience sudden reminders of the person who died that can cause a temporary resurgence of their grief and associated emotions. These grief triggers can result from questions or comments, sights, sounds, or smells—anything that reminds grieving children of the person that died. Anniversary reactions may also be seen around significant dates, such as the date of the death or the birthday of the deceased. Holidays and special occasions typically associated with family and loved ones may also be times when the absence of the deceased is more acutely felt. Caregivers should provide additional support around these times.

Healthy adaptation is associated with efforts to preserve long-term memories and connections with those who are significant in our lives that continue after their death. These continuing bonds, such as with deceased parents and other caregivers, should be encouraged, such as through talking about positive memories of the deceased, sharing stories about how a parent cared for or about the child, pointing out positive traits in the child that are similar to those of the deceased parent, serving foods that were associated with the deceased, or preserving important traditions that the child and parent had practiced. For children who were very young at the time of the death, family members can help create these positive memories through story-telling, sharing pictures and written materials, etc.

Professional Self-Care

It is distressing to witness the distress of grieving children. Children who are migrants or refugees face a wide range of significant challenges which are compounded greatly by the death of someone close to them. Professionals and volunteers who work with refugee and migrant children are generally empathic, compassionate, and mission-driven. As they provide support and assistance to grieving children in this context, they are apt to feel the grieving children's distress personally—their histories are upsetting, their experiences will often be something that children should never have experienced, and their stories poignant. The grief of children can also uncover feelings related to prior personal losses even among well-trained professionals. Those offering support and assistance may feel powerless to replace what is missing after the death of someone children have lost or to somehow compensate for their trauma and loss—the helping adults need to appreciate and accept that these are not reasonable goals. Helping adults should remain attuned to their own reactions and needs for personal and professional self-care, seek and accept support for themselves, and recognize the positive impact of the support and assistance that they can provide to grieving children.

Free Resources

The Promoting Adjustment and Helping Children Cope webpage on the American Academy of Pediatrics Children and Disasters website provides a range of free resources, including materials for assisting grieving children in the context of a disaster, at www.aap.org/disasters/adjustment.

The Coalition to Support Grieving Students (www.grievingstudents.org) provides a wide range of video-based and print materials on supporting grieving children that are endorsed by over 100 professional organizations. Free materials for parents and other caring adults are available for download and can be ordered at no cost. For example: "After a Loved One Dies" is a guide that reviews how children grieve and how parents and other caring adults can help them better understand and adjust to a death—https://www.schoolcrisiscenter.org/resources/loved-one-dies/.

The American Academy of Pediatrics (AAP) developed a clinical report to offer practical suggestions for pediatricians and other child healthcare providers on how to support grieving children and families and is relevant for all professionals working with grieving children. The clinical report (Schonfeld DJ, Demaria T, Committee on Psychosocial Aspects of Child and Family Health, and Disaster Preparedness Advisory Council: Supporting the grieving child and family. *Pediatrics* 2016, 138(3): e20162147. doi: https://doi.org/10.1542/peds.2016-2147) can be accessed at https://www.schoolcrisiscenter.org/resources/aap-guidelines-bereavement/.

Reference

1. Chung S, Foltin G, Schonfeld DJ, editors. Pediatric disaster preparedness and response topical collection. Itasca, IL: American Academy of Pediatrics; 2019.

David J. Schonfeld, MD a developmental-behavioral pediatrician, founded the National Center for School Crisis and Bereavement (www.schoolcrisiscenter.org) at CHLA. For 30 years, he has supported schools after crises, including COVID-19 pandemic, shootings in Parkland, FL, Santa Clarita and Corning, CA, Newtown, CT, Benton, KY, Las Vegas, NV, Marysville, WA, Osaka, Japan, Aurora and Platte Canyon, CO, Chardon, OH, and Townville, SC; hurricanes Maria (San Juan), Sandy (NYC/NJ), Katrina (New Orleans), and Ike (Galveston); tornadoes in Joplin, MO and Alabama; wildfires in Butte and Sonoma Counties, CA, Sevierville, TN; and the Sichuan earthquake. His school-based research (e.g., funded by NICHD, NIMH, NIDA, MCHB, WT Grant) involves children's understanding of and adjustment to serious illness and death and school-based interventions to promote adjustment and risk prevention. He is a member of the National Biodefense Science Board and former Commissioner for the National Commission on Children and Disasters and the Sandy Hook Advisory Commission.

Unaccompanied Minors

Saleh M. Al Salehi

Introduction

Unaccompanied minors are children below the age of 18 years who are separated from their parents, caretaker, or legal guardian. Children constitute at least 25% of most communities and will be affected when disasters strike, regardless of the type or location of a disaster. They will need proper help and support both during and after the event. Since children are expected to be away from their families at day care or school during the week, this may add to the concerns of possible separation, making them more vulnerable. This is especially true in countries with poor infrastructure which may also lack community or school disaster plans. When children are escaping from the potential danger of a disaster they easily become lost. Parents may be harmed during the emergency and be unable to initiate the search for their children.

Unaccompanied minors in disaster situations are likely to be frightened and fragile. Their basic needs may be unmet; they may be subject to abuse, or even taken by human traffickers to another community or country. They may suffer physical injuries and/or be psychologically traumatized. Unaccompanied children and adolescents found in refugee camps are likely to suffer discrimination and neglect. Some may be attempting to care for younger siblings.

When children are separated from parents but accompanied by another family member, they are called separated children. Separated children are expected to be in safe hands and receiving proper care, unlike unaccompanied children.

A plan to provide care for unaccompanied minors is of utmost importance. Children's rights are guaranteed by international conventions which must be observed particularly when dealing with unaccompanied children. These conventions include the right to: [1–3].

S. M. Al Salehi (✉)
Princes Nourah bint Abdulrahman University, Riyadh, Saudi Arabia
e-mail: salsalhi@kaauh.edu.sa

© Springer Nature Switzerland AG 2021
C. Harkensee et al. (eds.), *Child Refugee and Migrant Health*,
https://doi.org/10.1007/978-3-030-74906-4_7

- A name, legal identity, and birth registration.
- Physical and legal protection.
- Not to be separated from their parents.
- Provision for their basic needs.
- Care and assistance appropriate to their age and developmental needs.

These rights must always be faithfully observed and especially highlighted during disasters. Where unaccompanied minors are involved, the risk of neglect or abuse is greatest. Discussions about these rights should be culturally sensitive and should involve leaders in the refugee community.

Risk and Vulnerability

Although all unaccompanied minors are vulnerable to dangers brought on by disasters, very young children, girls, and the disabled are at greatest risk. Risks include direct effects of the humanitarian crises such as physical injuries, being trapped in wreckage or buildings, confusion, panic, fear, and becoming lost while running from danger. Consequences of disasters also include lack of food, destruction of homes, and death of caregivers or family. These vulnerable children may suffer anxiety, depression, forced relocation, or multiple types of abuse. They may even be abducted for purposes of human trafficking.

Helping Unaccompanied Minors

The following measures shall be undertaken for unaccompanied minors:

- Immediate protection and care for those at highest risk:
  - Children under 5 years.
  - Girls.
  - Disabled children.
  - Minority children in the community.
- Relief workers should inquire about systems to care for unaccompanied minors:
  - designated shelters,
  - safety precautions,
  - food and water,
  - clothing,
  - medical care,
  - education and play spaces,
  - reunification efforts,
  - vetting of interim caretakers.
- Medical Relief workers should give priority to unaccompanied minors in their clinical work.

Documentation and Confidentiality

The entire process of helping separated or unaccompanied children must be documented, including:

- Each child's identity: name, age, sex, body characteristics—including photos.
- Known details of parents, caregivers, or legal guardians.
- The child's sources of food, clothing, and housing.
- The child's health condition at first encounter.
- Any attempts to reunify children with family.
- Any accidents, injuries, neglect, or abuse including actions taken.
- Any communication inside a country or across borders.
- Foster family and adoption efforts.
- Death, including cause and where the child is buried.

Confidentiality is a basic right for unaccompanied children; their dignity must be preserved.

Children should not be exposed to media. Their personal information must not be leaked to any organization that may harm them or to persons who recruit child soldiers, beggars, or children for sex trafficking.

Tracing and Family Reunification

In humanitarian emergencies, responsibility for tracing and reunification of families lies with the International Committee of the Red Cross [4].

The best treatment for a lost and anxious child is feeling the arms of parents; all efforts must be made to reunify children with their families as soon as possible. All systems and policies must make this goal a priority. At any stage of the crisis, once parents verify a child's identification, and the child recognizes parents, they should be reunited.

When disasters occur, parents will go to the school or daycare to fetch their children. If families are unable to reach a school or daycare in time, it may be necessary to move children from under responsibility of school officials to unify them with parents following these steps:

- Most children will recognize their parents or family members from a distance.
- Verification must be carried out for every child.
- Verification is critically important for every child making sure he/she is in the right hands.
- It is necessary to follow local government laws or policies in line with children's rights.
- Reunification will be with one or both parents. If this is not possible, the child should be placed with other family members willing to take responsibility.

Identity of and relationship with other family members must also be verified and duly documented.

- The local community will help significantly in the verification process.
- Tracing of the family for an unaccompanied child should start as soon as possible using available resources and following international guidelines [5].
- Tracing may involve a great deal of collaboration between local agencies, NGOs, and countries.
- When tracing is successful, an assessment should verify that family reunification is in the best interests of the child. In cases where there are serious concerns, it may be necessary to involve the appropriate local authorities, existing welfare systems, other agencies and local communities for any further action or future support required.
- When early reunification is not possible, children must be allowed to communicate with their parents or family members as much as possible. When direct communication is impossible, Red Cross services should be requested.
- When unaccompanied children have been involved in armed violence against their own community, reunification of these children must consider the need to shield them against persecution, discrimination, targeted attacks, and further recruitment.
- The International Committee of the Red Cross, the National Red Cross, and the Red Crescent Society all have a mandate to trace across international borders. Nongovernmental agencies and any other implementing partners should therefore coordinate all cross-border tracing with these organizations, and work through UNHCR in the case of refugees.
- When parents or legal guardians cannot be found, children will need to stay for long periods of time in shelters, or be placed in foster families for interim care.
- Foster families can be utilized in compliance with a very strong legal framework.
- Adoption is not allowed during the acute phase of disasters. When considered at later stages it must follow the international law and conventions of children rights.

Follow-up:
- It is critical to keep track of children who are unified with their families.
- Community support for families in need is important.
- Health follow-up for reunified children is important, especially for those with chronic medical problems or disabilities.
- When children are given to foster or adoptive families, follow-up is essential and must continue as long as it takes to make sure that children are well cared for and happy.

Measures to Prevent Separation of Children from Families

It is important that children be in the minds and hearts of officials and professionals when planning disaster management. Care for unaccompanied minors must be included in disaster management plans of all community systems including schools, government agencies, health systems, and child protection organizations. At the same time, families should be encouraged to have their own disaster plan that includes a means of communication and a reunification process.

A "ready-to-go" bag for infants should be available in all homes in anticipation of disasters or the need for emergency evacuation. This bag should include milk, diapers, clothes, identification, and communication means.

Disabled minors must receive proper attention either at home, at intervention centers, or other residential homes. Their diagnosis, essential medications, and caregiver information must be clearly identified in special tags. At the same time, governments and NGOs should have plans to shelter and provide proper care for them when disasters strike. Their staff should be trained to guide children to safe assembly areas or shelters in a timely manner.

All efforts should be made to keep children with their caretakers. School children must be handed over to their parents as soon as possible, or kept safe in a designated space with proper identification measures made to avoid confusion during disasters. They should be under direct adult supervision with escorts whenever they move until they are handed to their families.

Government agencies and NGOs must incorporate separation prevention strategies in their disaster plans. They must monitor their guidelines to comply with a child's right not to be separated from their family, and the importance of early family reunification when they have been separated. Staff must be trained to handle this issue with sensitivity and vigilance. Government agencies should communicate their national disaster plans with the community and conduct solid awareness campaigns at all societal levels. It is of critical importance that all government and NGO policies do not include any statement that may lead to a child's separation from their family.

Evacuation Situations

If these evacuation activities are not well-planned, chaos may ensue and the most vulnerable will be affected negatively, either by direct injuries or by getting lost or abducted. While evacuating children in emergency situations the following should be observed:

- Properly educate and *inform* all children, according to developmental age, in a reassuring tone and describe what should be happening and where they are being taken. Also, children must be given the chance to call family and notify them.

- Proper *identification* of all children by names and other means; this should include who oversees them and how and by whom they are transported. Children must be tagged with ID's that are clear and visible.
- Take note of and provide care for *high-risk* groups during evacuation; identify those at risk to people managing the evacuation in order to assure special arrangements for their care during and after transport to the receiving venue.
- Care during *transport* is very important since children may be lost or board the wrong vehicle. There should be frequent counting and children should be calmed as much as possible.
- Receiving *shelters* should be ready and organized in a way that will provide safety and security to all children, taking into account age and sex while allocating space to children. Also, the shelter should be accessible for the disabled and have resources for their care. Managing the shelter is of critical importance to preserve children's rights and provide optimal care until they are reunited with their legal guardians.

Management

Reunification

- The best therapy any lost child can be given is to be reunited with family, and all efforts should be made to find a parent or family member of the unaccompanied child to comfort him and improve his mental well-being.
- Post names of separated children in places where they might be recognized, and network with others (NGO's, government agencies, and health centers).
- Establish or adopt guidelines to deal with unaccompanied children. It is of great importance to systemize work and insure proper implementation of child-friendly practices.
- Keep a secure comprehensive database containing children's names, pictures, and status. This is a key element to increase the likelihood of reunification.

Healthcare

Unaccompanied children may need urgent or typical medical care, which will depend on an initial assessment of each child's situation. There should be a focus on life-threatening treatable conditions such as dehydration or infection.

- *Assessment* should include but not be limited to the following:
  - Basic identification information (name, age, school level, family address, known medical conditions, medication, allergy, etc.)
  - Vital signs: look for signs of dehydration, fever, or respiratory problems.
  - Weight, height, and head circumference: look for signs of malnutrition.

- Scan skin for fresh or old scars that may signify acute injury or maltreatment.
- Psychosocial: observe the child's state of mind, level of resiliency, and coping abilities. Also learn about the child's family status (names, address, phone, last known location, and if their condition/situation is known).
- Note any mental or behavioral disturbances and the level of severity.

– *Treatment:*

- Children's health must be maintained during evacuation, to include continuing treatment for physical injuries, dehydration, respiratory or gastrointestinal problems, and care for children with chronic conditions such as diabetes or asthma.
- Follow best infection control practices to reduce cross infections and prevent disease outbreaks as much as possible, especially in shelters and refugee camps.
- Nutritional needs must be provided since most unaccompanied children will suffer from lack of food and may be intimidated by larger children who take their food.
- Psychosocial support for evacuated children is of great importance; relief workers should have skills in reassurance and comfort care for unaccompanied minors. Treatment of panic attacks, severe anxiety, depression or PTSD should be provided by trained and experienced professionals.
- Reinstate positive routines such as school and playtime as soon as possible after safe shelter is allocated.

Summary

Unaccompanied children are to be expected after any humanitarian emergency. The physical and mental effects on these children will vary depending on both the severity of the disaster and the pre-disaster infrastructure in the community. Ideally, communities should have policies and plans to care for unaccompanied minors prior to a disaster, including plans for shelter, food, water, schooling, and health services.

Allocating teams or agencies to deal with unaccompanied children is of great importance. These teams will establish a functional network of help and support for, and a solid communication system with, other care providers, government and international agencies.

Finally, providing a secure, supportive environment, such as school routines, is critical for the general well-being of unaccompanied children, and reuniting these children with their families should be the highest priority of all.

References

1. The Convention on the Rights of the Child (1989) and its two Optional Protocols (2000). https://www.unicef.org/child-rights-convention, accessed December 18, 2020.

2. The four Geneva Conventions (1949) and their two Additional Protocols (1977). https://www. icrc.org/en/doc/war-and-law/treaties-customary-law/geneva-conventions/, accessed December 18, 2020.
3. The Convention relating to the Status of Refugees (1951) and its Protocol (1967). https://www. unhcr.org/1951-refugee-convention.html, accessed December 18, 2020.
4. Inter-agency guiding principles on unaccompanied and separated children, International Committee of the Red Cross https://www.icrc.org, accessed December 18, 2020.
5. https://www.fema.gov/media-library/assets/documents/182218, accessed December 18, 2020.

Saleh M. Al Salehi, MD is an Assistant Professor, Consultant in developmental and behavioral pediatrics and the Associate Medical Director of Child Development Center at King Abdullah Bin Abdulaziz University Hospital (KAAUH), Princess Nourah University, Saudi Arabia. He also is a CBAHI Surveyor, the Chairman of the National Scientific Committee for Developmental Disorders at Saudi Health Council, the Chairman of the Scientific Committee for National Autism Registry at Saudi Health Council, and the Chairman of the National Scientific Committee for autism Accreditation Program at CBAHI.

How to Help Parents and Other Caretakers

8

Marlene Goodfriend

Introduction

Leaving one's familiar surroundings and resettling in a new location is always a stressful event. When unplanned and the result of a humanitarian crisis, the associated stress and anxiety can be overwhelming. No one including infants, children, and their caretakers is immune from the stress of a displacement or resettlement. The impact on parents/caretakers affects the care of their children resulting in nonintentional neglect or misunderstanding of children's needs. Children react to the extreme changes in their life circumstances and share their parents' distress. Their reactions frequently mirror their parents' feelings. Figure 8.1 is a picture a child drew while her mother was talking to a counselor. The family had recently fled Cote d'Ivoire to Liberia. The mother was verbalizing her distress to the counselor while the child waiting for her mother in a separate room expressed her feelings through a drawing. Note the tears in the mother's eyes. At the same time, caring parents can mediate the effects of a traumatic event for their children. This chapter will address how to help parents help their children during the immediate, intermediate, and long-term periods following a humanitarian disaster and displacement to a refugee camp or resettlement to a foreign country.

Approach to Helping Children Cope

To help parents and children, it is important to keep in mind similarities and especially differences in how they experience and manifest reactions to events. Adults are able to express their feelings with words and facial expressions. Children experience similar feelings as their parents. They express their feelings through behaviors that vary according to age and development. For example, a 3-year old who has

M. Goodfriend (✉)
Medecins Sans Frontieres, Jacksonville, FL, USA

© Springer Nature Switzerland AG 2021

C. Harkensee et al. (eds.), *Child Refugee and Migrant Health*,
https://doi.org/10.1007/978-3-030-74906-4_8

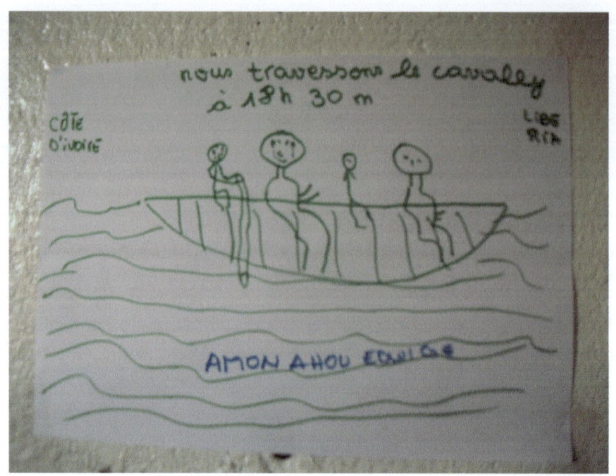

Fig. 8.1 Drawing of a child from Cote d'Ivoire

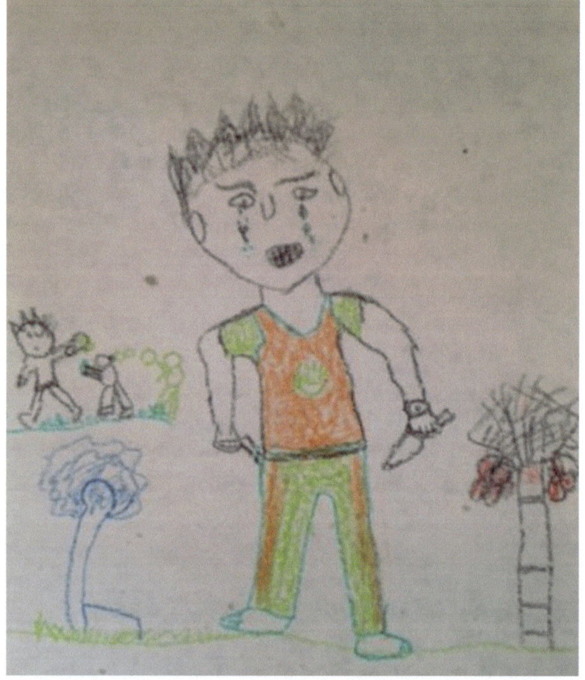

Fig. 8.2 Drawing from a Rohingya child

lived through a conflict situation and displacement might become clingy to a parent/caretaker whereas her 9-year-old brother, previously not a bed wetter, develops night-time enuresis. Other children might not outwardly exhibit a reaction to the traumatic event; they continue playing but their play reenacts the event. Children displaced in Syria who had witnessed beheadings reenacted the beheadings in their play. Other children might appear fine but have nightmares, frightening thoughts, or physiological symptoms of anxiety such as rapid heart rate. Figure 8.2 drawn by a boy outwardly doing well, depicts the attack on his Rohingya community in Myanmar and his feelings about the event. Both parents and children develop explanations for what has happened. Parents might explain an event as God's will, a frequent explanation for the earthquake in Haiti in 2010, or according to the sociopolitical climate of the country such as the Rohingya people not being accepted in Myanmar. Children, on the other hand, can be egotistical in their thinking and see themselves as the cause of bad events. "If I had gone to school, I could have prevented the death of my friend during the earthquake." Adults and children do better post-disaster when connected to mutually caring others. . Adults have more control in reestablishing interconnectedness with others and with community. Children rely on others to establish these connections and provide a secure environment.

The immediate period post-disaster is typically the initial 4–6 weeks post-event. Immediate interventions include the provision of basic needs, such as shelter, food, water, sanitation, medical care, and clothing, ensuring safety, supporting familial interconnectedness, and helping people calm themselves [1]. The WHO guideline *Psychological first aid: guide for field workers (2011)* describes psychological interventions during the immediate period. Anyone can do these interventions; you do not need to be a professional mental health worker; you do need to be a caring human being. PFA (psychological first aid) involves recognizing people in distress, listening to what they need, and linking them with services. *Look-Listen-Link* [2] It is important in each context to know which organizations do what. Emphasis is on keeping families together and referring unaccompanied minors to agencies that offer care and protection. Mental health interventions include support of coping skills, i.e., behaviors that help adults and children adjust to a new and stressful situation. Calming interventions such as deep breathing or progressive muscle relaxation are helpful during this period. Adults and children can learn these exercises, and do them together. Consider the cultural context. Prayer might help in one setting, meditation in another. Connection with supportive others and ability to calm oneself can prevent the later emergence of post-traumatic stress disorder [1]. Parents/caretakers can help calm their children by holding, reassurance of being together, and distracting activities, such as drawing, helping a parent cook, hearing a story, and singing. Advise parents to protect children from media coverage of the event. Establishing a routine provides a sense of security and normality for children [3]. Figure 8.3 depicts culturally appropriate drawings used in Ethiopia to educate parents in a refugee camp on the importance of developing a routine and comforting their children. Consider using simple visual aids to convey messages.

During resettlement in a new country, familiarize parents where to buy groceries, attend a church or mosque, find a doctor or dentist, and how to enroll children in school. It is especially important that families know where they can connect with others from the same culture.

In summary, in the immediate 4–6 weeks post-displacement or resettlement, focus on provision of basic needs, connection between children and parents/caretakers, establishing a routine as soon as possible, and helping parents/caretakers calm themselves and their children (Fig. 8.4).

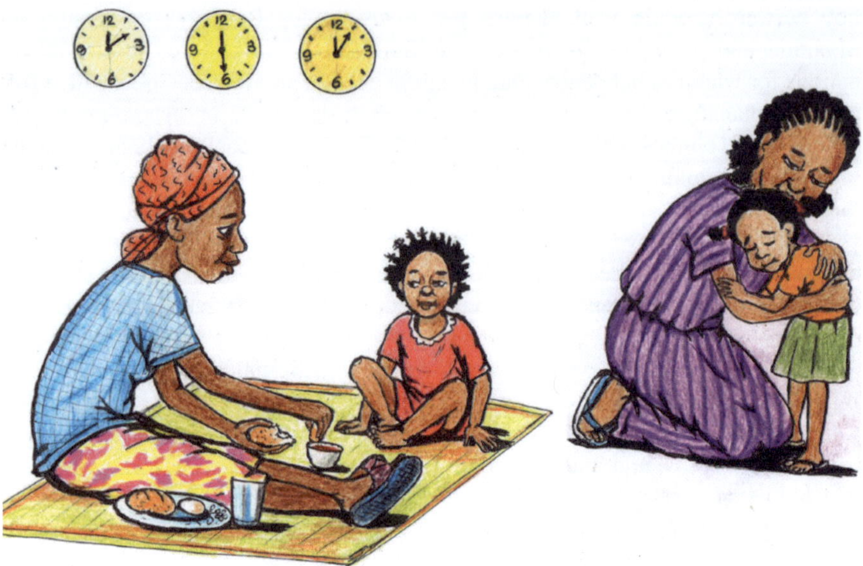

Fig. 8.3 Educational material from a refugee camp in Ethiopia

Fig. 8.4 Immediate phase interventions

Immediate Phase Interventions

✓ Basic needs
✓ Connecting parents and children
✓ Protection of unaccompanied minors
✓ Establishing a routine
✓ Calming activities
✓ Avoiding media exposure
✓ Mapping of services-who does what

The intermediate period usually begins 4–6 weeks post-displacement. Ideally, families have shelter, food, water, and begin to establish a routine to their newfound existence. In the case of resettlement, conditions are usually better than in a refugee camp but still a time of major adjustment. Whereas the majority of people stabilize and do not manifest a severe mental health disorder, many continue to experience symptoms of stress. Children can exhibit worrisome behaviors. Parents require explanations as to the meaning of their children's behaviors. In a camp setting, it is beneficial to gather parents/caretakers of children of specific age groups, such as early-middle childhood and adolescence, in order to address problems typical of these periods [4]. Be familiar with the common behavioral problems in the specific context. For example, in the Middle East children previously in control of their urine at night frequently regress and have night-time enuresis. This is less common in Africa. In all contexts, parents need to understand that new and worrisome behaviors are the child's expression of distress. The children are not bad or trying to get

Fig. 8.5 Common behaviors in reaction to stress

Early-middle childhood

✓   Irritability, crying

✓   Temper tantrums

✓   Withdrawal

✓   Aggression

✓   Defiance

✓   Nightmares

✓   Eating disturbance

✓   Somatic complaints

✓   Regression/delay in development

✓   Re-enactment of events

✓   Difficulty concentrating

✓   Decline in school performance

Adolescence

✓   Irritability

✓   Apathy

✓   Re-enactments or flashbacks

✓   Sleep disorders

✓   Appetite disturbance

✓   Delinquent behaviors

✓   Substance use

✓   Somatic complaints

✓   Poor school performance

attention. See Fig. 8.5 for common behaviors in early-middle childhood and in adolescence that occur during stressful events [4].

Example *A family fled Syria to a refugee camp in Jordan. The 9-year-old son, previously a good student and dry at night, developed night-time enuresis and did not concentrate at school or complete his school work. His father accused him of acting like a baby. The father beat him when he wet his bed or brought home failing grades. The father realized during a psychoeducation session that his son's behaviors were a reaction to losing the life they had in Syria. His son missed his friends, school, and home. Life felt strange and insecure. He the father felt the same way. On realizing this, he stopped punishing his son.*

Educate parents what they can do to help their children and not yell at or punish the child. Encourage parents to talk about what happened according to what the child can understand, to talk about the future, and emphasize the family is together and the parent will care for the child [5]. Children are not helpless; they have coping skills. Parents/caretakers can promote and support these skills. Children feel empowered when they can control themselves and be of help to their family. Older children benefit from helping younger children, for example, reading to them, or organizing games. Group activities such as sports, drawing, writing singing, dancing, storytelling provide normalcy and stimulation for children. Parents also need stimulation and support and can benefit from tea groups, sports (football), craft activities (knitting, local crafts), and reactivation of cultural events such as holiday celebrations.

Figure 8.6 lists psychoeducation messages to deliver to parents on how they can help their children.

Examples *Following the 2010 7.0 earthquake in Haiti, a children's hospital provided "comfort kits" to children with instructions to parents on how to use the materials (a finger puppet, notebook, crayons, party blower, bubbles). Both parents and children enjoyed this tool. Parents and children together can create their own comfort kit of fun and calming activities.*

In a project in Syria, parents requested to aid workers: "Do something for our children who are playing war." The response of the aid organization was to build playgrounds that provided fun and distraction for the children and brought relief to the parents.

Especially in a refugee camp, there are vulnerable groups who require more attention and support in adjusting to camp life. These groups include unaccompanied minors, orphans, single parent households, and families with children who have developmental delays. Orphans and unaccompanied minors require referral to protection agencies such as UNICEF or ICRC. If placed with foster families, the families require support and education on how to connect with children who are now in their care. Families with developmentally delayed children face challenges in any environment, and particularly in a camp setting. Parents can benefit from support groups with other parents facing similar challenges, and advice on appropriate stimulation and care of their developmentally delayed child [4]. Single parent

- ✓ Understand new and worrisome behaviors as a reaction to stress
- ✓ Reassure children the family will stay together
- ✓ Reassure children parents will care for them
- ✓ Spend time together
- ✓ Explain to children what has happened using a language they can understand
- ✓ Encourage stimulating and developmentally appropriate activities

Fig. 8.6 Psychoeducation messages for parents

households, usually mothers, benefit from group activities with other parents and linkage with services for their children such as day care, play activities, and school. These activities provide a welcome break from the demands of parenting alone.

A mapping of services includes identifying the location of community centers, child friendly spaces for play, sports, and other activities, safe spaces for breastfeeding, as well as agencies that provide protection for children, abused girls and women, and medical and other social support services. Resettlement can offer opportunities for care not previously available to families such as intervention for a developmentally delayed child and special educational programs [6].

Refugees are often exposed to potentially traumatic events. These events might include exposure to armed conflict, experiencing or witnessing physical and/or sexual abuse, detention, threatened or actual separation of families, trafficking, and the list is endless. The initial reactions to a potentially traumatic event are often described as a normal reaction to an abnormal event, or acute stress reaction. With psychoeducation and support of coping mechanisms, the majority of people are resilient and able to proceed with their lives [7].

Adults and children with ongoing symptoms including depression, anxiety, and symptoms of post-traumatic stress disorder require linkage with mental health and psychiatric services. Criteria for PTSD (post-traumatic stress disorder) involve several weeks of symptoms following a traumatic event including reexperiencing or reenactment of the event, hyperarousal, and avoidance of reminders of the event [7]. Hence, PTSD is not diagnosed during the immediate period post-displacement. A child or adult who develops persistent symptoms that interfere with life activities requires a mental health evaluation and intervention. Mapping should include available mental health and psychiatric services.

Many families spend months to years in a refugee camp waiting for resettlement. This can be a time of disappointment and frustration. Parents worry that their children will not have opportunities for education and advancement in life. Camp schools can be overcrowded and difficult learning environments. Parents are depressed due to concerns about money, lack of work, and their futures. These frustrations often lead to family conflict including violence and disintegration of relationships between husband and wife and parents and children. Ongoing psychoeducation messages about positive coping and availability of mental health services that offer counseling, psychiatric treatment, and support groups are especially important. Frequently, parents and children initially experience a "honeymoon" phase with resettlement and a resurgence of mental distress a few months later. Other issues for families during resettlement include learning a new language and adjusting to a new culture. Even in the direst circumstances, keep in mind that children like to play and their parents/caretakers enjoy social activities and a spiritual life. Community centers that offer culturally familiar activities and opportunities for socialization and spiritual houses such as churches or mosques can be sources of hope and comfort [6]. See Fig. 8.7 for interventions for helping parents and families during the intermediate-later phase of a displacement or during resettlement.

Intermediate-Later PhaseInterventions

✓ Ongoing psychoeducation to parents about behaviors and needs of their children
✓ Support of positive coping strategies
✓ Psychosocial stimulating activities for children and their parents
✓ Reactivation of community activities
✓ Ongoing mapping of safe spaces, social, medical and mental health services
✓ Counselling for children and parents who have moderate-severe mental health symptoms which interfere with life activities

Fig. 8.7 Intermediate-later phase interventions

References

1. Hobfoll SE, et al. Five essential elements of immediate and mid-term mass trauma intervention: empirical evidence. Psychiatry. 2007;70(4):283–315. https://www.researchgate.net/publication/5668133_Five_Essential_Elements_of_Immediate_and_Mid-Term_Mass_Trauma_Intervention_Empirical Evidence
2. Psychological first aid: guide for field workers, WHO, 2011. https://www.who.int/mental_health/publications/guide_field_workers/en/
3. Olness K, Torjesen K, Mandalakas A. Helping the children in disaster. Health Frontiers 2013.
4. Compiled by Goodfriend M S, Mental Health and Psychosocial Support for Children, Medecins Sans Frontieres, 2016. (Internal document).
5. Healthychildren.org, American Academy of Pediatrics, Talking to Children About Tragedies & Other News Events.
6. Linton JM, Green A, Council on Community Pediatrics. Providing Care for Children in immigrant families. Pediatrics. 2019;144:3. https://doi.org/10.1542/peds.2019-2077.
7. mhGAP Humanitarian Intervention Guide (mhGAP-HIG), World Health Organization and UNHCR, 2015. https://www.who.int/mental_health/publications/mhgap_hig/en/

Marlene Goodfriend, MD is trained as a pediatrician and as a psychiatrist. She has worked with vulnerable populations both in the United States and in the resource poor world for more than 40 years. She recently worked as a mental health advisor with the humanitarian organization Médecins Sans Frontières. Throughout her career, she has participated in the care of refugee children and their families in the United States, the Middle East, Southeast Asia, and sub-Saharan Africa including in conflict/post-conflict settings and refugee camps. She has developed psychosocial programs, trained colleagues, and delivered patient care. What has touched her deeply is the resilience of the children and families who experience the most dire circumstances and their openness and receptivity to our help.

Coping with Cultural Differences

9

Karen Olness

Introduction

Culture is defined as a way of life for a group of people, that is, how they work; how they relax; their values, prejudices, and biases; and the way they interact with one another. *Cultural norms* are the ethical, moral, or traditional principles of a given society and include unwritten definitions of health, sickness, and what is considered normal. Concepts about social self, culture, and cultural norms change over generations of families and over different settings. Persons of the same ethnic group may have very different cultures or cultural norms. Consider, for example, the different cultures of a Syrian farmer living in a rural area of Syria and an ethnically Syrian man in England who has a doctorate in economics, and lives in a wealthy area of London. The man in England may retain some ethnic traditions for special occasions but his cultural norms are likely to be quite different from those of the farmer in Syria. There is an assumption that a relief worker who belongs to the same ethnic group as the patient has more understanding and can relate more easily to the situation of the patient. If the relief worker has lived in the same area for a prolonged period and is fluent in the local language, this may be true. But if the relief worker is three or four generations removed from where her family originated, she may have fewer connections than someone of a different ethnic group who is fluent in the language and has been living for years as the same area as the patient.

Most persons belong to more than one "mini culture." For example, pediatricians may belong to the mini cultures of pediatricians, the mini culture of their sexual identity, the mini culture of their sports team or hobby groups as well as to the country in which they live. It is helpful to attempt to connect with others via a shared mini culture when ethnicity is different.

K. Olness (✉)
Department of Pediatrics, Case Western Reserve University, Cleveland, OH, USA
e-mail: karen.olness@case.edu

© Springer Nature Switzerland AG 2021
C. Harkensee et al. (eds.), *Child Refugee and Migrant Health*,
https://doi.org/10.1007/978-3-030-74906-4_9

Impacts on Health Care

Child health providers working in a refugee camp or in a clinic for resettled children will encounter different types of cross-cultural situations in everyday practice. Whether overtly demonstrated or not, children and families carry a cultural framework with them into each patient-physician encounter. Similarly, physicians bring and apply their own cultural frames of reference into patient care. As a result, there might be misunderstandings or conflicting beliefs related to infant care, nutrition, child discipline, herbal or other traditional treatments, and parental roles.

There are cultures in which people believe that it is usual to offer some type of bribe or incentive in order to get something. Among displaced populations, this might lead to offering bribes to relief workers in order to get more food or medication, or an earlier appointment time. A relief worker may be offended by such an offer, not recognizing that this is a standard operating procedure in some cultures.

Culture often has far-reaching impacts upon perceptions of mental health care. For example, different cultures may have different understandings about what causes emotional, behavioral, or mental health difficulties. Different cultures may have greater mistrust and fear of diagnosis or treatment for mental health problems, preferring alternative traditional healer or faith-based approaches [1, 2].

It is likely that some families will bring their children to both western medicine practitioners and traditional healers within the community. The information about the traditional treatment may not be shared. Clinicians need to ask, without judgment, about the use of traditional treatments and be aware of the possibility of negative drug interactions with herbs or other supplements [3].

In some cultures, the status of interpreters affects what information is provided by a patient and how information is conveyed to the physician. If the patient is of higher or lower social status than the interpreter, an awkward situation may result. The interpreter might not wish to ask certain questions and the patient may be uncomfortable speaking with the interpreter [4].

How to Work with Cultural Differences

It is important to learn about a family's cultural beliefs and customs. Doing so may help explain behaviors that might otherwise be interpreted as negative or nonadherent. Gathering information about a family's ethnic group affiliation, language, and dietary preferences may take a short time but learning about a family's values and beliefs may take much longer. Individual providers should also assess how their own social and cultural health beliefs influence their responses to patients.

Relief health workers should acknowledge their need for cultural humility, recognize their inability to fully understand another culture, and be open to new ideas or approaches. They can study differing viewpoints and decide which ones might be harmful to children and which ones are of little consequence. Then they might choose their battles. They may find it helpful to talk about specific diagnostic or treatment issues with leaders in a specific family or refugee camp and work out compromises.

It is important that medical relief workers recognize that the most important agenda for displaced families is to be resettled and that this agenda may interfere with the agenda of the relief workers. See the example in the appendix.

There are training programs to increase sensitivity among people toward varying cultural norms and values. Relief workers may benefit from a cross-cultural game called BaFaBaFa [5, 6]. This is usually played in groups but an online version will be available. The American Academy of Pediatrics has developed a practical "Culturally Effective Care" Toolkit [7].

Conclusion

It is important that pediatric relief workers be aware of differences in culture and cultural norms among colleagues and patients. These differences have important implications for decision-making with respect to the physical and mental health of children and their families.

Case Example for Culture Chapter

"Differing Expectations"

In 1980 our family, including four children, ages 11, 12, 13, and 14, spent 6 months living near and working in a Lao refugee camp in Thailand. All members of the family had tasks each day in the refugee camp including my husband who taught English as a second language to groups of refugees.

Most humans tend to attribute some of their own expectations and values to others.

Medical relief workers assume that health care is very important in a refugee area and that it is also important to refugees. They might also assume that being on time is important to everyone. The following vignette was written by my husband, Hakon Torjesen [8].

"By 3:45 PM the clinic work was finished and the students (all refugees who were nurses) were just beginning to wander in. This was 3:30 "Lao time" and we had talked about that together in class. The nurses knew that before long they would have to start living by western time. And we laughed.

We had no specific curriculum. Our goals were to learn spoken English and to learn about living in western countries. Our program was to pick a topic and talk about it in English until we had enough phrases to write a drill on the blackboard. Then we would practice the drill and memorize it. In recent lessons, we had practiced going to restaurants. Today it would be dinner in the town. We could go to McDonald's or to the Holiday Inn. We wrote some typical menu items on the board. And we talked about the typical cost of our evening for a family likely living on one or two minimum wage jobs.

"What'll you have?"

"Pepsi, hamburger, French fry," said Ponsi, the careful one. We talked about the western custom of ordering food and drink—in that order—and agreed that it made as little sense as ordering the drink first.

"One beer, one cheeseburger," said Souba, the extrovert.

"We don't sell beer at MacDonald's. Try the Holiday Inn." His bride, Dongmali, went straight to the Holiday Inn and ignored their menu.

"Omelette, Champagne," she blurted.

Most of the class had been sobered by our cost analysis. Plain hamburgers were the solid favorite.

The rationale for offering English and orientation classes at the hospital and clinic is a simple matter of reciprocity. Westerners have descended on the camp hospital obsessed with improving the quality of health care, and discover a Lao medical staff whose obsession, not at all surprisingly, is a continent away! So we share our obsessions, and everybody wins."

References

1. Hufford DJ. Folk medicine and health culture in contemporary society. Prim Care. 1997;24(4):723–41.
2. Krajewski-Jaime ER. Folk-healing among Mexican-American families as a consideration in the delivery of child welfare and child health care services. Child Welfare. 1991;70(2):157–67.
3. Flores G. Culture, ethnicity, and linguistic issues in pediatric care: urgent priorities and unanswered questions. Ambul Pediatr. 2004;4(4):276–82.
4. Olness K. Cultural aspects in working with Lao refugees. Minn Med. 1979;62(12):871–4.
5. Shirts RG. BaFá BaFá: a cross-cultural simulation. Del Mar, CA: Simile; 1977.
6. www.simulationtrainingsystems.com Accessed September 30, 2020.
7. Cora-Bramble D. Providing culturally effective care (*Culturally Effective Care Toolkit*). Am Acad Pediatr. https://www.aap.org/en-us/professional-resources/practice-transformation/managing-patients/Pages/effective-care.aspx. Accessed August 25, 2020
8. Torjesen H, Olness K, Torjesen E. The gift of the refugees. MN: Eden Prairie; 1981.

Karen Olness, MD is board certified in Developmental and Behavioral Pediatrics and Professor Emerita of Pediatrics, Global Health and Diseases at Case Western Reserve University (CWRU) in Ohio. She has been a field worker, helping children in humanitarian emergencies in many countries. In 1996 she initiated programs at CWRU to train relief workers about the special needs of children in disasters. These workshops have been replicated in many resource-poor settings. She is past chair of the Global Child Health Section of the American Academy of Pediatrics (AAP) and the Technical Advisory Group on Children in Humanitarian Emergencies of the IPA. She is past President of the Society for Developmental and Behavioral Pediatrics. She has more than 150 publications and has received many awards from universities and professional organizations.

B. Emily Esmaili

Overview

Clinics serving refugee and migrant children vary in size, structure, and level of financial support. As such, considerations and challenges will differ greatly across the range of clinical models. However, whether you work in a large federally funded clinic in urban America or a small NGO clinic in rural Uganda, similar threads run through many migrant clinics. The importance of trauma-informed care, the critical role of social workers or case managers, and the essential need for local partnerships, for example, are aspects that hold true across locations and organizations.

Trauma-Informed Care

The effect of trauma upon healthcare utilization, for both chronic and acute health needs, has been well demonstrated [1, 2]. It is upon healthcare providers to recognize and minimize these effects where at all possible, from intake staff to lab technicians to security personnel. Providing trauma-informed care may be as simple as offering to leave the door slightly ajar to minimize feelings of captivity or claustrophobia, or remembering to have caregivers nearby at all times, especially when doing physical exams. In addition, it is important to encourage self-care of all clinic staff in order to minimize secondary trauma and prevent compassion fatigue.

While the care of refugee and migrant children must involve addressing mental and behavioral health concerns, these conversations do not necessarily need to be had on the first clinical encounter. Establishing rapport and building trust take time, especially in these children with transitory and often traumatic pasts. Many of these

B. E. Esmaili (✉)
Duke Global Health Institute, Duke University, Durham, NC, USA

Lincoln Community Health Center, Durham, NC, USA
e-mail: bee6@duke.edu

© Springer Nature Switzerland AG 2021
C. Harkensee et al. (eds.), *Child Refugee and Migrant Health*,
https://doi.org/10.1007/978-3-030-74906-4_10

children-on-the-move have not had consistent medical homes and familiar health-care providers in years—if ever—and winning their trust can be a prolonged process, but worthwhile nonetheless. Establishing a safe, dependable medical home can guard against care that is fragmented, duplicative, and often fails at prevention.

Providing trained medical interpreters is another important aspect of trauma-informed care. In addition to ensuring that needs, concerns and responses are effectively communicated, interpreters can serve as cultural brokers, liaising between individuals from potentially very different backgrounds. If possible, it is important to confirm that the family is comfortable proceeding with a particular interpreter, to make sure they will be able to communicate freely.

Small, simple measures can go a long way. For example, learning to say "Hello," "How are you," and "Open your mouth please" in several languages can put an anxious child at ease and help build rapport with caregivers. Also, waiting rooms outfitted with multilingual reading materials and culturally acceptable toys will be much more welcoming to children and families from different backgrounds.

Public Health and Preventive Health Considerations

Requirements for medical and infectious disease screening and immunizations vary depending on clinic location, government resources, trending epidemiology, and a child's immigration status. For example, many refugee children in the US will have received some vaccines through the Vaccination Program for US-bound refugees, which is supported by the CDC and Department of State. Migrant children arriving through less organized immigration routes may present without any documentation of immunization status, nor any health records at all. Refugee and migrant children alike are advised to follow national immunization schedules, such as those outlined by the CDC's Advisory Committee on Immunization Practices, and demonstration of full vaccination status is a requirement for citizenship in many countries such as the US. For most up-to-date information on immunization and infectious disease screening recommendations, refer to resources listed at the end of the chapter including CDC guidelines, the *AAP Redbook*, and relevant policy statements from the American Academy of Pediatrics [3, 4]. With public health and preventive health considerations recommendations and requirements in mind, it is important to note that all immunizations and laboratory testing need not be done during the first clinic visit, which is often already quite frightening and re-traumatizing for a newly arrived child, as long as close follow-up is feasible.

While some clinics will only provide the minimum basic screening services to refugee and migrant populations, others may have sufficient resources to also link patients to ongoing preventive and primary care services. The same general preventive measures that are routinely offered to local children should be offered to refugee or migrant children, such as developmental assessments, nutritional counseling, and anticipatory guidance, on an ongoing basis. When establishing care with a newly arrived refugee or migrant child, it is important to obtain a full medical and surgical history—which may require multiple rounds of questioning in different ways, over multiple visits. For example, was the child born prematurely? Was he/she seriously ill in the past, or ever require hospitalization or surgery? Was the child ever malnourished? Details of a child's early history, in particular, could explain current cognitive impairments or behavioral problems. Be aware that caregivers may be reticent to share information about serious illnesses in the past (or present), perhaps due to fear of judgment, stigmatization of certain diseases, guilt, or fear of other possible repercussions. It may take several clinic visits to earn sufficient trust to flesh out a child's entire story.

At each visit, special attention should be paid to behavioral issues, such as adjustment and possible bullying at school or around the camp, which may manifest differently over time. In addition, newcomers should be screened for problems, such as iron-deficiency anemia, elevated lead levels, and vitamin D deficiency, which are common among pediatric migrant populations globally and can sometimes manifest as behavior and/or developmental problems such as inattention, learning disabilities, and mood disorders. Please refer to the guidelines listed at the end of the chapter for full screening recommendations.

The concept of regular preventive visits may be new to many families and thus require further and perhaps repeated explanation. Prior to resettlement, many children may not have experienced well visits or any sort of clinical encounter focused on health promotion and disease prevention. Thus, it is important to continually reiterate the importance of preventive visits and health-promoting behaviors, encouraging the development of healthy lifestyles as these children transition to their new home environments.

Ethical and Legal Considerations

Many countries will provide free healthcare for refugees and asylum seekers alike. According to the WHO, all resettled displaced persons should have access to comprehensive healthcare. In the US however one of the many points distinguishing registered refugees from other migrant groups is refugees' access to public benefits such as health insurance. Undocumented children or those without refugee status may be discouraged from seeking medical care due to financial barriers or fear of legal ramifications. Providers must continue to push back against these barriers by advocating for adequate healthcare for all children, regardless of citizenship or immigration status. Local resources such as asylum clinics or pro bono legal services may be available in certain areas and could provide valuable partnerships. In addition, many community health centers offer sliding-scale fees for patients without health insurance and are an important resource for children without coverage or whose coverage has lapsed.

Case Management and Clinic Flow

In addition to legal and financial barriers, refugee and migrant children experience a number of additional social challenges, often complex in nature. Their caregivers may lack transportation or protected time to take them to appointments. They may be allotted housing that is substandard or unsafe. Their caregivers may have different understandings of healthcare systems and different paradigms of health and wellness. Caregivers may carry culturally infused beliefs and stigmas against certain conditions, for example, not fully understanding the concept of a chronic condition or illness that has no cure, such as asthma or diabetes. Or, they may believe other conditions such as seizures are due to spirit possession and can thus only be treated by spiritual healers. These multidimensional barriers can collectively hinder a family's ability and/or willingness to navigate their current healthcare landscape.

A trained, culturally aware case manager or social worker can help overcome many of these barriers. In a new or less-resourced clinic, trained volunteers or community health workers can also serve this function. They can help arrange referral appointments and transportation, liaise with schools, employers, or housing managers, and offer information on clothing or food banks. On the individual level, case managers can be a tremendous help to a family learning to assimilate and navigate a new healthcare system, culture, and community. On the clinic level, case managers can enhance clinic flow by addressing these needs upfront, as well as helping patients find their way to the laboratory, radiology, or pharmacy departments. They can also help explore funding opportunities in order to expand clinic resources. And on the community level, they can help build relationships with local organizations such as refugee resettlement agencies, local youth groups, or church organizations.

Preemptively establishing systems and processes to ease clinic flow is essential to clinic efficiency and to improving the experience of staff and patients alike. Case managers and other ancillary staff who can assist with the nonmedical aspects of healthcare are critical members of the clinic team.

Building Partnerships and Building on Strengths

Meeting the many, complex needs that refugee and migrant children bring to your examining table will require collaboration and loads of creativity. Your clinic might not have mental health resources for non-English speaking children, for example, but the local public school system might have an arts-therapy program that could be beneficial. Local libraries might be willing to donate children's books, and student volunteers could be utilized to discuss the importance of early literacy. Determine the most pressing needs in your particular clinic situation and begin canvassing potential partners and resources. Be as specific as possible in desired interventions and seek to develop targeted programs for specified problems. For example, if worsening obesity is a trend among your Middle Eastern adolescent female patients, look for Arabic-speaking nutrition programs or culturally acceptable sports groups in your area.

The value of local partnership cannot be overstated. Resettlement agencies often can provide extended case management for high-risk families, classes in English or employment, and sometimes can provide volunteers to accompany patients to their appointments. Academic partnerships can be particularly useful, such as universities that have academic interests in migration issues, child health disparities, or refugee studies. Academic institutions can bring student volunteers, opportunities for grant funding and sponsorship, as well as consultation on clinical best practices and quality improvement. For example, Duke University Medical Center supports a community health clinic (Lincoln Community Health Center) in Durham, North Carolina, that cares for most refugees in that area. Duke provides a network of sub-specialty providers for referral when needed, at a steeply discounted cost, as well as a cadre of volunteer service-learners that benefit from the local/global clinical experience.

Amid the myriad challenges of running a clinic for refugee and migrant children, the hidden assets are also many. As most of these children have endured various forms of hardship and instability both before and during migration, they are often resilient, adaptable, and quite grateful for reliable medical care. Many cherish the doctor–patient relationship and look forward to provider visits as special social occasions. Many also come from families that uphold strong religious and/or cultural values and a sense of family cohesiveness, all of which can contribute to a strong set of moral values for the child. Finally, staff working in refugee or migrant clinics are often drawn to these positions out of a sense of personal responsibility, compassionate awareness, and sometimes personal experience as refugees or migrants themselves. These are all qualities that can greatly benefit care providers in meeting the unique health needs of refugee and migrant children, who are striving to resettle in their newest home.

Two Vignettes

Below are two vignettes of very different clinics serving refugee and migrant children, authored by editors of this book, each with different challenges at hand, and different resources and creative solutions to address them.

Case Study One: A Child Migrant and Refugee Service in Gateshead, UK

Gateshead, a city in the North East of England, has the second-highest proportion per population of resettled refugees and asylum seekers in the UK. Newly arriving migrants struggle with access to health care for a variety of reasons, including not speaking the language, not knowing the health system, and the system not considering their health needs.

The Gateshead Child Migrant and Refugee Service started in 2018 as a pilot project at Queen Elizabeth Hospital, belonging to and funded by the state-run

National Health Service (NHS) as a "new entry" clinic where children of refugees and asylum seeker families resettled in Gateshead would have a comprehensive health screening, have their health needs identified, and addressed either within the same service or by linking the family to another statutory or voluntary service in the area. Following a series of surveys, focus groups, and workshops with service users as well as providers, the clinic is evolving into a holistic service provider for migrant families, having learned that successful integration is the key to long-term physical and mental health of migrant families. The clinic builds on evidence-based guidance for the assessment of refugees [5, 6].

The purpose of the initial health screening is to identify all health needs and address these at the earliest opportunity. Approximately 45 min are spent with each new refugee child. The main elements of this visit include:

Identifying and Welcoming—The service works closely with the local Council (responsible for housing refugees and asylum seekers), housing companies, family doctors (GPs), and charities to identify and refer families. Families are then contacted by a migrant health nurse specialist and invited to attend a health screening appointment at the hospital. The service has encouraged local GP practices to join an initiative started by the NGO *Doctors of the World*, which promotes registration in primary care. Arriving in the hospital clinic, families are welcomed into a child-friendly waiting area by the specialist nurse, interpreter, and play specialist. The clinical assessment follows evidence-based guidelines for immigrant and refugee health [5].

A Comprehensive Personal and Family History—With the help of an interpreter, the clinic doctor explores any concerns the family has about their child, any current symptoms, details of the family's travel history, past medical history, family history, and health of all family members. Although the clinic cannot treat adults, the doctor gives recommendations to the family doctor to manage any health issues of the parents. Older children and teenagers are given the opportunity to talk to the doctor alone and are offered sexual health support or referral if desired.

Mental Health Assessment—All caregivers are asked a detailed history of mental health symptoms, history, exposures to trauma, concerns about behavior, and developmental milestone screening. This is started at the initial visit and explored further in subsequent visits if necessary. The doctor does ask specifically about exposure to trauma and how this affects the child and uses the Strengths and Difficulties Questionnaire (SDQ, freely available in several languages) to screen for mental health issues and inform decisions about follow-up [7, 8]. On arrival in the UK, families often feel extreme relief of starting a new life in a safe place and mental health symptoms may not be very prominent, though traumatic experiences often resurface after a period of resettlement.

Clinical Examination, Growth and Developmental Assessment—All children have their vital signs taken (heart rate, respiratory rate, oxygen saturation, blood pressure, temperature), a urine sample checked with a point-of-care test, and their weight and height measured (in younger children, and where malnutrition is suspected, mid-upper arm circumference (MUAC) is also obtained). The clinic uses WHO Anthro and Anthro+ to log children's growth parameters. Children then have a complete systems examination, focusing on common problems of refugee children: malnutrition, micronutrient deficiencies, dental decay, and features of parasitic infections and chronic infections.

Laboratory Tests—The following blood tests are obtained from all children during the initial screening:

- Full blood count.
- Kidney/liver function.
- Bone profile: Phosphate, Calcium, Alkaline phosphate.
- Thyroid function.
- Inflammatory markers (CRP, ESR).
- Micronutrient screen (iron, vitamins A, B12, D and E, folate, zinc).

Further investigations are obtained, depending on individual needs. Infection screens are tailored to exposure risks at the countries of origin, residence, and travel route, and may include a TB screening, hepatitis serologies, HIV testing, malaria testing, and Strongyloides and Schistosoma serologies. While a public health concern for host countries, the clinic found that management of infections is not the main health need of refugee and asylum-seeking families.

Comprehensive Recommendations—Families are provided with basic health recommendations, including information about available services in their native language. Specific written health recommendations are given to the family, the GP, the Council support worker, and any voluntary sector organization involved, keeping in mind patient confidentiality. The clinic uses social prescribing (where a doctor or nurse prescribes a social intervention with a health benefit, e.g., a physical activity program or a social worker visit) extensively to promote health and social integration. Common health problems identified include: malnutrition (stunting with undernutrition and obesity), nutritional deficiencies, mental health concerns, incomplete vaccinations, poor dentition, need for vision and hearing tests, and poor maternal health (e.g., multiple micronutrient deficiencies, especially with breastfeeding and having multiple children, and maternal depression). A major aspect of addressing health needs lies in the degree of social integration achieved by the family and helping overcome barriers inhibiting deeper integration. In addition to individual physical and mental health needs, the need for clinic follow-up is also determined by factors that inhibit integration (e.g., child's lack of access to education, lack of peer relationship experience, parental unemployment, poor housing, lack of language abilities, single parent, previous or current family experience of violence/racism, parental psychiatric diagnosis and/or disability). The clinic works closely with support workers and social workers to address issues of community integration.

Strategic Partnerships and Collaborations—Closely involving statutory services (e.g., primary, secondary, and tertiary healthcare, mental health services, local Council, social services, schools, employment services, public health departments), the voluntary sector (many specifically focused on the needs of refugees and asylum seekers, but also organizations providing general mental health care, children's education, food banks, cultural and religious organizations), and engagement with local as well as migrant communities and their leaders have been key to the success of this clinic. In the future, the service aims to be a community and primary care service for the entire family.

Case Study Two: A Mobile Clinic for Refugees in Kibungo, Rwanda

The mobile clinic was organized under the auspices of a large NGO to provide health care to refugees who were returning from their refugee camps in Tanzania to Rwanda, their country of origin. The NGO established a program in Kibungo to provide healthcare to returning refugees who were all of the same ethnic group.

The returning refugees traveled in long lines. UN Agencies provided trucks that were intended to provide rides to women and children but most trucks were taken over by young, healthy men. So most women and children walked. Many walked for days to reach their hometowns or villages.

There were three mobile clinic vehicles, two pickup trucks and one Land Rover. Drivers were local men who knew the area. Three NGO expatriate volunteer physicians (two pediatricians and one internist) and three volunteer expatriate nurses rode in the vehicles.

Each evening the NGO replaced supplies in the mobile clinic vehicles. These included standard medications, gloves, syringes, needles and small surgical kits from UN agencies, basic obstetric packs, and small amounts of intravenous fluids. NGO volunteers added water, nutritional biscuits, and germicidal solutions.

The three clinic vehicles left the small town early each morning to drive along the refugee routes, stopping at feeding stations where physicians and nurses would examine refugees who needed medical attention. They were often told about someone who had collapsed along the route and was too ill to travel; the vehicle would then go directly to that person and transport them to a nearby district hospital. Lost children were also picked up along the way and brought to a church where they were photographed for reunification purposes and fed. The children were cared for by nuns at the church while the International Committee of the Red Cross officials took responsibility for family reunification efforts. Children in this church who needed medical attention were seen by health staff from the mobile clinics.

Many children were examined alongside the road in the mobile clinics. A common problem was skin infections of their feet because most children walked barefoot. Other common problems were malaria, upper respiratory illnesses, diarrhea, and dehydration. Periodically, the clinic staff were informed about a mother about to give birth and many small infants were delivered alongside the road. Most likely maternal malnutrition coupled with the stress of long travel was triggering premature labor.

The mobile clinic vehicles returned to the house rented by the NGO each evening at sunset. During the several weeks that the mobile clinics were active in this area, there was substantial illness among the NGO volunteers including cerebral malaria, diarrhea, and food poisoning. Occasionally, these illnesses reduced the number of mobile clinics that could be staffed.

The local medical staff working in the district hospital represented a different ethnic group than the refugees and would often display outright discrimination against ill refugees. Expatriate health staff were sometimes frustrated by this clear discrimination; however, they had no authority in these local decisions. And thus the mobile clinic volunteers continued to care for Rwandan refugees in this difficult landscape, to the best of their ability.

Additional Resources

AAP Immigrant Child Health Toolkit: https://www.aap.org/en-us/advocacy-and-policy/aap-health-initiatives/Immigrant-Child-Health-Toolkit/Pages/Immigrant-Child-Health-Toolkit.aspx

CDC Refugee Health guidelines: https://www.cdc.gov/immigrantrefugeehealth/guidelines/domestic/checklist.html

AAP Red Book online: https://redbook.solutions.aap.org/redbook.aspx

MSF refugee health guidelines: http://refbooks.msf.org/msf_docs/en/refugee_health/rh.pdf

References

1. Raja S, Hasnain M, Hoersch M, Gove-Yin S, Rajagopalan C. Trauma informed care in medicine. Fam Community Health. 2015;38(3):216–26.
2. Brown JD, King MA, Wissow LS. The central role of relationships with trauma-informed integrated care for children and youth. Acad Pediatr. 2017;17(7):S94–101.
3. Linton JM, Green A. Providing care for children in immigrant families. Pediatrics. 2019;144(3):e20192077.
4. Kadir A, Shenoda S, Goldhagen J, Pitterman S. The effects of armed conflict on children. Pediatrics. 2018;142(6):e20182586.
5. Pottie K, Greenaway C, Feightner J, Welch V, Swinkels H, Rashid M, et al. Evidence-based clinical guidelines for immigrants and refugees. CMAJ. 2011;183(12):E824–925.
6. Pottie K, Mayhew AD, Morton RL, Greenaway C, Akl EA, Rahman P, et al. Prevention and assessment of infectious diseases among children and adult migrants arriving to the European Union/European economic association: a protocol for a suite of systematic reviews for public health and health systems. BMJ Open. 2017;7(9):e014608.
7. Zwi K, Rungan S, Woolfenden S, Woodland L, Palasanthiran P, Williams K. Refugee children and their health, development and Well-being over the first year of settlement: a longitudinal study. J Paediatr Child Health. 2017;53(9):841–9.
8. Zwi K, Woodland L, Williams K, Palasanthiran P, Rungan S, Jaffe A, et al. Protective factors for social-emotional Well-being of refugee children in the first three years of settlement in Australia. Arch Dis Child. 2018;103(3):261–8.

Emily Esmaili, DO, MA, FAAP is a pediatrician with global health experience both locally and internationally. After residency at Wake Forest Medical Center, she worked in Laos for 2 years as country coordinator and pediatric faculty for the NGO Health Frontiers. She then moved to Rwanda to serve as visiting pediatric faculty through Yale University and the Human Resources for Health program. While there, she helped start a "farm-to-bedside" nutrition program for food-insecure hospitalized children, which she later established as a 501c3, Growing Health, Inc. She then returned to the US to earn her masters in Global Bioethics and Science Policy from Duke University, followed by a fellowship in refugee child health also from Duke. Dr. Esmaili now works for Lincoln Community Health Center in Durham, NC, which serves primarily low-income, immigrant, and refugee children in the local community, where she also leads a grant-funded outreach program for refugee and immigrant families post-COVID. She has volunteered with humanitarian organizations in Greece, India, Nepal, Rwanda, and along the Thai-Burma border.

Part III

A Lifetime Perspective on Child Refugee and Migrant Health

Christian Harkensee

The humanitarian sector, seen either from a perspective of acute disaster relief or more long-term development of capacity and capability, has undergone substantial changes in recent years. Traditionally, humanitarian interventions were often short (such as in a disaster situation) or narrow and subject-focused (e.g., programs on HIV or nutrition) with little coordination between such programs ("vertical" approach). We now know humanitarian efforts are often closely interlinked, and that the impact of "vertical" programs can be very limited; while integration of several such programs at the same time amplifies the outcomes for each individually and all collectively ("horizontal" approach). The integration of HIV, tuberculosis, and nutrition programs in many Sub-Saharan African countries are good examples for this [1, 2].

This section introduces you to some themes which are commonly given low priority in humanitarian emergency responses because of their broad scope and long timelines: Maternal and child growth and nutrition, child development, prevention, and health promotion. These themes closely relate to the psychosocial aspects discussed in Part I of this book.

In this part, we aim to raise your awareness of two very important points: firstly, that disturbance of child growth and development has lifelong implications for the child; and secondly, that there is only a very short window of opportunity to rectify this. You may be familiar with the concept of "the first 1000 days," that it is during life in utero and the first two years thereafter, the phase of the most rapid growth and largest brain plasticity and development, that maternal and child malnutrition and physical and psychosocial trauma have the largest impact but also the largest potential for recovery [3]. Problems remaining unrecognized and untreated beyond this age may persist lifelong, such as stunting from malnutrition or cognitive impairment from iron deficiency. In any humanitarian setting, 1000 days is not a long time—considering that the majority of displaced people spend years or even decades

C. Harkensee
Queen Elizabeth Hospital Gateshead, Gateshead, UK

in temporary settlements. Considering maternal health, child growth and development, and health promotion as equally important to other emergency health measures could go a long way in securing the lifelong health and well-being of refugee and migrant children.

References

1. Wilkinson D. Tuberculosis and health sector reform: experience of integrating tuberculosis services into the district health system in rural South Africa [Planning and Practice]. Int J Tuberc Lung Dis. 1999;3(10):938–43.
2. Corbett EL, Marston B, Churchyard GJ, Cock KMD. Tuberculosis in sub-Saharan Africa: opportunities, challenges, and change in the era of antiretroviral treatment. Lancet. 2006;367(9514):926–37.
3. Innocenti UO of R-. The first 1,000 days of life: The brain's window of opportunity [Internet]. UNICEF-IRC. [cited 2021 Jan 20]. https://www.unicef-irc.org/article/958-the-first-1000-days-of-life-the-brains-window-of-opportunity.html

Christian Harkensee, MD PhD MSc DLSHTM, DiMM, MAcadMEd, MFPHC (RCSEd), FHEA, FRCPCH. Made his first humanitarian experience in Central America in 1987. Since, became a doctor (Humboldt University Berlin, Germany, 1997), pediatrician and pediatric infectious diseases and immunology specialist (UK, 2012), researcher (PhD in immunogenetics, UK, 2012), medical educator (2003), and mountain—and expedition doctor (2017). Humanitarian disaster relief, development, and capacity building work in many countries ever since; and currently leading a health service for refugee children and families in the North East of England.

Malnutrition

11

Christine Fernandes and Minh Tram Le

Definition of Malnutrition

Malnutrition is the result of an imbalance between intake of nutrients, and energy provided to the body, relative to its needs. Common reasons are more than a lack of food: it can be a combination of factors such as insufficient protein, energy and micronutrients intake, frequent infections or disease, poor care and feeding practices, inadequate health services, and/or poor water and sanitation. The lack of adequate breastfeeding practices alone results in almost 12% of all deaths among children under age 5. The term "malnutrition" refers to undernutrition (wasting, stunting, underweight), micronutrient deficiencies, overweight, and obesity.

Malnutrition violates a child's right to survival and development [1]. However, its consequences often remain invisible until it is too late. Malnutrition can present itself in many ways:

- A child who never reaches full height due to poverty, poor sanitation, lack of breastfeeding, and limited access to nutritious foods.
- A young woman who becomes anemic during her pregnancy and v birth to an underweight baby who later faces developmental delays.
- A child rendered blind by vitamin A deficiency.
- A child who becomes obese through overconsumption of energy-dense foods that are high in fat and sugars.
- A desperately thin and wasted child, at imminent risk of death.
- Physical and cognitive development delays as a result of malnutrition early in life, having individual, societal, and economic impacts.

C. Fernandes (✉)
Save the Children, Amman, Jordan
e-mail: christine.fernandes@savethechildren.org

M. T. Le
UNICEF Regional Office for South Asia (ROSA), Kathmandu, Nepal

© Springer Nature Switzerland AG 2021
C. Harkensee et al. (eds.), *Child Refugee and Migrant Health*,
https://doi.org/10.1007/978-3-030-74906-4_11

Around 45% of deaths among children under 5 years of age are linked to undernutrition [2] and mostly occur in low- and middle-income countries. For the last few years, rates of childhood overweight and obesity, often in conjunction with stunting, are also increasing in these countries. In the majority of cases, the effects of malnutrition are far more silent and occur over a longer time period: it stunts children's mental and physical growth, deprives them of essential vitamins and minerals, which makes them more susceptible to disease, illness, and even death.

Malnutrition is one of the most serious challenges in the world today. It is a principal contributing factor to global illness and death, and carries dire economic consequences. In addition to its worldwide impact, economic losses, as well as the physical, cognitive, and emotional outcomes of malnutrition afflict vulnerable populations the most, such as refugees, migrants, and internally displaced people (IDP), those living in poverty, women, and young children. Therefore, global efforts to put an end to malnutrition are imperative and require multiple resources as well as international and national commitment.

Chronic malnutrition or *stunting* (when a child is too short for his or her age) is a condition that develops when young children do not receive the correct balance of nutrients in the first 1000 days of life (from conception to the age of 2 years), resulting in stunted cognitive and physical development [3]. A child is considered stunted if their height-for-age is more than two standard deviations below the WHO Child Growth Standards median [4]. Chronic malnutrition early in life prevents children's bodies and brains from growing to reach their full potential, compromises their immune systems to fight off illnesses, and makes them more prone to degenerative diseases, obesity, and are more likely to die prematurely [5]. The damage caused by chronic malnutrition is irreversible and has far-reaching consequences, from impaired learning and school performance, to lower future earnings. Stunted children often come from the poorest households, making stunting a key marker of poverty and inequality. Globally, 144 million (21.3%) children under 5 years were stunted in 2019 [6]. The causes of chronic malnutrition are multifaceted and complex, and include poor maternal nutrition, suboptimal infant, and young child feeding including breastfeeding, limited access to a diverse diet, inadequate child care practices, lack of healthcare and availability of clean water, poor hygienic conditions and repeated illness such as diarrhea. Further, other underlying, indirect causes also impact chronic malnutrition such as social norms, gender dynamics, education attainment, the political economy, and overall equity. In 1990, UNICEF developed a causal framework that illustrates the varying immediate, underlying, and basic causes of malnutrition to better analyze and address the multi-sectoral gaps for improved nutrition (See Fig. 11.1).

Critically, chronic malnutrition can carry over to the next generation. For example, a stunted girl child will grow to be a poorly developed adolescent or adult, who will then become an undernourished pregnant mother, who is more likely to experience birth complications, poor intrauterine growth, premature birth, or a baby with low birth weight for gestational age. This baby, already facing physical complications, may then grow to also be stunted, creating an intergenerational cycle of chronic malnutrition, growth failure, poor health, and poverty. (See Fig. 11.2).

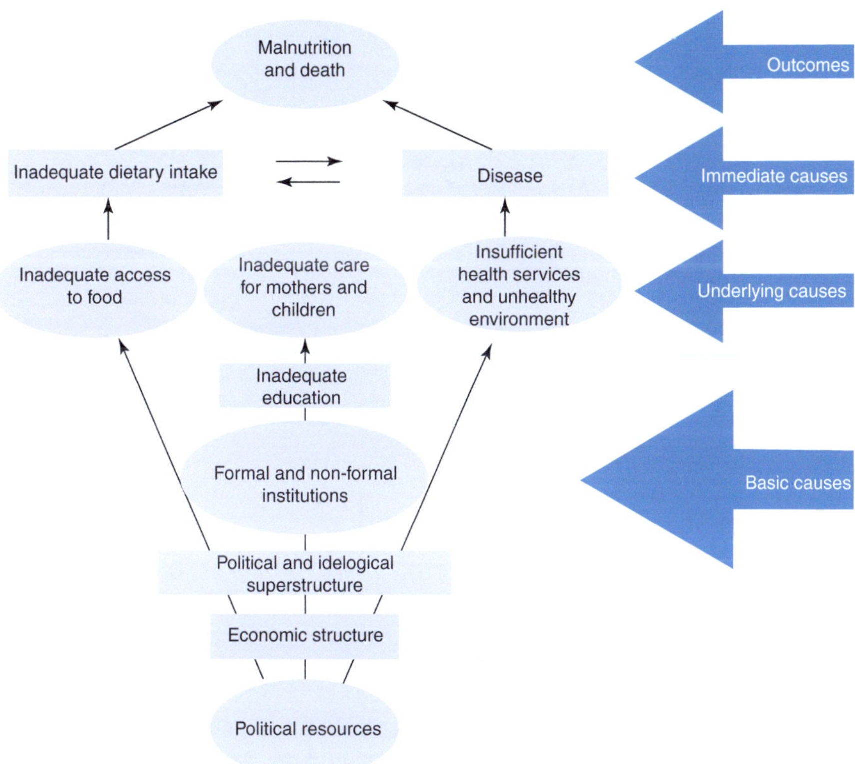

Fig. 11.1 UNICEF's conceptual framework for undernutrition [7]

Malnutrition throughout different stages of life, or the cycle of chronic malnutrition, has both immediate and permanent consequences. In the short term, maternal malnutrition increases the risks of morbidity and mortality. For example, stunting or underweight during pregnancy increases the risk of low birth weight, or small gestational age; obesity during pregnancy contributes to gestational diabetes, preeclampsia, and hemorrhaging; and both forms can lead to maternal and neonatal death. In the long-term, maternal malnutrition impacts poor development of the fetus, and can lead to metabolism and hormone adaptations in the womb that alter the structure and bodily functions of the neonate. When a mother's body is not able to provide nutrients through her bodily stores or the placenta, permanent negative effects can occur such as poor tissue growth, dysfunction of the organs and brain, as well as fetal hormone imbalance such as insulin production that contributes to type 2 diabetes, obesity later in life, and an increased risk of other challenges such as high blood pressure, lung function, coronary heart disease, and overall mortality [8, 9].

The first 1000 days of life, from conception until a child's second birthday, is a period for rapid growth and development physically, cognitively, and emotionally. Growth failure may occur in utero, and/or during infancy and young childhood due to suboptimal or no breastfeeding, poor complementary feeding of solid foods that

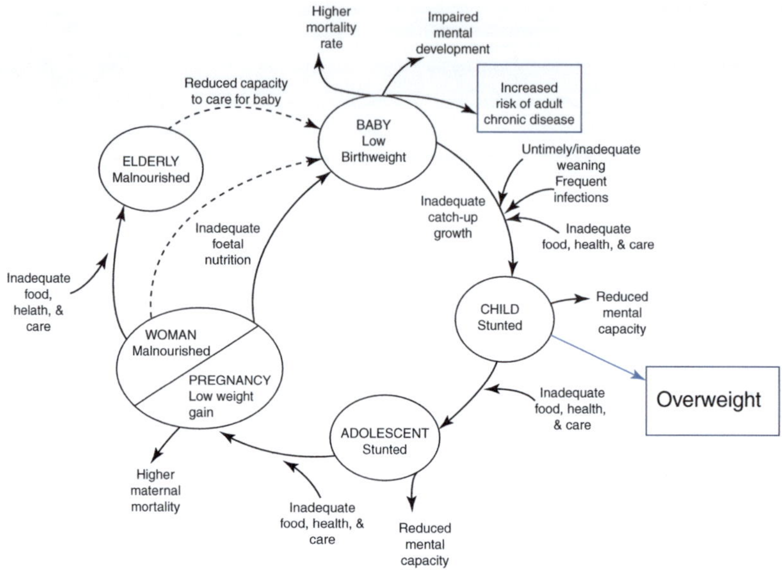

Source : United Nations Subcommittee on Nutrition Fourth Report on the World nutrition Situation, 2000 - modified

Fig. 11.2 Intergenerational cycle of malnutrition

are inadequate in quality and quantity, and repeated illnesses that hinder absorption such as diarrhea due to poor hygiene or unclean drinking water. If a child's diet and overall care remain poor during this window of time, the consequences of malnutrition can be irreversible later in life. Therefore, this period is seen as a critical time of both vulnerability and potential during which the foundations for lifelong health are laid [10].

Less monitored, but equally important, is *malnutrition in school-aged children*, also associated with high risks both physically and cognitively. Malnourished children between the ages of 4–14 years of age present with micronutrient deficiencies, wasting, stunting, and sometimes all three, due to poor household dietary diversity and recurring illness such as diarrhea and upper respiratory infections [11, 12]. In addition, studies demonstrate that hunger in school-aged children can exacerbate behavioral, emotional, and academic problems, in particular, aggression and anxiety [13].

Adolescence (from 10 to 19 years of age) is also a critical time for rapid growth and development, including accelerated linear and skeletal growth—commonly known as "catch-up" growth, as well as pubertal growth, and sexual maturation. Poor nutrition during adolescence leads to micronutrient deficiencies, being underweight or overweight, or stunted. Extra energy, protein, and micronutrients are needed for the adolescent body, and when adequate nutrition is lacking, physical growth, brain function, and hormonal development falters [14, 15]. Pregnancy during adolescence also has adverse nutritional consequences for a young mother. The additional energy and nutrients required for adolescent growth *and* fetal development are not sufficient, and therefore both the mother's and infant's bodies can potentially be compromised, such as causing stunting for both, high risks of eclampsia, puerperal endometritis, as well as systemic infections for the adolescent, preterm delivery, low birth weight, and higher infant mortality rates [14, 16].

Although chronic malnutrition is a term to describe a form of undernutrition, it does not exclude children who are also suffering from or at risk of other forms of malnutrition such as wasting or obesity. Children can be susceptible to multiple forms of malnutrition and may also ebb and flow between the various states, which increases risks to their health and life over time [6, 17].

Acute malnutrition, also known as *wasting*, is characterized by a massive loss of body fat and muscle tissue, detected by low weight for height of the child, a low mid-upper arm circumference (MUAC) and/or the presence of bilateral pitting edema. This form of malnutrition poses an immediate threat to child survival and is considered as a health emergency. Wasting is the crushing result of acute malnutrition and poses an immediate threat to survival. In 2019, 47 million children under 5 years old were wasted globally, and 14.3 million severely wasted [6]. Infants under 6 months who are severely acutely malnourished are defined by very low weight-for-length or bilateral pitting edema, though it is more difficult to identify signs of acute malnutrition in younger infants than older infants [18].

Acute malnutrition is defined in various ways with different names such as protein-energy malnutrition, wasting, kwashiorkor, or marasmus. Marasmus refers to children who are very thin for their height but do not have bilateral pitting edema. These children look almost elderly and their bodies are extremely thin even skeletal. Kwashiorkor refers to edematous malnutrition and can be verified by applying thumb pressure on top of both feet for a few seconds and checking if a pit or indentation on the feet is left after the thumbs are lifted. Without treatment, edema can spread to the legs and face, and the child appears puffy and is also found to have irritability, weakness, and lethargy. Skin lesions can be present, with thinning hair and enlarged liver. Both types of acute malnutrition compromise the body's vital functions and can lead to long-term effects, similar to those found in chronically malnourished children. Micronutrient deficiencies such as lack of iron, iodine, or vitamin A can accompany acute malnutrition, and these children are at greater risk of medical complications and death from illness or infections.

The currently accepted WHO definitions for wasting are based on anthropometric cut-offs and the presence of clinical signs:

- Moderate acute malnutrition (MAM) is defined by a weight-for-height z-score (WHZ) between -2 and -3, or a MUAC between 115 and 125 millimeters.
- Severe acute malnutrition (SAM) is defined by a WHZ < -3, a MUAC <115 millimeters, and/or the presence of bilateral pitting edema.
- We also refer to Global acute malnutrition (GAM) as moderate and severe acute malnutrition together. This is the indicator used for the measurement of the child nutritional status at a population level and reflects the severity of an emergency situation.

Using existing studies of case fatality rates in several countries, WHO has extrapolated mortality rates of children suffering from SAM. The results reflect a 5–20 times higher risk of death compared to well-nourished children. SAM can be a direct cause of child death, or it can act as an indirect cause by dramatically increasing the case fatality rate from common childhood illnesses such as diarrhea and pneumonia. Both stunting and wasting can share similar determinants, as acute malnutrition occurs mainly in families that have limited access to nutritious food and are living in unhygienic conditions, which also increases the risk of repeated infections. Thus, preventive programs are essential in the context of poverty and associated factors and must be implemented alongside treatment programs for children who already are suffering from wasting and need immediate care.

To prevent the development of child acute malnutrition, interventions targeting appropriate breastfeeding and complementary feeding practices are crucial. Similarly, disease prevention strategies particularly interventions addressing risks of diarrhea and respiratory infections are important. An integrated approach in the prevention of stunting and wasting together is the key to optimizing healthy growth in children and can significantly reduce child wasting.

Overnutrition, which includes *overweight and obesity*, is on the rise in almost every country in the world, including those with a high prevalence of stunting and wasting. Globally, an estimated 38.3 million children under 5 years old were overweight in 2019, 78% of them living in middle-income countries [6]. Many countries are now facing an emerging threat known as the *triple burden* of malnutrition: overnutrition, undernutrition, and micronutrient deficiencies, all three present in the same country. Undernutrition and overnutrition not only can coexist within the same country, but also at the community and household level, and even within the same individual. Stunted children, for example, face a greater risk of becoming overweight as adults [1]. The causes of undernutrition and overweight and obesity can also be similar. Economic status, inadequate diets, poor infant and young child feeding practices can lead to both undernutrition and overnutrition. In addition, an emerging and modern problem is related to the marketing and sales of unhealthy foods and drinks in every country with high impacts on young children and their families.

Because of often dire living situations in refugee and migrant camps, and uncertain access to basic and vital needs, such as clean drinking water, adequate food, hygiene, and shelter, refugee children's lives are even more at risk of malnutrition. We know that infants and young children are already more vulnerable because their nutritional status can rapidly change and deteriorate, but the environment in which they live during these displacements due to conflicts, natural disasters, or other catastrophes also contribute to the worsening of their health status and heighten their vulnerabilities. Similarly, lifestyle or cultural factors can affect nutritional status. Those can be gender-related (e.g., prioritizing food for men and boys in times of scarcity, leaving girls and women more at risk of malnutrition), cultural (e.g., mothers leaving their own food for their children and husband, putting themselves at risk), and economical (lack of access to diverse and nutritious food), and all are often exacerbated during times of emergency.

Developmental and Emotional Impact of Malnutrition

Maternal and child mental health and well-being is inextricably linked to the physical health and nutrition of a young child. Dependency of infants on their mothers, or primary caregivers, for nutritional care and emotional and physical stimulation is critical to a child's development. Interference of appropriate care and mother-baby connection often occurs during times of high stress, lack of food, unavailability of basic health care, as well as underlying factors such as poverty, lack of education, gender-based violence, and sociocultural norms. These disturbances impact the mental health and psychosocial well-being of both caregiver and young child therefore obstructing the full physical, intellectual, and emotional potential of a child—a pattern which can continue into adulthood.

Appropriate child care also includes adequate feeding and nurturing. A caregiver experiencing depression or stress is less likely to be emotionally and physically available for his or her child. Research into mothers experiencing depression and stress shows a correlation between maternal mental health and breastfeeding cessation. Nutrition assessments in refugee and displaced contexts have demonstrated that feeding and care are negatively impacted during situations that exacerbate maternal distress, seen as a decreased frequency of breastfeeding and deteriorated complementary feeding practices [19, 20]. Figure 11.3 demonstrates the important links between the lack of nutrition and care practices and its long-term consequences.

The interaction between lack of food and lack of stimulation

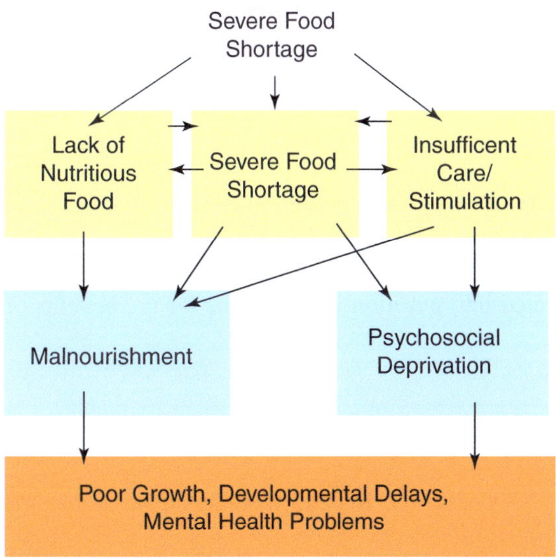

Fig. 11.3 Severe food shortage situations, Geneva, WHO, 2006

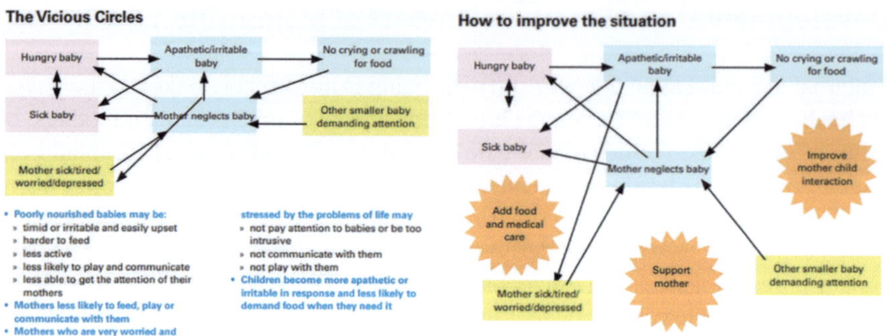

Fig. 11.4 Integrating ECD activities into nutrition programmes in emergencies: why, what, and how? WHO/UNICEF

Inadequate care and nurturing in infanthood over time put children at risk of toxic stress, which is prolonged exposure to stress that causes the child's body to remain in a stress response, leading to poor emotional and physical growth. The absence of appropriate care can be a vicious cycle. A young child or infant experiencing nutritional deficiencies and/or lack of emotional stimulation due to neglect may show reduced physical and cognitive activity and become apathetic (see Fig. 11.4). The caregiver may reduce the amount of stimulation provided to the child as the child stops responding to the caregiver, leading to permanent developmental delays and vulnerability to mental health issues.

In some nutrition interventions, caregivers are not only supported with feeding and nutrition education but also given information on infant development: Caregivers are shown various ways to engage with and stimulate their infants, to be responsive and better connect with their child. This is important to improve feeding practices, but also helps to reduce stress, which is critical in migrant and refugee crises. Nutrition interventions that incorporate Early Childhood Development (ECD) have been shown to improve maternal mood, in addition to strengthening the parent–infant relationship, leading to better infant health and development outcomes (Fig. 11.4). Similarly, interventions expressly designed to improve maternal mental health have a positive impact on infant health and development [21]. It is therefore critical that the well-being of caregivers is protected and supported as part of a nutrition response, and emotional, intellectual, and physical engagement between caregiver and child are incorporated into nutrition interventions for the benefits of both child and caregiver.

Nutrition Assessments

Malnutrition can be assessed at different levels to determine the nutritional status of individuals or population groups. Information about nutritional status is essential for the identification of critical nutrient deficiencies and emergencies that can help formulate recommendations for nutrient intake and inform the development of effective public health nutrition programs. A number of factors should be assessed such as anthropometric measurements, medical and family history, observations of the child's physical aspect and behavior, cultural practices, and socioeconomic status. Methods of nutrition assessments can be categorized into four different types: nutrition surveys, surveillance, screening, and interventions (monitoring).

Nutrition *surveys* are performed to assess the nutritional status of a selected population, identify the groups at risk of malnutrition or already malnourished, evaluate other health problems, and inform programming. Nutrition *surveillance* is a continuous and systematic collection and analysis of health and nutrition-related data, needed for the planning and implementation of nutrition programming. Data collection and analysis take place over a long period of time, which helps establish comparative trends and identify nutrition risk factors at the population level [22]. Nutrition *screening* is used to identify malnutrition at the individual level. During screening, measurements and other medical protocols are used. Nutrition *interventions* are carried out on populations or subgroups of the population at risk and are implemented after a nutrition screening or survey. This can be a method of nutrition assessment if an efficient monitoring framework is already set up and nutrition data are regularly collected and analyzed. Contextual and program information helps further explain improvements or deteriorations of nutritional status in the population and informs programming and policies.

Nutrition Assessment at the Population Level

At the onset of the emergency, a rapid situational analysis will help to establish whether the nutrition situation is deteriorating or stable, whether groups in the community have specific needs, and whether community members have specific skills or resources that can help prevent the deterioration of the situation. Situational analyses should review the state of nutrition before the emergency, including eating habits and livelihood practices, and compare the risks now that the emergency has arisen.

Where nutrition is a concern, the prevalence of acute malnutrition in children under 5 years old should be assessed, as child acute malnutrition is considered as a good indicator of recent changes in dietary intake and infection rates, and is also used to provide an indication of the nutritional status of the whole population. It is assessed using weight for height, MUAC, and bilateral pitting edema for children aged 6–59 months. Infants aged 0–6 months also need specific attention during these assessments. It is important to identify infants who are not being breastfed since infant formula supply can be unreliable, as well as dangerous due to lack of access to clean, boiled water and clean utensils for safe preparation of formula. If an infant is not being breastfed or if the caregiver is having breastfeeding difficulties, the mother or caregiver and the child should be referred immediately to providers trained on breastmilk substitute programming for further assessment, tailored support, and adherence to global guidelines for non-breastfed infants [23].

In contexts where nutrition security is a concern, a rapid assessment of the nutrition status of the refugee or migrant population should be conducted as soon as possible after the start of the emergency. This assessment will collect child anthropometric data and secondary data related to the nutrition situation, access to services and food sources, and key infant and child feeding practices. The number of people affected can be estimated, including the availability of local resources and the need for external assistance. Results of this initial rapid assessment indicate the need for a more in-depth assessment carried out after a few months, to reassess the situation and determine longer term needs and approaches.

Assessments should be designed, carried out, and supervised by nutrition workers with appropriate qualifications and relevant experience. If the nutrition situation is at risk, a more comprehensive nutrition survey should then be undertaken as soon as feasible, and no later than 3–6 months after the start of the emergency.

Assessment of Women's and Children's Diets

Assessing the diets of pregnant women and children against global recommendations is fundamental to both preventing and addressing malnutrition. UNICEF's Global Database (2019) lists a set of indicators to appropriately measure infant and young child feeding practices. They include [24]:

Indicator	Definition
Early initiation of breastfeeding	Percentage of newborns put to the breast within 1 h of birth
Exclusive breastfeeding	Percentage of infants 0–5 months of age who are fed exclusively with breast milk
Introduction of solid, semi-solid, or soft foods	Percentage of infants 6–8 months of age who receive solid, semi-solid, or soft foods
Minimum acceptable diet	Percentage of children 6–23 months of age who received a minimum acceptable diet (breastfed children 6–23 months of age who had at least the minimum dietary diversity and the minimum meal frequency during the previous day AND non-breastfed children 6–23 months of age who received at least two milk feedings and had at least the minimum dietary diversity not including milk feeds and the minimum meal frequency during the previous day)
Minimum diet diversity	Percentage of children 6–23 months of age who received a minimum diet diversity (number of children 6–23 months of age who received foods from ≥5 (out of 8) food groups during the previous day)
Minimum meal frequency	Percentage of children 6–23 months of age who received a minimum meal frequency (number of breastfed children 6–23 months of age who received solid, semi-solid, or soft foods the minimum number of times or more during the previous day and the number of non-breastfed children 6–23 months of age who received solid, semi-solid, or soft foods or milk feeds the minimum number of times or more during the previous day.)
Continued breastfeeding at 2 years	Percentage of children 20–23 months of age who are fed breast milk

Maternal Nutrition indicators include:

Indicator	Definition
Minimum dietary diversity for women of reproductive age (MDD-W) [25]	MDD-W is a dichotomous indicator of whether or not women 15–49 years of age have consumed at least five out of ten defined food groups the previous day or night. The proportion of women 15–49 years of age who reach this minimum in a population can be used as a proxy indicator for higher micronutrient adequacy, one important dimension of diet quality.
Proportion of pregnant women receiving iron and folic acid supplements [26]	Percentage of women with a birth in the last 2 years who received or bought iron/folic acid supplements for at least 6 months during their last pregnancy in amounts that were in accordance with recommended protocols.

Assessing the diets of infants and young children is important due to the vulnerability of the age group to morbidity and mortality, a time of rapid growth and development, as well as significant changes of the diet from birth to 6 months of age, 6–12 months, and 12–24 months that require support and protection. In addition, the young child is heavily dependent on the caregiver or mother for his or her diet, and with breastfeeding as a global recommendation for the duration of the 2 years, caregivers require additional support. To this end, IYCF assessments should be conducted with the primary caregiver of the child, even though the child 0–24 months is the target of the assessment. Assessing the diets of children can be carried out to:

- Determine nutrition and care risks such as growth faltering.
- Identify critical gaps, needs, and feeding challenges.
- Develop specific and contextualized nutrition support.
- Evaluate any changes in feeding practices.
- Understand feeding norms, beliefs, and cultural practices.

Methodologies include household surveys, rapid assessments, and focus group discussions, and should be representative of the population to the extent possible. In addition to collecting information on the IYCF standard indicators, responses need to be disaggregated by the age of the child, sex, and "type" such as a refugee and a displaced person. Key informant interviews, observation or "transect walks," desk reviews, Knowledge, Attitude, and Practice assessments, a barrier analysis, and IYCF questions added to a multi-sectoral assessment can also help build a bigger picture of the common infant and young child feeding practices. No matter the methodology, enumerators (those conducting the survey) need to be trained in the concepts of IYCF as well as learn how to probe for answers without swaying the responder (Guidance on the methodologies include [27–31]).

Assessment of Malnutrition in Children and Women

Chronic malnutrition is detected by measuring the height of the child and comparing it with his or her age. As part of growth monitoring programs, often weight and age are also assessed to determine whether the child is under or overweight. There are two anthropometric ways to assess acute malnutrition: measurement of weight in relation to height (WHZ) and measurement of the Mid-upper Arm Circumference (MUAC) using a specific measuring tape. Another important screening to diagnose child acute malnutrition is the presence of bilateral pitting edema. MUAC tape is also used to detect acute malnutrition in pregnant women and women who breastfeed. There are no agreed international cut-off points for MUAC for women, with national guidelines cut-offs ranging from 21 to 23 centimeters in different contexts.

There is evidence showing that those identified as being severely malnourished based upon MUAC as the anthropometric indicator are often different from those identified as being severely malnourished based on weight for height [32] with an overlap of around 40% with geographical variations. The two indicators do not always identify the same children and are both recommended by WHO in the detection of wasted children. Oftentimes, MUAC tape will be used for community level screening, and children referred to the hospital or outreach facilities will be screened again using both MUAC and weight for height measurements. Similarly, rapid nutrition assessments can be done using MUAC only, while more thorough assessments will be conducted using all measurements. The methodology mostly used for child malnutrition assessments is the SMART methodology (Standardized Monitoring and Assessment of Relief and Transitions) [33]. The SMART methodology is a recognized and improved survey method that balances simplicity (for rapid assessment of acute emergencies) and technical soundness, using MUAC, height and weight measurements, and providing information on both chronic and acute malnutrition in children and pregnant and lactating women. While emergencies tend to focus more on acute malnutrition, several experts and working groups over the past few years have been advocating for more attention given to children with stunting during emergencies, given the close association between both conditions and the association of severe stunting with higher mortality rates than moderate wasting [34].

Once children are identified as suffering from acute malnutrition, they need to be seen by a health worker to fully assess their medical situation, following the Integrated Management of Childhood Illness (IMCI) approach. The health worker should then determine whether they can be treated in the community with weekly visits to the health center, or whether referral to inpatient care is required when medical complications are present. Early detection, coupled with decentralized treatment to the community level has drastically increased the access to treatment for children affected with wasting over the past 15 years, making it possible to prevent the onset of life-threatening complications in wasted children.

Prevention of Malnutrition

Malnutrition is preventable. Investing in the prevention of malnutrition is essential to reducing morbidity and mortality, and is also beneficial to communities and society at large. The World Bank estimates that malnutrition caused the loss of national productivity and economic growth by as much as 11% in 2019 [35].

There are multiple approaches to prevention, mostly addressing the causes of malnutrition illustrated in UNICEF's Conceptual Framework that focuses on *nutrition-specific* interventions. They can include: improving access to high-quality foods and to healthcare, improving nutrition and health knowledge and practices of caregivers, promoting exclusive breastfeeding for the first 6 months of a child's life, supporting improved complementary feeding practices for all children aged 6–24 months with a focus on ensuring access to age-appropriate, diverse foods (using locally available foods as much as possible), and improving water and sanitation systems and hygiene practices to protect children against communicable diseases. These interventions often focus on children under 5 years of age as well as pregnant and lactating women, given their specific vulnerabilities to the detrimental consequences of malnutrition.

For immediate prevention in emergency situations, blanket supplementary feeding programs (BSFP), or mass distribution of specialized nutritious foods during critical times are provided for population groups who are at risk of acute malnutrition. These specialized foods include lipid-based nutrient supplements, such as *Plumpy'Doz*, or fortified blended foods, such as *Super Cereal Plus* for children, and *Super Cereal* for pregnant women, which contain a combination of energy, protein, vitamins, and minerals. BSFPs are often implemented at the onset of an emergency, population movement, when there is little food availability, high micronutrient deficiencies, or lack of access to treatment of acute malnutrition [36]. However, experts now promote the expanded scope of BSFP, such as its use in refugee operations to also prevent micronutrient deficiencies and stunting [37]. Key target groups are usually children 6–24 months, 6–59 months, and/or pregnant and lactating women (PLWs), depending on the circumstances, vulnerabilities, and availability of basic services. Blanket supplementary feeding means that admission is not based on individual nutritional status, but rather the context and nutritional risks, where the target group receives provision of the specialized foods for only a short period of time, usually a few months [38]. They can be provided as a standalone product or together with food distribution, for example. However, provision of appropriate materials/utensils, safe drinking water, and clear communication on the use and purpose of the products are key requirements of any distribution of a blanket supplementary feeding program.

> *If a new vaccine became available that could prevent one million or more child deaths a year and that was moreover cheap, safe, administered orally and required no cold chain, it would become an immediate public health imperative. Breastfeeding can do all this and more.*—The Lancet, 1994

A common immediate cause across all forms of malnutrition is a suboptimal diet, including inadequate breastfeeding for infants [39]. Just as the cycle of malnutrition can be broken in the first 1000 days of life through appropriate maternal nutrition and adequate infant and young child feeding practices, so too can malnutrition be prevented during this window of time with breastmilk and locally produced, affordable foods—a more sustainable solution. The World Health Organization and UNICEF recommend:

- Early initiation of breastfeeding within the first hour of birth.
- Exclusive breastfeeding for the first 6 months of life.
- Introduction of nutritionally adequate and safe complementary (solid) foods after 6 completed months, together with continued breastfeeding up to 2 years of age or beyond.

In fact, breastfeeding is *the most effective prevention intervention in the world for children under 5 years old,* saving 13% of children's lives every year, with the third most effective preventive intervention of complementary feeding saving 6% of all children per year [40].

Preventing maternal malnutrition during preconception, gestation, and postpartum/breastfeeding is crucial in the prevention of malnutrition in children. Even before pregnancy, appropriate nutrition such as the consumption of a variety of nutrient-dense food is important for reproductive health and reducing chronic diseases that can develop in a child's life. During pregnancy, a woman should eat a diverse diet, rich in protein, calcium, and other vitamins, up to an extra 300 calories per day, with additional supplements of folic acid and iron. Although current evidence shows that multiple micronutrient supplements given to pregnant women may reduce the risk of low birth weight and babies who are small for gestational age (SGA), compared with iron and folic acid supplementation alone, there remains evidence gaps, in addition to evidence of risk, and therefore the WHO does not currently recommend Micronutrient powders (MNPs) as a standard for pregnant women [41]. Breastfeeding women also need additional energy, liquid, and nutrients to help the body produce breastmilk, optimize the nutritional components of breastmilk, and ensure nutrient intake of the mother's body as well. It is recommended that pregnant and lactating women (PLWs) should consume approximately 500 additional calories more each day with healthy, diverse foods such as protein, other foods that are rich in iron, calcium, vitamin A, folic acid, with iodized salt.

The global Maternal, Infant, and Young Child Nutrition recommendations are a key set of tried and tested interventions that are life-saving, as well as critical to sustainable prevention of malnutrition both in the short and long-term and for the next generation. However, to protect, promote, and support these nutrition practices and allow for sustainability, *nutrition sensitive* approaches must also be considered and implemented, while addressing the basic and underlying causes of malnutrition. As mentioned above, malnutrition has many different causes occurring at different levels within a society. Therefore, malnutrition cannot be prevented through nutrition services alone. Multi-sectoral action that addresses underlying determinants

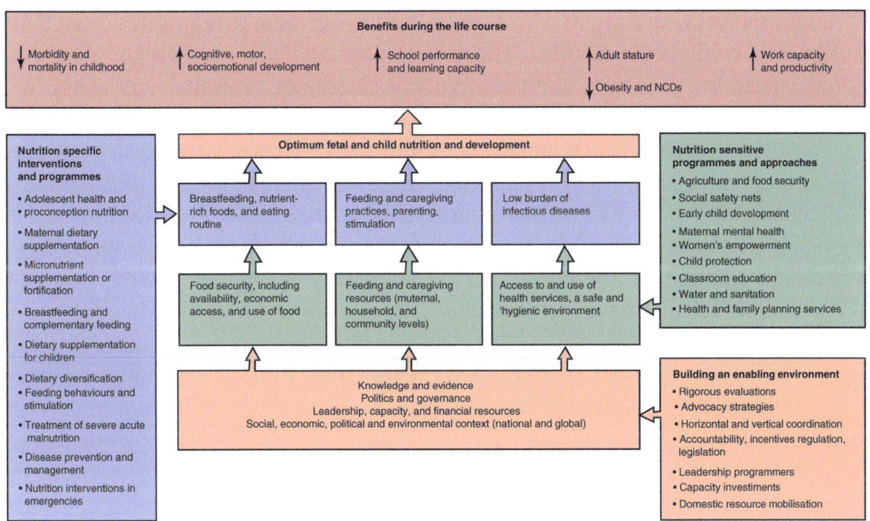

Fig. 11.5 Framework for actions to achieve optimum fetal and child nutrition and development, This article was published in The Lancet, Maternal and Child Nutrition Series, Copyright Elsevier (2013)

of malnutrition such as livelihoods, food security, access to clean water, gender equity, child protection, the mental health of caregivers, and basic education for all are just as critical as nutrition-specific actions. To further uphold prevention interventions, commitment by leaders, adoption of global policies, and guidelines that are put into legislation are needed at a national level to ensure an enabling environment is created for best nutritional outcomes. The Framework for Action in Fig. 11.5 provides a model of how an enabling environment underpins nutrition sensitive approaches, which strengthen nutrition-specific interventions for best nutrition and health outcomes that allow children to thrive.

Management of Acute Malnutrition

The *Community-based Management of Acute Malnutrition (CMAM) approach* has become the standard protocol for the treatment of acute malnutrition in children under 5 years and pregnant and lactating women. The approach is often adapted at the national level by governments in countries where the prevalence of malnutrition is high. The main components of the CMAM approach are:

- The early identification of children with moderate and severe acute malnutrition through *community level screening* with the use of a MUAC tape. The screening is done by community workers trained on the use of the tape and the detection of bilateral pitting edema. Most recently, research has proved that teaching mothers and caregivers on using MUAC tapes and allowing them to regularly screen their children could be as efficient. These screenings take place on a regular basis as the nutrition status of a child can quickly deteriorate. Families and caregivers also often know the community workers and regularly receive the relevant nutrition messages which empower them in seeking care when needed. Once a child is found to have SAM or MAM, he or she will be referred to the nearest health center where a more thorough medical assessment will be performed.

- The management of children at the outpatient level: the child can be referred following community screening or from an outpatient medical service or another center where his or her nutritional status was found to be at risk. Within the CMAM approach, two different services are provided:
  - Moderately malnourished children (MAM) will be enrolled in Supplementary Feeding programmes (SFP) and receive nutrient supplementation to prevent worsening of their status to severe malnutrition. Malnourished women who are pregnant or breastfeeding an infant aged less than 6 months will also be enrolled in SFP.
  - Severely malnourished children (SAM) presenting with no medical complications are also managed at the outpatient level, with weekly visits to monitor their health status and provide them with Ready-to-Use Therapeutic Food (RUTF). SAM children will also receive basic oral medications to treat infections at admission.
- Children with severe malnutrition and medical compilations are most effectively managed in specialized units in inpatient care, which require higher levels of care to treat their medical condition.

The greater proportion of children with severe acute malnutrition do not develop medical complications if they are detected early enough, and therefore can be treated at home. Inpatient units are resource-intensive and require skilled staff around the clock. Programs with community-based therapeutic care have been a revolution and have substantially reduced case fatality rates and increased coverage. With improved access to treatment, the case fatality rates of acute malnutrition can lower to 5%, both at community and facility level. The approach can be used in both emergency and non-emergency contexts where the prevalence of acute malnutrition is high, with increased efforts to integrate the approach to existing health systems.

Ready-to-Use Therapeutic Food

The success of the CMAM approach was possible thanks to the development and efficiency of Ready-to-Use Therapeutic Food (RUTF) such as *Plumpy Nut®* or *Eezeepaste®*. RUTF are soft foods classified in essential medicine lists in some countries and that can be consumed easily by children from the age of 6 months without adding water. It has a similar nutrient composition to F100, which is one of the therapeutic milks used in hospital settings for SAM cases with medical complications. RUTF, as per its name, is ready to be eaten by the child with no preparation required. Therefore, its use is safe in all settings, without refrigeration and even in areas where hygiene conditions are not optimal. The dose of RUTF depends on the weight of the child, and it is given until nutritional recovery.

Because RUTF must often be imported and can represent a considerable program cost, some settings instead use other therapeutic diets made of locally available nutrient-dense foods and ingredients with added micronutrient supplements. More research and trials are needed regarding the efficiency of these local recipes in the treatment of severe acute malnutrition. In addition, the production of WHO-compliant RUTF has increased over the last decades around the globe, with factories, for example, in India, South Africa, Ethiopia, etc., that help to decrease the cost of the product. Similarly, many countries and research institutes have been working on developing locally made recipes of RUTF using different ingredients (rice, chickpeas, soymilk, etc.) which could be more culturally appropriate depending on the contexts.

References

1. UNICEF. https://www.unicef.org/nutrition/index_faces-of-malnutrition.html
2. WHO. https://www.who.int/news-room/fact-sheets/detail/malnutrition
3. Valid Nutrition. https://www.validnutrition.org/malnutrition-definition/
4. World Health Organization. Global nutrition targets 2025: stunting policy brief (WHO/NMH/NHD/14.3). Geneva: World Health Organization; 2014.
5. Grillo LP, Gigante DP. Evidence for the association between early childhood stunting and metabolic syndrome. In: Preedy V, Patel V, editors. Handbook of famine, starvation, and nutrient deprivation. Cham: Springer; 2017. p. 1–17.
6. United Nations Children's Fund (UNICEF), World Health Organization, International Bank for Reconstruction and Development/The World Bank. Levels and trends in child malnutrition: key findings of the 2020 edition of the joint child malnutrition estimates. Geneva: World Health Organization; 2020.
7. Mason BJ. Keynote paper: measuring hunger and malnutrition. New Orleans: Tulane University; 2002.
8. Barker DJP. The malnourished baby and infant: relationship with type 2 diabetes. Br Med Bull. 2001;60(1):69–88. https://doi.org/10.1093/bmb/60.1.69.
9. Black RE et al. Maternal and child undernutrition and overweight in low-income and middle-income countries, Maternal and Child Nutrition, The Lancet, Published Online June 6, 2013. https://doi.org/10.1016/S0140-6736(13)60937-X.
10. Sullivan LM, Brumfield C. The first 1,000 days: nourishing America's future. The First 1,000 Days. Washington, D.C. 2016.
11. Mwaniki EW, Makokha AN. Nutrition status and associated factors among children in public primary schools in Dagoretti, Nairobi, Kenya. Afr Health Sci. 2013;13(1):39–46.
12. Aiga H, Abe K, Andrianome VN, et al. Risk factors for malnutrition among school-aged children: a cross-sectional study in rural Madagascar. BMC Public Health. 2019;19:773. https://doi.org/10.1186/s12889-019-7013-9.
13. Kleinman, R., et.al. Hunger in children in the United States: potential behavioral and emotional correlates. Pediatrics, 101(1), e3. 1998. https://pediatrics.aappublications.org/content/101/1/e3.
14. Christian P, Smith ER. Adolescent undernutrition: global burden, physiology, and nutritional risks. Ann Nutr Metab. 2018:316–28. https://doi.org/10.1159/000488865.

15. Luna B. Developmental changes in cognitive control through adolescence. Adv Child Dev Behav. 2009;37:233–78. https://doi.org/10.1016/s0065-2407(09)03706-9.
16. World Health Organization. Global health estimates 2015: deaths by cause, age, sex, by country and by region, 2000–2015. Geneva: WHO. p. 2016.
17. Wells JCK, et al. Beyond wasted and stunted—a major shift to fight under nutrition. Lancet. 2019;3(11):831–4.
18. WHO. https://www.who.int/elena/titles/full_recommendations/sam_management/en/index7.html
19. Prudhon C. Save the children. Assessment of infant and young child feeding practices among refugees on Lesvos Island, Greece—22 February-4 March. 2016.
20. Save the children, infant and young child feeding practices among IDPs and host communities in South Syria, Nawa, Mseifrah and Moarba, South Syria 11–21 January. 2018.
21. Rahman A, Fisher J, Bower P, Luchters S, Tran T, Taghi Yasamy M, Saxena S, and Waheed W. Interventions for common perinatal mood disorders in women in low- and middle-income countries: a systematic review and meta-analysis. Bulletin of the World Health Organisation. 2013. p. 593–601.
22. Mirjana Gurinović, Milica Zeković, Jelena Milešević, Marina Nikolić, Maria Glibetić. Nutritional Assessment. Reference Module in Food Science. Elsevier. 2017.
23. IFE Core Group. Infant feeding in emergencies: operational guidance for emergency relief staff and programme managers. Oxford. Vol 3. 2017.
24. A full list of IYCF indicators in UNICEF's expanded global database. https://data.unicef.org/topic/nutrition/infant-and-young-child-feeding/
25. FAO. Minimum dietary diversity for women: a guide to measurement, FAO, USAID's food and nutrition technical assistance III project (FANTA). Managed by FHI 360. Rome. 2016.
26. World Health Organization. Indicators for the global monitoring framework on maternal, infant and young child nutrition. WHO; 2014.
27. CARE. Infant and young child feeding practices, collecting and using data—A Step-by-Step Guide. 2010.
28. WHO/UNICEF. Indicators for assessing infant and young child feeding practice. Part 1 Definition. Part 2—Measurement. 2010.
29. Tech Rapid Response Team. Fact sheet on infant and young child feeding practices assessment in emergencies. 2016.
30. [Internet] Knowledge, attitude, and practice survey: https://www.spring-nutrition.org/publications/tool-summaries/kap-survey-model-knowledge-attitudes-and-practices
31. Kittle B. A practical guide to conducting a barrier analysis. New York, NY: Helen Keller International; 2013.
32. Hossain MI, et al. Comparison of mid upper arm circumference and weight-for-height z score for assessing acute malnutrition in Bangladeshi children aged 6-60 months: an analytical study. Am J Clin Nutr. 2017:1232–7.
33. SMART. https://smartmethodology.org/?doing_wp_cron=1595704433.32964301109313964843 75
34. Mates E, Shoham J, Khara T and Dolan C. Stunting in humanitarian and protracted crises. ENN Discussion Paper. 2017.
35. World Bank. https://www.worldbank.org/en/topic/nutrition/overview
36. UNHCR. Guidelines for Selective feeding: The Management of Malnutrition in Emergencies. Geneva. 2011.
37. UNHCR. Operational guidance on the use of fortified blended foods in blanket supplementary feeding programmes—An Addendum to the UNHCR 2011 Operational Guidance on the Use of Special Nutritional Products to Reduce Micronutrient Deficiencies and Malnutrition in Refugee Populations. Geneva. 2014.
38. World Food Program. Nutrition at the world food programme, programming for nutrition-specific interventions. WFP; 2012.
39. Global Nutrition Report 2018. https://globalnutritionreport.org/reports/global-nutrition-report-2018/

40. Jones G, et al. Series: child survival, how many child deaths can we prevent this year? Lancet. 2003;362(9377):65–71.
41. WHO. https://www.who.int/elena/titles/micronutrients_pregnancy/en/

Christine Fernandes, MSc is a Maternal, Infant, and Young Child Nutrition specialist with significant experience in humanitarian contexts ranging from fieldwork to global policy and guidance development. She is a member of the Infant Feeding in Emergencies (IFE) Core Group, based in Oxford, UK, and was on the editorial board to produce the Operational Guidance on Infant Feeding in Emergencies (Version 3.0, 2017), in which the revisions she spearheaded were heavily influenced by nutrition contexts in the Middle East. Areas of focus include training curricula on Infant and Young Child Feeding in Emergencies (IYCF-E), management of breast milk substitutes, complementary feeding program design, and IYCF-E technical support to the nutrition clusters for improved emergency response.

Minh Tram Le is a public health nutritionist with more than 10 years of experience in development and humanitarian settings. She has worked with different non-governmental organizations (Action Contre la Faim, Save the Children) as a nutrition adviser in contexts including emergency responses (Pakistan floods, Afghanistan conflict, European refugee and migrant crisis, Horn of Africa drought, Rohingyas' crisis, etc.). She is currently working as a nutrition specialist with UNICEF with a focus on child wasting and nutrition in emergencies in the South Asian region.

Food Security

12

Zoë Bell, Christine Fernandes, and Minh Tram Le

Background

The concept of food security and food insecurity is quite complex, it can be understood at different levels; the (inter)national, household, and individual level. The most commonly used definition of food insecurity is when "people do not have adequate physical and economic access to sufficient, safe and nutritious foods that meet their dietary needs and preferences for an active and healthy life" [1]. Put another way, food insecurity is when there are not readily available nutritious, safe foods that can be obtained in socially acceptable ways and are culturally appropriate or personally acceptable.

Figure 12.1 depicts the four components required for food security: access, availability, utilization, and stability that can be applied at (inter)national, household, or individual level. *Availability* refers to a reliable supply of sufficient quality and quantity food, i.e., in a shop or food market. This depends on shops and food markets existing, imports, food stocks, food aid, and domestic production. *Access* refers to the ability of people to both financially and physically obtain food. This depends on physical, social, and economic factors, market infrastructure, purchasing power, income, and transport. *Utilization* refers to adequate dietary intake of food that the body can metabolize. This depends on food safety, food hygiene, food quality, proper food preparation, and nutritional knowledge. *Stability* refers to long-lasting,

Z. Bell (✉)
Newcastle University, Baddiley Clark Building, Population Health Sciences Institute, Newcastle, UK
e-mail: z.bell2@ncl.ac.uk

C. Fernandes
Save the Children, Amman, Jordan
e-mail: christine.fernandes@savethechildren.org

M. T. Le
UNICEF Regional Office for South Asia (ROSA), Kathmandu, Nepal

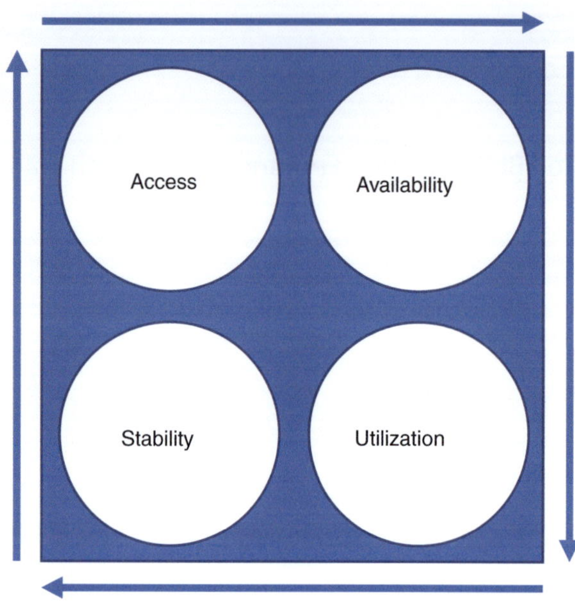

Fig. 12.1 Four components of the concept of food security; access, availability, utilization, and stability

permanent access to food, i.e., all components are maintained over time. Food insecurity can be experienced episodically (i.e., a few weeks of the year) or chronically (i.e., every month) as well as experienced differently by different people within a household (i.e., a mother may experience it differently to a child in the same household) [2]. Experiences range from worrying about the ability to obtain food, to experiencing hunger when food security is very low. Coping strategies and interventions can amend the severity of the experience of food insecurity.

Experiences of Food Insecurity

In refugee settings, reasons for food insecurity can be multiple. People may have lost all their belongings and income due to displacements and be entirely dependent on any external assistance provided. In this case, it is important to properly estimate and respond to the needs, as per the population's culture, demography (gender, age groups) medical history, etc. Even if the population is partially relying on external assistance, it is important to ensure that all nutritional needs are covered to prevent deficiencies and malnutrition, and that assistance properly responds to the special needs of the most vulnerable (infants and young children, pregnant and breastfeeding women, elderly, people with disease or disabilities, etc.).

During the last [12 months/ 30 days], was there a time when, because of lack of money or other resources:

1. You [or others in your household] were worried you would not have enough food to eat?

2. You [or others in your household] were unable to eat healthy and nutritious food?

3. You [or others in your household] ate only a few kinds of foods?

4. You [or others in your household] had to skip a meal?

5. You [or others in your household] ate less than you thought you should?

6. Your household ran out of food?

7. You [or others in your household] were hungry but did not eat?

8. You [or others in your household] went without eating for a whole day?

Fig. 12.2 The Food Insecurity Experience Scale eight question module developed for global use, from Food and Agriculture Organisation [3]

Assessing Food Insecurity

Measuring food insecurity at the household and individual level requires capturing the four components of food insecurity [4]. Dietary recalls can be used alongside questions such as "Do you eat less food than you would like due to a lack of money?". However, several technical tools measuring the existence, occurrence, and severity of food insecurity exist. The Food Insecurity Experiences Scale (FIES) was developed and validated for global use [3]. Asking eight questions about food-related behaviors and experiences, the tool identifies the severity of food insecurity experienced by a household or individual. Questions relate either to the last 12 months or 30 days. Figure 12.2 shows the eight questions from the FIES. Responses from questions are analyzed together to measure the severity of food insecurity. Small-scale use (i.e., not national level) uses the raw score between 0 and 8. Lower scores correspond to less severe food insecurity.

What Can you Do with the Information?

This data can provide rationale for setting up a local project addressing food insecurity and help inform its procedures and practices. Collecting this data with researchers could help inform local policy or advocacy work.

Who Should Ask?

For local community projects a senior volunteer or project coordinator is best suited, or a trained researcher.

Where Should you Ask?

It is important that questions relating to food insecurity are asked on an individual basis, and not in big groups. This acknowledges the sensitivity of the topic and limits feelings of embarrassment, stigma, and shame. Ideally, the person asked will handle the food for the household. Commonly, this will be a woman, especially in households with children.

Case Studies

This section of the chapter provides four case studies each addressing food insecurity. The first two case studies are national, humanitarian interventions addressing food insecurity. The following two case studies are examples of best practice of local, community responses to addressing food insecurity in Gateshead, UK.

Case Study One—Food Assistance in Refugee Settings

South Sudanese refugee crisis, Northern Uganda camps.

Description

Ongoing civil war in South Sudan has led to one of the largest influxes of the South Sudanese population to neighboring countries in 2016. More than a million people fled the conflict and were displaced in Northern Uganda, in different settings and camps. Considered one of the largest refugee crises, the high number of people fleeing South Sudan forced local authorities to install and expand existing refugee sites.

A few days and weeks after the first arrivals, the situation in the camps was scarce. During the initial assessments, the population was asking for the most basic provision of food and water. Many men stayed behind and were involved in the conflict, resulting in a large proportion of the population being women and children (more than 80% at the beginning of the crisis). Local authorities and humanitarian organizations urgently responded to the need by providing food and water assistance to the population.

Food Assistance and Gardening

At the onset of the emergency and because of pressing needs to respond, food rations were distributed in newly established camps. Each ration was composed of wheat and maize, lentils, peas, and vegetable oil. For households with children between the ages of 6 and 24 months, specialized nutritious foods were also provided (called blanket supplementary food under the form of high-energy biscuits—usually for newly displaced situations). Food rations were also distributed in schools set up in the camps for school-aged children. In addition, cash transfers were also provided once markets were operational again to allow households to choose food that was culturally appropriate and be more independent.

Due to a large number of people and incessant arrivals in already overcrowded camps, the food assistance approach was quickly overwhelmed and deemed insufficient. More advocacy towards setting up cash assistance instead of food distribution started, to avoid negative coping mechanisms in camps such as selling items or prioritizing some households' members because of food shortage.

After many months and realizing, that the situation was prolonging with no prospects for many to return to South Sudan, some households received pieces of land from local authorities to cultivate their own garden. Although this represented only a small portion of the refugee population, it allowed some families to plant some vegetables to increase household food security. In some cases, this additional food helped families supplementing their food rations. However, some of the challenges encountered were access to water (particularly underground water) and ensuring that lands were fertile. This pushed many families to move from one camp to the other, even trying to leave the camps (which was difficult for administrative purpose), hoping to find better living conditions for them and their children.

Way Forward

The situation in the South Sudanese refugee camps of Northern Uganda remains dire because of the large population in the camps and a decrease in financial assistance over the years. However, community support plays a vital role. Plots of land allocated to households, although sometimes too small and not allocated to all, provide some relief to families in addition to the food and cash assistance.

Case Study Two—Food Assistance for Internally Displaced and Refugee Pregnant and Lactating Women (PLW) and Children 6–24 Months

Syria Crisis, Northeast Syria Camps, 2020.

Description

In the protracted emergency of Syria, almost 10 years of conflict and violence caused loss of access to basic services such as food, clean water, shelter, and health care for millions of people. In the Northeast of Syria, regional conflict caused the displacement of hundreds of thousands of people, mostly women and children, to flee or be transferred to IDP and Refugee camps in the governorates of Al-Hassakeh, Raqqa, and Dier-Ez-Zor—all of them dependent on aid for basic services. By 2020, the devaluation of the Syrian pound greatly inflated the cost of food in the markets, further limiting access to a quality diet for all households such as fruits, vegetables, and animal sources. After almost a decade of conflict and depleted resources, chronic malnutrition (stunting) began to rise to WHO "high" thresholds, micronutrient deficiencies climbed, where 1 in every 3 pregnant women was anemic, as well as over 40% of all children 6–24 months, and within 1 year (from 2018 to 2019) maternal acute malnutrition increased fivefold. Yet, access to diverse foods was still a challenge.

Food Assistance

In the camps of Northeast Syria, food security actors provided vulnerable households with food baskets containing staple items such as vegetable oil, sugar, rice, pasta, lentils, tomato paste, flour, salt, tea, dried chickpeas, and zaatar (mix of spices, herbs, and sesame seeds). However, this provision only covered partial needs, and families would have to supplement other foods such as fresh fruit or vegetables, meat, or eggs, which was difficult due to lack of livelihoods/income and high prices in the market.

Pregnant women and children 0–2 years were some of the most physically vulnerable to food insecurity in Syria. A food and nutrition intervention in Areesha Camp of Al-Hassakeh governorate prioritized all pregnant and lactating women (who were also mothers of children 0–24 months) with food vouchers for a 6-month duration. Following analysis of the food basket content in Areesha camp, the vouchers were initially restricted to fruits and vegetables to cover gaps in micronutrients. However, following a market assessment, it had been decided that restricting the voucher to specific products with specific amounts (kg) posed logistical constraints such as availability for different vendors or seasonality of the products. Therefore, it was decided to implement a value voucher modality where mothers were able to choose the products they needed with the specific amount they received. Mothers were provided with vouchers of 20 USD per month. Knowing that families did not have access to refrigerators to properly store products, mothers were able to redeem 5 USD vouchers from selected vendor shops on a weekly basis.

Strategically, all pregnant and lactating women receiving vouchers were already accessing maternal and infant nutrition support in a Mother Baby Area (MBA) with daily counseling and education by skilled staff. Nutrition actors focussed on the importance of dietary diversity during pregnancy, in a child's diet after 6 months of age, and the criticality of breastfeeding during food insecure contexts. In addition, nutrition messages related to foods containing Vitamin A, C, and iron, were printed directly on the vouchers, and voucher distribution was only carried out at the MBA during nutrition sessions to ensure mothers were receiving support to both *access and utilization* of food.

Way Forward

Food insecurity continues to be a concern in Syria, and since the COVID-19 pandemic, has only worsened. Humanitarian actors are now recognizing that food assistance through food baskets is necessary for certain food insecure contexts, but in the long term, access to fresh and animal source foods is critical to ensure adequate health and nutrition of the population. Therefore, unrestricted cash and vouchers are now beginning to be a more accepted food security intervention, especially when it is combined with health and nutrition behavior change support. Evidence shows that food security programs have more nutritional impact if access to food is combined with nutrition education. However, more analysis on modalities in humanitarian contexts needs to be conducted. In Syria, food security assistance with cash and vouchers are being scaled up but more information on the outcomes of integration with nutrition programs and health services (such as Antenatal Care/Postnatal Care) are required.

Case Study Three and Four—Food Assistance in a High-Income Country

By the end of 2018, the UK had resettled around 14,000 Syrian refugees [5]. National statistics show that the UK welcomed around 30,000 asylum applications in 2019 [5]. A person arriving in the UK awaiting a decision on an asylum claim does not have the same rights as a British citizen. Asylum seekers are not allowed to work until they have received refugee status which can take up to 6 months. This precarious situation means many asylum seekers and refugees in the UK are more vulnerable to food insecurity.

In the UK, asylum claims can fall under various schemes such as the unaccompanied asylum-seeking children (UASC), the Syrian Vulnerable Persons Resettlement Scheme (SVPRS) or resettlement schemes for those The United Nations Refugee Agency (UNHCR) have referred as being in greatest need of assistance [5]. After claiming asylum in the UK, if a person has no finances, they can also apply for support from the Home Office via the Dispersal programme. The Dispersal programme is a process where the Home Office moves asylum seekers living in destitution to local authorities across the UK, and Central Government provides local authorities funding to support housing of asylum seekers and refugees. Gateshead Council, in the Northeast of England, has voluntarily participated in the program since it started in 2000 and has housed several thousand asylum seekers [5]. In Gateshead, organizations have been set up in response to help settlement and integration, and improve access to food for asylum seekers and refugees.

Case Study Three—Bensham Community Food Co-Operative (BCFC) Food Assistance in Gateshead, UK

Bensham CFC is a community-led venture set up for the benefit of the local community and run on a not-for-profit basis. It primarily serves Bensham's refugee community, although welcomes all. Bensham CFC has a non-paying membership scheme. Membership does not require "proof-of-need," i.e., people do not have to provide reasons for accessing the food cooperative, reducing any potential stigma or embarrassment.

Bensham CFC runs a weekly service. It intends to supplement a household's food supply to provide balanced meals, rather than be the main source of food for a household. Bensham CFC rely predominantly on public donations of nonperishable food items that can be stored for a long time without the need for refrigeration. However, BCFC places emphasis on providing fresh produce. To obtain fresh produce, BCFC is linked with larger supermarket chains and local allotments who pass on their surplus fresh produce. Food Co-Operatives often have to supplement donations, buying food with their own funds. Bensham CFC does this through a subscription with a charity called FareShare. A FareShare subscription ensures delivery of weekly or bi-weekly variety of fresh produce. For BCFC, providing foods that are culturally appropriate is important, so they ask for specific donations of rice, lentils, chickpeas, and other pulses and types of oils and herbs and spices to meet the needs of their members. Figure 12.3 provides an example of some of the food BCFC offers.

Way Forward

Providing access to food on a weekly basis with a focus on fresh produce helps people get a step closer to eating enough healthy, quality foods that form a balanced meal. Bensham CFC recognises that refugees and asylum seekers experiencing food insecurity are experiencing multiple aspects of poverty. Therefore, they have evolved to meet needs beyond food, for example, providing free clothes, toys and furniture. Community spaces such as BCFC offer more than nutritional benefits. As Irna says "this place helps my family, more than food, they are so lovely, and this place is like home." They provide a space where people can share experiences with others in similar situations. Volunteering opportunities help increase self-esteem, confidence, and sense of purpose. This model provides an opportunity for people to be a part of the solution by volunteering themselves and donating back when they are able to do so. The community nature of a food cooperative means anyone is welcome. As volunteer Lena put it, "it is a place full of kindness and peace and with people who have a big heart." Table 12.1 in the appendix of this chapter provides questions to prompt those contemplating opening a food-co-operative. Further guidance on food co-operatives can be found at the Sustain website that provides toolkit to help set-up a food co-operative, and locate others in the UK [6].

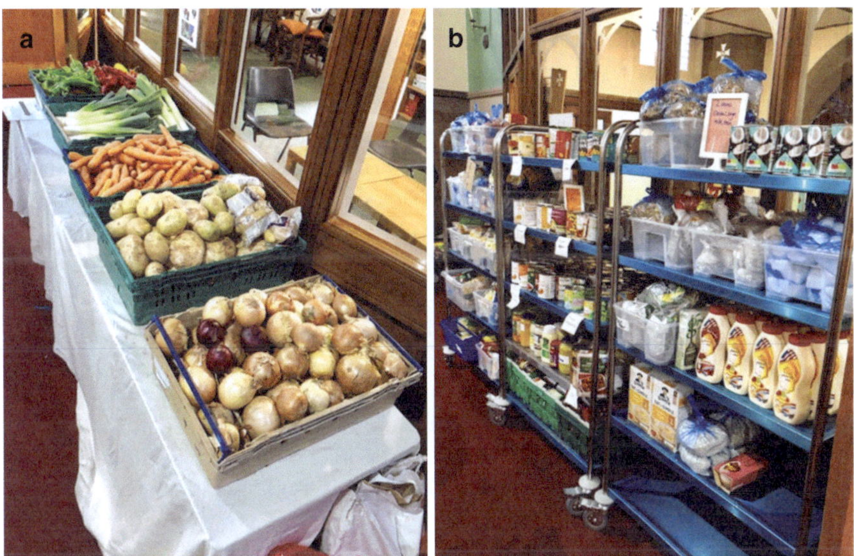

Fig. 12.3 Food on offer at Bensham Food Co-Operative. (**a**) Fresh vegetables on offer onions, potatoes, carrots, leeks, green, yellow and red peppers (**b**) Tinned fruit, vegetables, and beans, coconut milk, oats, pasta, flour, and sugar

Case Study Four—The Comfrey Project Food Assistance and Gardening in Gateshead, UK

The Comfrey project was founded in 2001 and received charitable status in 2002. Starting as a pilot project offering one session a week on an allotment, the project has expanded. In 2016, the project had three sites with 21,000 sq. feet of land under cultivation. Set in the same local authority as BCFC, this project provides a different approach to addressing food insecurity, primarily through its community gardening space.

Food Assistance and Gardening

The Comfrey Project works with refugees and those seeking asylum. Their community gardening space is on land previously used by Gateshead local authority but was left neglected. Refugees volunteer at The Comfrey Project to maintain the garden and keep local, seasonal produce growing all year round. Volunteers also maintain the beehives producing local honey and cook food grown in the garden to provide hot lunches for everyone taking part in an activity that morning. This cooking aspect is beneficial because it provides an opportunity to practice cooking and eating different locally grown fruits and vegetables. This helps diversify diets and introduce more affordable options; affordability or availability of ingredients native to home can be an issue for refugees. It also has environmental and health benefits too as people are eating seasonal foods, which can mean less need for chemical substances.

Warmer seasons result in excess leftover food which can be taken home. Other seasons require a contingency plan to continue running lunchtime cooking activities. This might involve using project funds to purchase surplus food or support from local business. The Comfrey Project is supported by local businesses providing surplus vegetables. This is particularly useful in winter. Investing in a freezer allows the project to have frozen vegetables in the winter months that are just as nutritious. Also, investing in indoor gardening equipment such as electric propagators helps grow more vegetables and fruit earlier compared to if they waited for the spring months in the UK when it is ok to go out into the garden space.

The range of fresh produce provided by the community garden depends on what is grown, which depends on numerous factors including size of gardening space available, season, soil type, budget size, among other things. Having a volunteer or paid member of staff knowledgeable on gardening is useful as they can teach people a variety of growing techniques, discuss the benefits of growing food, and offer advice on garden growing and management.

Way Forward

Food insecurity continues to be an issue for refugees and asylum seekers in the UK. Local projects, like The Comfrey Project are being recognised as playing a vital role in adddressing food insecurity. Their wider benefits are also recognised. Community gardening is very important in terms of community integration. Growing, cooking, and sharing food provides a vehicle for people to share learn about one another's culture, bringing people together through a common activity. One volunteer at the Comfrey Project said "when you are working with the earth, everywhere you go feels like home" showing how getting involved offers much more than food. Volunteers at the Comfrey Project have experienced how the project's gardening space brings a sense of community, inclusivity, and belonging. They have decided to "give back" by venturing into a "mobile" garden so they can visit different streets in their area and connect with neighbors. For those setting up a community gardening space, Table 12.1 provides thought-provoking questions to inspire its creation.

Conclusion

This chapter has provided insight into the issue of food insecurity for migrating children and their families. Each case study is unique, taking on the shape of its location and people, developing within its means to meet the needs of its community. This chapter will hopefully have inspired creation or evolvment of local community projects addressing food insecurity.

Acknowledgments We thank Bensham Community Food Co-Operative and The Comfrey Project for their contribution to this chapter.

Appendix

Table 12.1 Questions to inspire creation and evolution of community food co-operatives and community gardening projects in response to local food insecurity

	Food cooperative	Community gardening
Description	Create a set of principles 1. Write a description of the envisaged project 2. Write a mission statement/ethos/set of values the project acts in accordance with	
Location	• What is an ideal venue? List features to help a search, i.e., kitchen, non-faith based • What spaces are available in the local community, when? • What facilities does the space offer? • Is there storage space in the facility, or will the project need to "move in and out" every session? • What are the running costs of the project?	• What spaces of land are available in the area? • Who owns or has previously used it? • Is the space accessible to project members? • What facilities does the space offer in addition to gardening space? • What is the cost of the land (and facilities)? • What tools are required to grow food? • What are the running costs of the gardening project?
What is provided	• How will food be sourced; what contacts does the project have to collect and donate food? • Is there a collection point for people to drop food donations? • When can supermarket donations be collected? • Will fresh produce be collected? • Does the venue have storage space? • Are there food hygiene, health, and safety guidelines that need action? • Are there regulations regarding the handling of food donated from shops? • Is there a system to track food coming in and out and expiry dates? • Has the venue got the capacity to provide refreshments or hot food?	• What produce will be able to be grown in the gardening space from season to season? • What gardening roles are offered at the project? • What other activities will be provided? • What talents/skills do those using the services have? Could they facilitate an activity or volunteer? • Has the venue got the capacity to provide refreshments or hot food?

(continued)

Table 12.1 (continued)

	Food cooperative	Community gardening
Volunteers	• List volunteer roles that are needed • Will there be volunteer job descriptions listing the role and responsibility? • Will there be team meetings? • Will there be volunteer training for each role? • What about volunteer rotas?	• List volunteer roles that are needed • Will there be volunteer job descriptions listing the role and responsibility? • Will there be volunteer training for each role? • What about volunteer rotas? • Will there be team meetings? • What about linking with voluntary organizations to find someone with gardening knowledge, or is there a local volunteer?
Considerations	• Are there policies on abusing the system or inappropriate behavior? • Are there policies on the amount of food provided, i.e., per person, household? • Are there policies for dealing with allergies/dietary requirements? • Are links with other organizations possible, e.g., a council employee who can help asylum seekers with their specific cases? • Are there other ways to expand to meet people's needs?	• Are there policies on how to share excess grown produce in a fair way? • Are there plans in place for seasons when produce is not as fruitful, e.g., winter months? What equipment could help mitigate these obstacles when gardening? • Are there local businesses to collaborate with? If so, in what ways? • Are there ways to expand to meet people's needs?

References

1. Food and Agriculture Organization of the United Nations. 1996. Declaration on world food security.
2. Kendall A, Olson CM, Frongillo EA Jr. Validation of the Radimer/Cornell measures of hunger and food insecurity. J Nutr. 1995;125(11):2793–801. https://doi.org/10.1093/jn/125.11.2793.
3. Food and Agriculture Organization of the United Nations. 2015. Rome: Food and Agriculture Organization. Voices of the hungry. http://www.fao.org/in-action/voices-of-the-hungry/en/#.XMxIG3KWyUk. Reproduced with permission.
4. Campbell C. Food insecurity: a nutritional outcome or a predictor variable? J Nutr. 1991;121(3):408–15.
5. Gateshead Council. 2018. Gateshead JSNA—Refugees and Asylum Seeker. Joint Strategic Needs Assessment. https://www.gatesheadjsna.org.uk/article/10448/What-the-data-tells-us. Accessed 02 September 2020.
6. Sustain. 2018. Food co-ops toolkit. https://www.sustainweb.org/foodcoopstoolkit/. Accessed 01 September 2020.

Zoë Bell, BSc, MSc is a doctoral student within the Population Health Sciences Institute at Newcastle University, England. She is currently completing her PhD focusing on food insecurity and its nutritional impact amongst women and children; with a particular focus on the first 1000 days. She has a BSc in Biomedical Sciences (University of Southampton) and an MSc in Human Nutrition (University of Surrey).

Christine Fernandes, BA UCLA, MSc   is a Maternal, Infant, and Young Child Nutrition specialist for Save the Children with significant experience in humanitarian contexts ranging from fieldwork, such as nutrition counseling with mothers and infants during emergencies, to global policy and guidance development. She is a member of the Infant Feeding in Emergencies (IFE) Core Group, based in Oxford, UK, and was on the editorial board to produce the Operational Guidance on Infant Feeding in Emergencies (Version 3.0, 2017), in which the revisions she spearheaded were heavily influenced by nutrition contexts in the Middle East. Areas of focus include training curricula on IYCF-E, breast milk substitute program management, complementary feeding program design for the first 1000 days, and technical support to nutrition clusters (UNICEF and UNOCHA) in the Middle East region.

Minh Tram Le   is a public health nutritionist with more than 10 years of experience in development and humanitarian settings. She has worked with several non-governmental organizations (Action Contre la Faim, Save the Children) as a nutrition adviser in different contexts including emergency responses (Pakistan floods, Afghanistan conflict, European refugee and migrant crisis, Horn of Africa drought, Rohingyas' crisis, etc.). She is currently working as a nutrition specialist with UNICEF with a focus on child wasting and nutrition in emergencies in the South Asian region.

Child Development and Developmental Concerns

13

Ramzi Nasir

Background: Child Development for the Nonspecialist Health Professional

Pediatric Health Professionals and Child Development: Why Is this Relevant?

The past few decades have seen a shift in why caregivers seek medical advice for their children. As childhood mortality due to infectious disease has dropped, there is a rise in noncommunicable diseases presenting as a main area of concern. A significant percentage of these visits relate to concerns about children's development and behavior.

Even in refugee camps and humanitarian settings, once the acute crisis is over, a large number of concerns are related to children's development, behavior, and school-related concerns. The role of the health care provider is to be able to take a history and perform a basic assessment, know when to be concerned, investigate for medical causes, assess the child within the context of the family, reassure, monitor, and/or provide recommendations.

Using this Chapter

The focus of this chapter is to give a brief overview of this topic, and introduce some guidelines to support nonspecialist health professionals working in the field. This chapter builds on principles outlined in the *MhGAP intervention Guide (developed by the World Health Organization's Mental Health Gap Action*

R. Nasir (✉)
Royal Free London NHS Foundation Trust, London, UK

The Portland Hospital, London, UK

© Springer Nature Switzerland AG 2021
C. Harkensee et al. (eds.), *Child Refugee and Migrant Health*,
https://doi.org/10.1007/978-3-030-74906-4_13

Programme) [1], which is a concise and simple to use guidance for the assessment and management of mental health, neurological, and substance use disorders (including developmental disorders) in nonspecialized health settings. Additionally, recognizing the limitation on resources in humanitarian settings, an additional guidance was further developed to be used in humanitarian settings (MhGAP-Humanitarian Intervention Guide) [2]. Information in this section is complementary to the WHO guidance and may be used by the reader to further develop their knowledge. In addition to this chapter, additional resources are recommended to readers interested in expanding their knowledge on this topic include: *Disabled Village Children* [3] which brings a wealth of practical and resourceful suggestions for individuals working in low resource settings and *Where There Is No Child Psychiatrist* [4].

Definitions

Child development is the learning process that every child goes through to enable him/her to master important skills for life. The term "child development" indicates advancement of the child in all areas of human functioning. The most crucial period for child development starts at conception and continues through the preschool years (roughly 2–5 years of age). This is a period of rapid brain growth and reconfiguration of neuronal connections shaped by biological and environmental factors that set the trajectory of the individual's growth and development into adulthood. Identifying children with developmental difficulties in these early years is a priority as early supports and interventions are associated with improved outcomes later in life. While emphasizing the importance of the early years, it is important not to forget the needs of older children and young adults whose brains are still developing and can still benefit from supports and interventions.

What Are Developmental Milestones and Developmental Domains?

Developmental milestones is a practical framework to understand and monitor the developmental process. It is based on the fact that children usually acquire their developmental skills in a gradual sequential order with earlier skills promoting the development of subsequent skills. For example, a child first is able to say single words before being able to speak in sentences, or a child is first able to sit upright (develop strength of the trunk) before they are able to stand up or walk (requires more coordination of muscles).

Developmental milestones are often thought of as occurring in separate domains. This is an arbitrary (but familiar) way to organize symptoms and information observed or provided by caregivers. Below is one example of classification that may be useful to a broad range of health professionals in refugee and humanitarian settings. The reader may wish to use different classifications depending on the setting (e.g., many countries have their own specific guidance on how to monitor children's development). The reader will note this framework is imperfect (for example, children often present with overlapping delays in multiple domains which may also change with different ages).

Domains of Development (for the Purpose of this Chapter)

Social/Emotional: Children bond early with their caregivers and continue to develop the skill to initiate and respond to social interactions. These skills are closely linked to their ability to regulate their emotions and make emotional connections with others.

Communication: Children acquire communication skills in a predictable order. These skills include the ability to speak, understand, and use nonverbal communication strategies (e.g., eye contact, hand gestures).

Cognition (problem-solving, learning, thinking, independence skills): Children with cognitive difficulties may present as younger than their chronological age in the way they behave, play, understand instructions, or acquire independence skills (e.g., toileting, dressing, eating). As these children grow older, they may have difficulties assisting with chores/responsibilities in the home or learning in school.

Movement (posture/movement of body and limb): Children acquire motor skills in a predictable order. As children grow, their ability to control their posture, move in their environment and use their limbs continues to develop.

What Are Developmental Concerns?

For the purpose of this chapter, we will use the general term *Developmental Concerns* to describe any delays, disorders, or resultant disability. The definitions of these specific terms are outlined below, but in refugee and humanitarian settings it is often difficult to differentiate them and a general term (concerns) is more appropriate to avoid misunderstandings.

Developmental delay is a nonspecific term that suggests a child is developing behind his peers.

Developmental Disorders suggest a clear deviation from the typical trajectory of milestones that is likely to continue throughout the child's life.

Developmental Disability: Disability is a complex term with both medical and social implications. The UN Convention on the Rights of Persons with Disabilities provides a globally agreed on definition: *Persons with disabilities include those who have long-term physical, mental, intellectual, or sensory impairments which in interaction with various barriers may hinder their full and effective participation in society on an equal basis with others* [5].

Many national governments and nongovernmental agencies have their own methods of classifying levels of disability as a means to allocate various services or financial supports. Based on the above, children with developmental delays or disorders may or may not be classified as disabled.

When to Be Concerned about a Child's Development

Children do not present with a label but a variety of concerns either directly observed, or more often raised by caregivers or others in the community who have an opportunity to observe the child (e.g., teachers or social workers). In general, caregivers are usually the first to notice differences in their child's development and any concerns they express should be taken seriously. In certain situations, caregivers might also play down the child's difficulties for a variety of reasons, and not share their concerns until a certain amount of trust has been built with the healthcare worker. Sometimes, children are brought to professionals because of concerns about behaviors or recurrent health problems without specific mention of the developmental delays.

Assessing Children's Development

In well-developed health care systems, clinicians have access to infrastructure that allows for early identification of risk factors and developmental concerns. Developmental surveillance requires a stable ongoing relationship between a child/family and healthcare professionals and the use of standardized assessment and screening tools. Clinicians working in such settings should use local procedures and guidance on developmental surveillance and screening [6, 7] (also see Chap. 1.2. "What Are the Drivers of Good and Ill Health in Refugee Children and their Families?" in this book for additional details). The review by Marlow et al. provides additional information on developmental screening tools developed for specific low- and middle-income country settings that may be used in specific refugee populations [8].

In less advanced healthcare systems (where most refugees are encountered), children and families may encounter health care professionals sporadically (e.g., acute illness, immunization campaigns, refeeding programs for malnutrition). These encounters can still provide an opportunity to enquire about children's development and make a difference for the child or family. A step-by-step approach is recommended including obtaining a history (through interview with caregivers and other sources), examination/observation of the child and finally interpreting findings and recommending interventions.

Using Developmental Milestones Checklist Charts

Developmental milestone checklist charts are commonly used as a tool to inform caregivers and professionals about expected trajectories of development. An example of a checklist by the US Centers for Disease Control is provided in the Appendix. Recent research revealed significant variability between different checklists and there may also be cultural variations that limit the use of such lists in refugee settings [9]. Developmental check lists are not an evidence-based tool to assess children's development and are not a substitute for standardized developmental monitoring and surveillance tool (see above). Therefore, it is recommended that such a list only be used as a guidance on trajectories of development, but not as a definitive means to diagnose developmental delay or as a way to ask yes/no questions of caregivers (instead, the open-ended interview approach described above is recommended).

Approach to Assess a Child with Developmental Concerns

In contrast to more acute medical assessments, which are often focused more on acute physical symptoms and signs, a child developmental assessment is more holistic, encompassing physical, developmental, psychological, and social aspects of health. For a comprehensive and structured assessment, it is important to think about set up and preparation of clinical encounters. Key elements of the assessment include obtaining a detailed history from the caregiver, observing and examining the child, considering diagnoses, differential diagnoses and investigations, and planning and agreeing on a management plan with the caregiver. Although this seems a logical sequence, for experienced clinicians these elements often intercalate and merge.

Considerations when Setting up and Starting a Clinical Encounter

The Physical Setting: Even in a busy and chaotic clinic/hospital, it is possible to establish a child and disability friendly clinical area can make the child and family feel calm and welcome and facilitate the clinical encounter. Some children with developmental concerns may be over sensitive to loud noise (e.g., from other children waiting), bright lights, or crowded environments. It can be useful to have a low sensory room or section of the waiting area that is quiet and soothing. Ask caregivers to tell you what helps and what stresses the child.

Observing child behavior and parent-child interactions: Before initiating interaction with the child, observe how the child and caregiver interact and respond to one another. This can provide hints at areas of strength or challenges in the relationship that need to be explored further.

Clinician/child encounter: (see also Table 13.1 *on examples of what to observe):* If appropriate to the health care professional's role, a child should be initially approached in a reassuring manner in the company of their caregivers. Most children feel reassured if held by or are near their usual caregiver. It is important to be respectful to the child and treat them with dignity as this sends an important message to caregivers who may hold negative biases towards the child.

In many situations, children may be reluctant to play or interact during initial health care assessments. Ask the caregiver if the child is acting like their usual self before drawing conclusions.

Table 13.1 Examples of questions and observations when assessing children with developmental concerns

Focus/developmental domain	What to ask (remember to start with open-ended questions)	What to observe	Notes
General: Establish the age or approximate age of the child [11]	Ask to see official documents and verify the date of birth with caregivers. You may need to ask specific questions about historic or natural events around the time of birth to further verify a birth date	Some children might appear younger than chronological age due to malnutrition/stunting. Some adolescents might appear older than their chronological age (e.g., adolescents with precocious development of facial/body hair)	In some settings, caregivers may not know a child's birth date, or a child might not be accompanied by their caregivers (e.g., orphaned children or unaccompanied adolescents). In some settings, official documents may not be a reliable means of confirming age. In contexts where age is a factor in granting asylum rights (e.g., determining if a child is younger or older than 18 years), there is controversy about the use of investigations for age determination—Such as bone—Age x-rays or dental exams (as these are often imprecise) [12]
Social/emotional	Do you have concerns about how your child interacts or plays with others? How does your child interact with the main caregivers? Do they recognize the main caregivers? What about other close adults, children? What about school? How does your child respond to strangers? Tell me about their friends? Is it easy or difficult to make friends? What do they do together? Who does your child play with? Do they prefer to play alone or with others? Can they share/take turns? What games/toys do they enjoy? What happens if they lose at a competitive game? Tell me about their imagination (e.g., pretend playing with toys or role-play)	Observe how the child interacts with caregivers, siblings. How he/she looks to them for reassurance, seeking comfort in an unfamiliar setting How do they respond when you smile, offer a toy? Do they check in with caregivers?	It is common for children to be shy or quiet with unfamiliar adults Do not overwhelm a child with your greetings or trying to interact with them and let them first get used to your presence Ask caregivers how the child's behavior with you compares with their behavior in more comfortable settings Do not over-interpret the child's behavior with you, especially if you have not known them for a long time

Communication **Topics of inquiry include:** Speaking/vocalizations Understanding and listening Nonverbal communication (e.g., use of eye contact and gestures)	Do you have concerns about how your child communicates? How does your child communicate? How do they tell you what they want (e.g., food)? How do they request things they cannot access (e.g., food or toy that is on a shelf)? Do they use words/sounds? How do they respond when you call their name? Do they understand what you are saying? Do they understand more when you gesture/show them? Do they use gestures? Do they look at you when requesting or showing you things?	How does the child use words/sounds, gestures, eye contact to communicate (e.g., request, ask questions, show interest in something)	Some children use words/sounds but these may not be used to communicate (e.g., talking or babbling to themselves while playing). Gestures include: Pointing to things that are close or far away, shaking head to say "no" or "yes", open and closing palm to ask for something, extending the arms to describe that an object is "big"
Cognition (problem-solving)	Is your child aware of their environment/other people around them? Can they solve new problems? Do they remember and learn from past experiences? What does your child play with? How does she play or find out how the toys work?	Does the child understand instructions (simple or multistep)? Can the child solve jigsaw puzzles or matching games?	Children with language difficulties may have difficulties understanding verbal instructions (and so appear to also have reduced abstract thinking skills). Try to minimize the use of language and use pictures or gestures when giving instructions
Cognition (independent living skills) **Topics of inquiry include:** Feeding: Hygiene: Toileting: Sleep: Safety: Expected household or community chores	How does your child eat, wash hands/brush teeth, go to the toilet? How does this compare to other children in your community? Do you have concerns about your child's sleep? How do they fall asleep? Do they wake up frequently? How much supervision does your child need to stay safe?		Notice overlap with other domains (e.g., using utensils requires both understanding, memory, and fine motor skills).

(continued)

Table 13.1 (continued)

Focus/developmental domain	What to ask (remember to start with open-ended questions)	What to observe	Notes
Cognition (school readiness and academic learning)	Do you have concerns about your child's learning or memory? Are you able to teach them new things (e.g., names of people, songs, colors, shapes, letters, numbers)? How are they doing in school? What do teachers say?	Assess children's knowledge of colors, shapes, numbers, letters, or academic concepts (depending on age)	Do not over-interpret difficulties if a child has not been exposed to instruction
Movement	Fine motor: Do you have concerns about how your child uses their hands? How does your child use their hands? Gross motor: Do you have any concerns about how your child moves, crawls, walks, runs, climbs stairs? Do you have concerns about their coordination?	How does the child manipulate toys, buttons, crayons? Drawings/writing How does the child walk, run, etc.	Be careful introducing small toys to children who still put objects in their mouth (choking hazard). Be careful when interpreting the quality of writing and drawings in children who have not had previous opportunities to draw
Behavioral profile: Topics of inquiry include: Temperament/ personality Response to frustration (emotional regulation) Attention and perseverance Safety awareness Unusual behaviors	Tell me about your child's personality. How does your child react to frustration, stress, difficult tasks? How much supervision does your child need? Does your child engage in any behaviors that are unusual or different than most other children in your community?	Is the child shy, outgoing? How do they adjust to new setting? How do they adjust to change (e.g., when it is time to come in to the examination area, or time to leave) Is the child calm or overactive? How much supervision do they need to stay safe? Any unusual behaviors (see also autism section)	Do not over-interpret how the child responds in the clinical setting, especially if this is a new environment for them

Vision (poor vision can impact all areas of development, so it is important to assess if the child sees well or not)	Do you think your child sees well?	For vision assessment, see if the child can – Look at your eyes – Follow a moving object with the head and eyes – Grab an object – Recognize familiar people	*Additional professional assessment is typically needed if concerns are noted*
Hearing (poor hearing can impact all areas of development, so it is important to assess if the child hears well or not)	Do you think your child hears well?	For hearing assessment, see if the child can: – Turn head to see someone behind them when they speak – Show reaction to loud noise – Make a lot of different sounds (Tata, dada, baba), if an infant	*Additional professional assessment is typically needed if concerns are noted*

Using drawing tools, toys, and fun activities are an effective way to engage children. Through play, clinicians can observe how children communicate, problem solve, use their hands, regulate their emotions, and relate to their caregivers. Useful tools include crayons/pencils (or even sticks can be used to make marks in the sand), blocks (bricks), cause and effect toys (that make noise or lights), soap bubbles, cars, toy animals, rattles that make sounds, toys for pretend play (e.g., eating utensils). You may have to make your own toys [3].

Most children are wary when meeting strangers and will take time to warm up. Allow them to explore the room and toys before engaging them. Ask the caregivers to play with their children and then you can join in. Note that in many health care settings, caregivers do not expect health professionals to play with children and see them in a more paternalistic role. Explain to caregivers that play is an excellent and nonthreatening way to assess and communicate with children.

This context also allows the professional to observe how the child and parent communicate and interact. Observe if the caregiver is caring, kind, patient or appears aloof, angry, or impatient with the child.

Interviewing Children Without Their Caregivers: It may be appropriate in certain circumstances to interview children/adolescents separate from their caregivers. Using chaperones in such situations (e.g., another professional) is good practice as it can be reassuring to families and avoids any potential misunderstandings or misinterpretation of the nature of the interview or assessment.

Using Interpreters: Local healthcare workers or interpreters are usually a helpful resource to avoid misunderstandings or biases. However, it is important to note that some families may not wish to disclose sensitive information to an interpreter from their own community and may prefer to communicate via alternative resources (e.g., an interpretation telephone line or someone from outside their immediate community). Please see Chap. 3, Sect. "Methodology: The Nicaragua and Colombia Experiences", for further details on working with interpreters.

Including the Child in the Interview: Ask the caregivers if they think it is appropriate for the child to be in the room during the caregiver interview. Some children may have some awareness of their difficulties and misinterpret the interview as a form of criticism or judgment. In such situations, it is best to have them wait in a separate area with a responsible member of the family or clinical staff.

Communicating with Educators and Early Childhood Development Professionals: Teachers and other professionals in the educational sector can provide valuable information on children, their learning and behavior. It is important however to be aware that such reporting may not be reliable in setting where teachers are less experienced or if they are not familiar with the local culture and customs of displaced children which can lead to inappropriate academic expectations (too high or too low) or inaccurate interpretation of behaviors (e.g., misinterpreting reduced eye contact with adults as a form of social withdrawal rather than a culturally appropriate sign of respect) [10].

Approach to Obtaining a History

If within the health care provider's skill set, a comprehensive developmental and medical history should be collected. For how to take a detailed medical history, see Chap. 1.

Building Rapport, Exploring Caregiver's Concerns

Introduce yourself and the purpose of the interview. Explain this is different than a medical interview and that you are very interested in what the caregiver is worried about and what they think. Acknowledge you are an expert in your profession, but the caregiver knows the child well and you value their observations and opinion. This may be an unfamiliar concept in many settings where the public may show much more deference to the health care professional.

Caregiver Priorities and Interpretation

Ask caregivers what they or other family members think is going on? Ask conversationally how this problem is impacting the child and family and what are their most urgent needs. If not familiar with the culture, health care professionals should enquire sensitively about unique cultural beliefs or interpretations (but remain focused on the specific beliefs and interpretations of the family rather than be biased by general cultural factors). Examples of unfamiliar beliefs may include the concept of magic, spells, evil eye, etc.

Taking a Developmental–Behavioral History

A caregiver might have clear concerns or may not be able to articulate their concern and the health care provider can seek further clarification. Health care providers should strive to use an open-ended conversational style during the interview. For example, rather than asking how many words a child can use, it is more natural and informative to ask *"how does your child communicates with you?, how do they tell you what they want or need?"*, *"do you have concerns about how your child communicates, plays, thinks, learns etc."* In the event the healthcare provider is not familiar with the local culture or traditions, it is helpful to ask how the child functions compared to other children in the family or community.

Try to collect information on key developmental domains (see Table 13.1, for examples).

Risk and Resilience Factors

While taking a history, enquire about risk factors (biomedical and psychosocial attributes that increase the risk of a child have developmental concerns) and resilience factors (protective factors that reduce risk or allow the child to respond to intervention) (see Table 13.2).

What Are your Child's Strengths?

Questions looking for a child's positive attributes (e.g., what do you like about your child? what things are they good at?) are important part of the clinical interview and

Table 13.2 Examples of Risk and Resilience Factors: (Adapted from Aites and Schonwald [13] and Walker et al. [14])

Risk factors	Resilience factors
Antenatal exposures (e.g., infections, alcohol, drugs, environmental toxins)	Strong connections with at least one supportive and dependable adult caregiver.
Maternal death, ill health (e.g., folate, iron deficiency)	Active caregiver-child engagement.
Birth complications (e.g., prematurity, asphyxia, low birth weight)	Opportunities to safely interact with other children
Perinatal infections (e.g., encephalitis, meningitis)	School attendance
Chronic health conditions	
Undernutrition (iodine, zinc, iron, other micronutrients).	
Environmental toxins (e.g., lead, methyl mercury, arsenic, manganese)	
Neurogenetic syndromes (e.g., down syndrome, fragile X syndrome)	
Adverse childhood experiences	
Caregiver factors (poverty, mental health, unemployment, limited education)	
Adolescent parents	
Consanguinity	
Short birth spacing	
Lack of appropriate child care	
Unintended pregnancy	
Excessive television/media exposure (this is a debatable topic, but in the author's experience there is a correlation although not a clear causation of delays in development and excessive media exposure)	

can help the caregiver have a balanced view of the child's strengths and difficulties. It also helps the clinician assess the parent's attitude towards their child and what types of supports they may need.

Psychosocial and Family History

General Assessment

Healthcare professionals are used to taking detailed family and psychosocial histories. It is important to build a picture of this social and physical environment by asking about family, school, play areas, possible employment, and other social settings the child frequents. In addition to basic information, it is useful to ask specific questions about the living environment, the role of trauma, and environmental exposures.

The Living Space

It is important to ask about the living space, overcrowding, sleep areas, safety concerns (e.g., going to communal outdoor toilets at night, or co-sleeping with nonfamily members).

Quality of Caregiving

Responsive care giving is a term used to describe the adult's attentiveness to the child's needs (e.g., need for stimulation, comfort, reassurance nourishment, etc.). Limited caregiver responsiveness is associated with delays in cognitive and social-emotional development. Reduced responsive caregiving can be associated with lack of knowledge on this crucial component of caregiving, caregiver mental health difficulties (e.g., exposure to traumatic experiences, postpartum depression), or absence of a consistent responsive caregiver (e.g., in certain institutional settings or in cases of family disruption due to war). Information on the quality of the caregiver's response can be gained by asking about the daily routine and what the child/caregiver do together (e.g., do they play games, read books), how daily tasks are conducted (e.g., feeding, bathing), and if the child is often exposed to electronic media (e.g., mobile phones, iPads) to keep them entertained or quiet. In addition to caregiver factors, some children with developmental delays can be extremely passive and difficult to engage, which makes it difficult for the parent to be consistently available and stimulating to the child. It is therefore important to note your concerns but not make a quick value judgment as to why caregivers may not be responsive.

Ask about Maltreatment and Psychological Trauma

Traumatized caregivers may be less responsive or respond inappropriately to their children, and this may exacerbate their children's trauma reactions. Trauma is often thought of as occurring during escape from harrowing situation, but often individuals report traumatic symptoms in response to the hardship of adjusting to life in a new country despite being physically safe [7]. Traumatized children can present with behavioral changes (e.g., withdrawal or anger/defiance) and may also present as developmentally delayed (e.g., not speaking, failing grades in school, bedwetting). Contrary to some misconceptions, children with developmental delays and disorders are at higher risk for experiencing trauma, grief, and ill treatment [15].

In the context of a general interview, enquiring about trauma should be done in a sensitive and indirect manner to avoid further traumatization (for example, asking open-ended questions and following the interviewee's lead: "What was your experience or you child's experience like during migration?", rather than direct and intrusive questioning). It is enough at this stage for the clinician to have a sense of the potential impact of the parent or child's trauma without going into specific details (further referrals can be made for psychological support). If possible, enquire about the child's function before experiencing trauma and how they are now.

Children may be traumatized by witnessing or experiencing violence related to the humanitarian situation. Unique situations in war settings include sexual exploitation by armed groups or coercion to contribute to the war effort (e.g., as fighters, messengers, brides, or concubines). It is also important to keep in mind that even in non-humanitarian settings children with developmental concerns are at higher risk for maltreatment and neglect.

It is important to be aware of harmful cultural practices (e.g., honor killings, child marriage, or female genital mutilation) and obtain the advice of professionals in the child protection sector on appropriate screening and prevention strategies.

Please see also Chaps. 5 and 9 (Trauma and PTSD) and (Coping with Cultural Differences).

Environmental Exposures Specific to Humanitarian Settings

In humanitarian settings children may be exposed to environmental injury from weapons (e.g., nontraumatic ballistic injury that leads to concussion-like symptoms, explosive mines; chemical, biological, or nuclear weapons). All of these may impact health and developmental progress. This information may not be known to caregivers but may be well known within the context of the conflict.

Medical History and Examination

Occasionally, developmental concerns can be caused by an underlying medical condition. Children should be assessed for treatable health conditions that can cooccur with or contribute to developmental concerns (e.g., malnutrition (see also Chap. 11), parasitic infestation, epilepsy, anemia, thyroid disease, chronic infections, gestational prematurity) or that might recur in the family (e.g., genetic condition or environmental exposures). (See section below on cooccurring medical conditions).

Hearing and Vision impairment may often contribute to learning and communication difficulties. See Table 13.1 for possible ways to assess hearing and vision if appropriate professional resources are not available.

A medical history includes a pregnancy history of the mother, the birth history, nutritional history (in particular the first 2 years of life), previous illnesses, injuries, treatments, operations and hospital stays, current and previous medication, allergies, and family history.

A medical examination of all systems (central and peripheral nervous systems, cardiovascular, respiratory, gastrointestinal and urogenital systems, skin) and assessment of growth parameters (height, weight, mid-upper arm circumference, and head circumference) should be conducted.

Arriving at a Differential Diagnosis Formulation

By considering all the information obtained from the history and assessment, it is possible to summarize what are areas of difficulty and strength in a particular child. Even if you are not able to arrive at a specific diagnosis, defining the areas of difficulties and other family and social factors allows you to think rationally about further investigations, interventions, and referrals. If available and feasible, initiate diagnostic assessments and laboratory investigations to look for underlying causes or medical comorbidities. Prioritize investigations that can impact management and the life of the child. (e.g., reversible or partially reversible conditions like malnutrition, iron deficiency, or hypothyroidism). Although caregivers may hope to get definitive answers as to what causes their child's condition, resource limitations, or unavailability of diagnostic tests often makes it necessary to focus on investigating for treatable conditions only, and concentrate on a more functional diagnosis and assessment that can help to determine the most helpful interventions.

Genetic and environmental factors contributing to developmental disorders are complex and should only be discussed with families by trained, culturally competent individuals and in the setting where long-term follow-up and support are available. Inappropriate discussions can have negative effects (e.g., a parent blaming themselves or the other parent and lead to further psychosocial difficulties).

Interventions and Supports

Health professionals (within the scope of their skills and remit) can support families in several ways: *Support caregivers to understand the child's condition and needs.*

Developmental conditions are often life-long conditions. Young children who are under-stimulated may catch up with increased caregiver involvement and enrollment in Early Childhood Development (ECD) settings, but it is often difficult to predict who will catch up and who will not. When not sure of a specific diagnosis or prognosis, it is still useful to summarize the child's difficulties and what are recommended next steps.

It is important to understand different types of caregiver reactions that may include grief, anger, guilt, or relief to finally understand what the child needs.

Help caregivers understand that behavioral challenges are often due to frustration, anxiety, or a way for the child to communicate their needs. They should not take this personally and they should not punish the child inappropriately (see Appendix 2 for further discussion of behavioral management strategies).

Help caregivers understand their child's strengths and what they like about them: For example, persistence, kindness, and certain areas of ability. If parents are unable to come up with anything positive about the child, ask them to reflect on that and let you know the next time they see you.

Speak to the child or help caregivers communicate with their child. Many children with developmental concerns (especially as they grow older) wonder why they have more difficulties than other children. Help a child understand that all people have areas of strengths and areas of difficulties. Help them identify these areas (especially their own strengths). This is an important first step to develop self-esteem and self-advocacy skills.

Support Caregivers to Be Responsive to the Child's Needs

Encourage caregivers to be attentive to their children's emotional and nurturing needs. Some caregivers may feel their role is simply limited to feeding and assuring the child is clean. Emphasize the importance of talking and playing with the child as a way to promote brain development. Refer caregivers to additional community supports (e.g., mental health supports, or parent training workshops) as needed. In many cases, improving the caregiving environment and additional stimulation can significantly improve developmental outcomes.

Advise the Family What they Can Do at Home to Support their Child's Development

Speech Delay: Read to the child regularly in an engaging animated style. Ask her questions and encourage her to comment, point, and share in turning pages. If books are not available, tell stories from memory and use gestures, pictures, or objects in the home environment to illustrate the story.

Speak regularly to the child, commenting on what you and they are doing/observing using simple language. Do not correct the child when they make a mistake but restate what they want to say (e.g., if the child uses an unclear word when requesting water, do not correct her, but you may say "You want water, here is some water".

Understanding and Problem-Solving Skills: Break down learning, do not lose your patience, use pictures and picture schedules, and frequent reminders. Pay attention that noncompliance is not being "naughty" but may occur because a child is not able or does not understand what is required of them.

Independent Living Skills: Break down tasks into their individual components and give positive reinforcement. Teach about safety, sexual health, and menstruation.

Motor Delay: Adjust the environment to facilitate the child's movement (e.g., remove physical obstacles, adapt tools (e.g., pencils, eating utensils for easy manipulation, and employ ramps for wheelchair access). Try to get them to do as much as possible for themselves.

Supporting Child's Mental Health and Self-esteem: Emphasize the child's strengths, engage them in activities that they enjoy and are good at (e.g., special clubs if available). Advocate for inclusion (e.g., in safe play areas) and protection from bullying.

Respite Care for Caregivers: Ideally, families should receive appropriate supports and training to care for their children. Temporary placement solutions can include foster care arrangements or brief respite breaks and can be helpful where children require intensive care and monitoring due to either behavioral or developmental needs. Such decisions are complex and require multidisciplinary input from various professionals (e.g., health, education, and social care).

Behavioral Management: Advise caregivers that behavior is often a form of communication and advise them on appropriate strategies to support positive behaviors and discourage negative behaviors (see Appendix 2).

Address Potentially Harmful Cultural or Personal Beliefs: Some common cultural attributions to explain the cause of developmental disorders may be harmful (e.g., Magic and superstition), and may lead to caregivers to pursue interventions/practices that may hurt the child. In a nonjudgmental manner, ask caregivers what they and other members of their community (e.g., family or community elders) think caused their child's difficulties and what interventions they may be seeking within their community. Learn more about the local culture from trusted colleagues or community members.

Encourage Enrollment in Educational Settings

In addition to schools for older children, Early Childhood Development activities are often available in humanitarian settings and can provide a stimulating, nurturing environment for children in addition to caregiver support. It is important for health-care workers to liaise with colleagues in the Education sector to understand available services and referral procedures. The Interagency Network on Education in Emergencies website can also be consulted to understand more on education in emergency settings (https://inee.org/).

For young children, It is also recommended that health professionals investigate local access to the World Health Organization *Caregiver Skills Training Program (CST)*. This is an increasingly available program composed of a series of individualized and group interventions targeting caregivers of children with developmental disorders and delays. The focus is on *"training the caregiver on how to use everyday play and home activities and routines as opportunities for learning and development."* [16].

Seeking Additional Supports

Referrals: Children with developmental concerns and their families often have broad-ranging needs beyond what can be offered in the healthcare setting, so it is important for health professionals to understand the roles and referral pathways to different professionals and services.

In humanitarian emergency settings, the humanitarian response is coordinated in the form of sectors (each composed of groups or "clusters" of humanitarian organizations, both UN and non-UN). Children with developmental concerns may have needs that require coordination between different sectors. For example, a child with learning difficulties and mobility issues may have needs related to malnutrition (Nutrition sector), accessible housing and toilets (Shelter and Water, Sanitation and Hygiene sectors), inclusive education (Education sector) and neglect by caregivers (Protection sector). It is important for health care professionals to be able to refer and coordinate care within this framework.

In other settings (e.g., resettlement programs) health professionals will need to learn about different referral pathways related to the context.

Using Telehealth: Telehealth is emerging as a valuable tool to seeking advice from specialists in the field of child development. Some organizations (e.g., Doctors without Borders) have their own official telehealth platforms. In other cases, informal advice can be arranged. Professional organizations, such as the *International Developmental Pediatrics* Association and the *Society for Developmental Behavioral Pediatrics*, among others can provide links with experienced practitioners available to engage in remote consultation.

Advocacy and Long-Term Planning

Inclusion/Empowerment: Community Based Rehabilitation (CBR) describes an approach across a variety of settings (including the humanitarian setting) that aims to improve equality for individuals with disability in all spheres of society. CBR projects are implemented through efforts of people with disability, their families, and a variety of other organizations/services (https://www.who.int/disabilities/cbr/en/) [17]. Health care providers can enquire about existing CBR programs in their setting or may even contribute to the creation of such programs.

Supporting Resettlement Applications: Some countries prioritize asylum seekers with disability or special health circumstances. Healthcare professionals can be helpful by providing documentation that can support asylum seeking applications.

Combatting Discrimination: As a trusted and respected source in the community, the health care provider can impact the attitude of parents, families, and communities regarding children's disabilities.

In conversations with caregivers, always use the child's first name and consciously emphasize their areas of strengths and their right to health and happiness as enshrined in international law. Emphasize the same principles in your work within the health sector, other humanitarian organizations, governments, etc.

Health care providers can also present a positive image of individuals with disabilities by employing those with disability in their organization.

Consider a Long-term Plan: Arrange for long-term care and monitoring (e.g., provide family with a summary of child's condition so that other professionals may follow up appropriately at the next stage in the family's journey).

Prevention and Mitigation

Prevention and mitigation of developmental concerns involve broad public health measures such as promoting maternal health, education, immunization, prevention of malnutrition, and supporting families provide a nurturing environment for children (e.g., through Early Childhood Development—ECD programs). Healthcare providers can contribute to any of these activities through direct involvement in specific projects or through broader advocacy (e.g., engaging in and promoting activities related to the Nurturing Care Framework) [18].

Special Clinical Topics

Autism Spectrum Disorder (ASD)

Children with ASD display a wide range of speech and social communication difficulties as the main feature. They additionally show a range of unusual, repetitive behaviors, unusual or intense interests, and often unusual responses to sensory stimuli. These challenges can predispose to heightened vulnerability in humanitarian settings (see Table 13.3) and may be mitigated if recognized early.

Table 13.3 Children with ASD in humanitarian settings

Clinical Feature	Potential Vulnerability	Examples of Intervention/Support[a]
Social communication difficulties (limited interest/ability to interact with caregivers, other children; limited ability to communicate using speech, eye contact, or gesture).	• Unable to communicate distress • Unable to understand reassurances • Unable to communicate pain, health concerns, maltreatment	Specialized speech and behavioral interventions, picture communication, social stories
Difficulties adapting to change or new situations	Distress with minor or major changes (e.g., change in caregiver, displacement, loss of favorite toy)	Preparing them in advance for anticipated change. Use of social stories. Maintaining other routines as much as possible.
Unusual sensory responses e.g., hypersensitivity to noise, lights, mouthing nonfood objects, skin and oral sensitivity to various textures, food items/flavors.	• Difficulties getting on public transport, going into clinic, refusing to take medication • Stress in clinic due to lights and sounds (e.g., fluorescent lights) • Overwhelmed by smells/sounds in toilet/ shower facilities • There is an increased risk of malnutrition or micronutrient deficiency when children have restricted diets (e.g., iron deficiency causing anemia, vitamin D deficiency causing rickets)	• Ear defenders for children with sensitivity to noises • Sunglasses, or reduce light exposure when sensitive to lights (e.g., fluorescent lights) • Safe chewy toys for children who mouth objects • Limit exposure to unpleasant textures • Camouflage medication (e.g., hide in food— Although many children can still detect its presence) and consider alternative routes of administration • Advocate for separate hygiene facilities (or special times to access toilets) • Nutritional supplements and behavioral strategies to encourage trying new foods for children with restricted diets (see appendix)
Self-injury/aggression.	Often occurs as a response to frustration or inability to communicate needs.	Understanding and addressing the underlying reason for the behavior

[a]See Appendix 2 for more discussion of behavioral supports

The Interplay between Health and Development

Health and Development are intimately connected in several ways (see Table 13.4 for examples):

(a) Health Conditions can have a direct impact on development (e.g., health conditions impacting brain or neuromuscular function).
(b) Health conditions can lead to loss of developmental opportunities (e.g., school absences, frequent hospitalizations, medical procedures, hospice care for terminally ill children):
(c) Developmental difficulties complicate management of acute or chronic health conditions (e.g., difficulty taking a history or performing a medical exam, children with sensory difficulties can struggle to take medication, nutritional supplements, or participating in rehabilitation after limb injury), refusing to wear glasses for treatment of squint or amblyopia, refusing to wear hearing aids, some children may have a high threshold for pain responses leading to delayed recognition of sickle cell crisis or other injuries).
(d) Accidental or nonaccidental injury can occur due to maltreatment or low safety awareness (e.g., in hyperactive or impulsive children).
(e) Late diagnosis of treatable conditions may occur due to difficulty reporting symptoms or neglect by caregivers.

Table 13.4 Examples of the Interplay between Health Conditions and Developmental Concerns (not a comprehensive list)

Health condition	Examples of developmental/behavioral comorbidity	Other comments
Psychiatric/mental health	Children with developmental difficulties are at higher risk of mental health difficulties (e.g., anxiety, depression, post-traumatic stress) [15]	Emotional distress and mental health problems in children can often manifest as irritability, disruptive/ aggressive behavior, bedwetting, withdrawal, sleep and feeding difficulties
Neurological: Congenital infections Vaccine preventable diseases Brain injury related to prematurity/birth asphyxia Meningitis/encephalitis (e.g., bacterial/ viral (e.g., HIV, HSV)/cerebral malaria and other parasitic infections). Brain injury related to kernicterus (neonatal jaundice) [19, 20] Hereditary neuromuscular disorders (e.g., Duchenne muscular dystrophy) Hereditary metabolic syndromes Genetic syndromes Epilepsy syndromes	Cerebral palsy Motor delay and/or regression Learning/intellectual difficulties Attention difficulties, impulsivity, and hyperactivity	Vaccine preventable illness include measles, mumps, rubella, diptheria, tetanus, polio, bacterial meningitis)
Musculoskeletal Congenital hip dislocation Traumatic limb injuries	Motor delay	Indirect consequence of limited mobility is inability to explore the environment which may impact learning
Visual impairment Visual impairment (variable causes can be isolated or associated with other health and developmental challenges)	Motor delay due to inability to see the environment. Nonverbal communication difficulties (e.g., eye contact/use of gesture)	Blind children can display behaviors overlapping those with autistic children (e.g., poor eye contact, repetitive motor behaviors). Trachoma (due to infection) and vitamin A deficiency are common preventable causes of blindness in low and middle income countries

Table 13.4 (continued)

Health condition	Examples of developmental/behavioral comorbidity	Other comments
Deafness (variable causes can be isolated or associated with other health and developmental challenges)	Speech and language delay	Hearing impaired children often have normal cognition. Early intervention (e.g., supplying hearing aids, or teaching sign language) are essential to maximize communication skills and reduce the risk of academic and occupational underachievement
Dental: Dental decay	Difficulties with feeding and speech development due to dental decay and discomfort	Dental decay is common in children with developmental difficulties (for example, due to milk bottle caries, difficulties implementing tooth brushing). Some medications (e.g., used to treat epilepsy) can cause gum overgrowth which can contribute to dental decay.
Endocrine disorders: Congenital hypothyroidism	Delays in all domains of development (global developmental delay)	Congenital and acquired hypothyroidism is common in regions where iodine deficiency is endemic (often manifesting as goiter in adults) [21]
Respiratory Central sleep Apnea Obstructive sleep Apnea Recurrent aspiration	Sleep disruption due to apnea often results in difficulties with daytime behaviors (difficulties with attention, learning, disruptive behavior) Children with difficulties in oral-motor control have difficulties sucking, chewing or swallowing leading to recurrent aspiration pneumonia	Central sleep apnea can be associated with some neurogenetic syndromes and brain abnormalities Obstructive sleep apnea is often associated with tonsillar/adenoidal hypertrophy, obesity, and congenital malformations of the oral cavity
Cardiovascular Syndromic and non-syndromic congenital heart disease Acquired heart disease (e.g., rheumatic fever)	Variable association with delays in development	Children with congenital heart disease are at higher risk of developmental difficulties, some related to chronic hypoxemia and others related to cooccurring issues (e.g., undiagnosed Williams syndrome, 22q.11 deletion syndrome, Down syndrome). Children with rheumatic fever may develop self-limited difficulties with involuntary movements of the body (Sydenhams' chorea) that can impact mobility and use of limbs. Neuropsychiatric symptoms such as obsessive and compulsive behaviors have also been reported

Gastrointestinal Constipation Diarrhea Gastoesophageal reflux	Irritability and challenging behaviors due to inability to communicate pain	Reduced gastric motility secondary to hypotonia contributes to constipation. Restricted feeding patterns in some children (e.g., commonly in children with autism) can predispose to constipation/diarrhea
Nutritional Malnutrition Obesity Pica	Global delays in development are associated with general malnutrition and specific micronutrient deficiency Children who are excessively obese can have difficulties with mobility Pica is commonly encountered in children with developmental delays. It is often a manifestation of developmental delay and immature behaviors, but can also be a manifestation of iron deficiency. Children with pica are predisposed to environmental intoxication (e.g., lead intoxication from contaminated soil or paint chips) which can further impact development	Common nutritional causes of developmental delay include perinatal iron deficiency [22], iodine deficiency (leading to congenital hypothyroidism) [21] Children with difficulties in oral-motor control have difficulties sucking, chewing, or swallowing leading to malnutrition Children with autism Spectrum disorder and restricted feeding habits are at risk for malnutrition Parasitic gastrointestinal infections are a common cause of malnutrition and micronutrient deficiencies in low- and middle-income countries
Dermatological Eczema Other rashes and skin findings	Discomfort due to itching can present as behavioral irritability and sleep disruption. Eczema can also be a manifestation of genetic or metabolic conditions associated with developmental delays (e.g., conditions resulting in zinc or biotin deficiency)	Specific skin rashes or lesions can provide a clue to the presence of specific genetic or metabolic conditions (e.g., neuro-cutaneous disorders such as Neurofibromatosis I or tuberous sclerosis). Healthcare professionals should document these findings and seek further advice if they are uncertain about the cause

(continued)

Table 13.4 (continued)

Health condition	Examples of developmental/behavioral comorbidity	Other comments
Hematological Nutritional anemias (e.g., iron deficiency, vitamin deficiencies). Anemia syndromes (e.g., sickle cell, thalassemia)	Variable association with developmental delays. Recurrent hospitalizations may be associated with reduced stimulation and school attendance	Iron deficiency in young children (especially in the perinatal period and often associated with iron deficiency in the mother) is associated with poor developmental outcomes. Iron deficiency can also impact brain development even in the absence of anemia [22]. Iron deficiency in older children may cause fatigue, difficulties with sleep, attention, and focus. Cerebral infarcts in sickle cell disease may manifest as learning difficulties and other neurological symptoms
Liver/kidney disease	Chronic illness/hospitalization can impact child's energy level and school attendance resulting in reduced stimulation and socialization	

Appendix 1

Age	Social/emotional	Language/communication	Cognition (problem-solving)	Movement	Red flags for concern
2 months	o Begins to smile at people o Can briefly calm himself (may bring hands to mouth and suck on hand) o Tries to look at the parent	o Coos, makes gurgling sounds o Turns head toward sounds	o Pays attention to faces o Begins to follow things with eyes and recognize people at a distance o Begins to act bored (cries, fussy) if activity does not change	o Can hold head up and begins to push up when lying on tummy o Makes smoother movements with arms and legs	o Does not respond to loud sounds o Does not watch things as they move o does not smile at people o Does not bring hands to mouth o Cannot hold head up when pushing up when on tummy
4 months	o Smiles spontaneously, especially at people o Likes to play with people and might cry when playing stops o Copies some movements and facial expressions, like smiling or frowning	o Begins to babble o Babbles with expression and copies sounds he hears o Cries in different ways to show hunger, pain, or being tired	o Lets you know if she is happy or sad o Responds to affection o Reaches for a toy with one hand o Uses hands and eyes together, such as seeing a toy and reaching for it o Follows moving things with eyes from side to side o Watches faces closely o Recognizes familiar people and things at a distance	o Holds head steady, unsupported o Pushes down on legs when feet are on a hard surface o May be able to roll over from tummy to back o Can hold a toy and shake it and swing at dangling toys o Brings hands to mouth o When lying on stomach, pushes up to elbows	o Does not watch things as they move o Does not smile at people o Cannot hold head steady o Does not coo or make sounds o Does not bring things to mouth o Does not push down with legs when feet are placed on a hard surface o Has trouble moving one or both eyes in all directions

Age	Social/emotional	Language/communication	Cognition (problem-solving)	Movement	Red flags for concern
6 months	o Knows familiar faces and begins to know if someone is a stranger o Likes to play with others, especially parents o Responds to other people's emotions and often seems happy o Likes to look at self in a mirror	o Responds to sounds by making sounds o Strings vowels together when babbling ("ah," "eh," "oh") and likes taking turns with parent while making sounds o Responds to own name o Makes sounds to show joy and displeasure o Begins to say consonant sounds (jabbering with "m," "b")	o Looks around at things nearby o Brings things to mouth o Shows curiosity about things and tries to get things that are out of reach o Begins to pass things from one hand to the other	o Rolls over in both directions (front to back, back to front) o Begins to sit without support o When standing, supports weight on legs and might bounce o Rocks back-and-forth, sometimes crawling backward before moving forward	o Does not try to get things that are in reach o Shows no affection for caregivers o Does not respond to sounds around him o Has difficulty getting things to mouth o Does not make vowel sounds ("ah," "eh," "oh") o Does not roll over in either direction o Does not laugh or make squealing sounds o Seems very stiff, with tight muscles o Seems very floppy, like a rag doll

Age	Social/emotional	Language/communication	Cognition (problem-solving)	Movement	Red flags for concern
9 months	o May be afraid of strangers o May be clingy with familiar adults o Has favorite toys	o Understands "no" o Makes a lot of different sounds like "mamamama" and "babababa" o Copies sounds and gestures of others o Uses fingers to point at things	o Watches the path of something as it falls o Looks for things he sees you hide o Plays peek-a-boo o Puts things in her mouth o Moves things smoothly from one hand to the other o Picks up things like cereal o's between thumb and index finger	o Stands, holding on o Can get into sitting position o Sits without support o Pulls to stand o Crawls	o Does not bear weight on legs with support o Does not sit with help o Does not babble ("mama," "baba," "dada") o Does not play any games involving back-and-forth play o Does not respond to own name o Does not seem to recognize familiar people o Does not look where you point o Does not transfer toys from one hand to the other

Age	Social/emotional	Language/communication	Cognition (problem-solving)	Movement	Red flags for concern
12 months	o Is shy or nervous with strangers o Cries when mom or dad leaves o Has favorite things and people o Shows fear in some situations o Hands you a book when he wants to hear a story o Repeats sounds or actions to get attention o Puts out arm or leg to help with dressing o Plays games such as "peek-a-boo" and "pat-a-cake"	o Responds to simple spoken requests o Uses simple gestures, like shaking head "no" or waving "bye-bye" o Makes sounds with changes in tone (sounds more like speech) o Says "mama" and "dada" and exclamations like "uh-oh!" o Tries to say words you say	o Explores things in different ways, like shaking, banging, throwing o Finds hidden things easily o Looks at the right picture or thing when it is named o Copies gestures o Starts to use things correctly; for example, drinks from a cup, brushes hair o Bangs two things together o Puts things in a container, takes things out of a container o Lets things go without help o Pokes with index (pointer) finger o Follows simple directions like "pick up the toy"	o Gets to a sitting position without help o Pulls up to stand, walks holding on to furniture ("cruising") o May take a few steps without holding on o May stand alone	o Does not crawl o Cannot stand when supported o Does not search for things that she sees you hide. o Does not say single words like "mama" or "dada" o Does not learn gestures like waving or shaking head o Does not point to things o Loses skills he once had

Age	Social/emotional	Language/communication	Cognition (problem-solving)	Movement	Red flags for concern
18 months	o Likes to hand things to others as play o May have temper tantrums o May be afraid of strangers o Shows affection to familiar people o Plays simple pretend, such as feeding a doll o May cling to caregivers in new situations o Points to show others something interesting o Explores alone but with parent close by	o Says several single words o Says and shakes head "no" o Points to show someone what he wants	o Knows what ordinary things are for; for example, telephone, brush, spoon o Points to get the attention of others o Shows interest in a doll or stuffed animal by pretending to feed o Points to one body part o Scribbles on his own o Can follow one-step verbal commands without any gestures; for example, sits when you say "sit down"	o Walks alone o May walk up steps and run o Pulls toys while walking o Can help undress herself o Drinks from a cup o Eats with a spoon	o Does not point to show things to others o Cannot walk o Does not know what familiar things are for o Does not copy others o Does not gain new words o Does not have at least six words o Does not notice or mind when a caregiver leaves or returns o Loses skills he once had

Age	Social/emotional	Language/communication	Cognition (problem-solving)	Movement	Red flags for concern
2 years	o Copies others, especially adults and older children o Gets excited when with other children o Shows more and more independence o Shows defiant behavior (doing what he has been told not to) o Plays mainly beside other children but is beginning to include other children, such as in chase games	o Points to things or pictures when they are named o Knows names of familiar people and body parts o Says sentences with two to four words o Follows simple instructions o Repeats words overheard in conversation o Points to things in a book	o Finds things even when hidden under two or three covers o Begins to sort shapes and colors o Completes sentences and rhymes in familiar books o Plays simple make-believe games o Builds towers of four or more blocks o Might use one hand more than the other o Follows two-step instructions such as "pick up your shoes and put them in the closet." o Names items in a picture book such as a cat, bird, or dog	o Stands on tiptoe o Kicks a ball o Begins to run o Climbs onto and down from furniture without help o Walks up and down stairs holding on o Throws ball overhand o Makes or copies straight lines and circles	o Does not use two-word phrases (for example, "drink milk") o Does not know what to do with common things, like a brush, phone, fork, spoon o Does not copy actions and words o Does not follow simple instructions o Does not walk steadily o Loses skills she once had

Age	Social/emotional	Language/communication	Cognition (problem-solving)	Movement	Red flags for concern
3 years	o Copies adults and friends o Shows affection for friends without prompting o Takes turns in games o Shows concern for a crying friend o Understands the idea of "mine" and "his" or "hers" o Shows a wide range of emotions o Separates easily from mom and dad o May get upset with major changes in routine o Dresses and undresses self	o Follows instructions with two or three steps o Can name most familiar things o Understands words like "in," "on," and "under" o Says first name, age, and sex o Names a friend o Says words like "I," "me," "we," and "you" and some plurals (cars, dogs, cats) o Talks well enough for strangers to understand most of the time o Carries on a conversation using two to three sentences	o Can work toys with buttons, levers, and moving parts o Plays make-believe with dolls, animals, and people o Does puzzles with three or four pieces o Understands what "two" means o Copies a circle with pencil or crayon o Turns book pages one at a time o Builds towers of more than six blocks o Screws and unscrews jar lids or turns door handle	o Climbs well o Runs easily o Pedals a tricycle (3-wheel bike) o Walks up and down stairs, one foot on each step	o Falls down a lot or has trouble with stairs o Drools or has very unclear speech o Cannot work simple toys (such as peg boards, simple puzzles, turning handle) o Does not speak in sentences o Does not understand simple instructions o Does not play pretend or make-believe o Does not want to play with other children or with toys o Does not make eye contact o Loses skills he once had

Age	Social/emotional	Language/communication	Cognition (problem-solving)	Movement	Red flags for concern
4 years	o Enjoys doing new things o Plays "mom" and "Dad" o Is more and more creative with make-believe play o Would rather play with other children than by himself o Cooperates with other children o Often cannot tell what is real and what is make-believe o Talks about what she likes and what she is interested in	o Knows some basic rules of grammar, such as correctly using "he" and "she" o Sings a song or says a poem from memory such as the "itsy Bitsy spider" or the "wheels on the bus" o Tells stories o Can say first and last name	o Names some colors and some numbers o Understands the idea of counting o Starts to understand time o Remembers parts of a story o Understands the idea of "same" and "different" o Draws a person with two to four body parts o Uses scissors o Starts to copy some capital letters o Plays board or card games o Tells you what he thinks is going to happen next in a book	o Hops and stands on one foot up to 2 s o Catches a bounced ball most of the time o Pours, cuts with supervision, and mashes own food	o Cannot jump in place o Has trouble scribbling o Shows no interest in interactive games or make-believe o Ignores other children or does not respond to people outside the family o Resists dressing, sleeping, and using the toilet o Cannot retell a favorite story o Does not follow 3-part commands o Does not understand "same" and "different" o Does not use "me" and "you" correctly o Speaks unclearly o Loses skills he once had

Age	Social/emotional	Language/communication	Cognition (problem-solving)	Movement	Red flags for concern
5 years	o Wants to please friends o Wants to be like friends o More likely to agree with rules o Likes to sing, dance, and act o Is aware of gender o Can tell what is real and what is make-believe o Shows more independence (for example, may visit a next-door neighbor by himself [adult supervision is still needed]) o Is sometimes demanding and sometimes very cooperative	o Speaks very clearly o Tells a simple story using full sentences o Uses future tense; for example, "grandma will be here." o Says name and address	o Counts 10 or more things o Can draw a person with at least six body parts o Can print some letters or numbers o Copies a triangle and other geometric shapes o Knows about things used every day, like money and food	o Stands on one foot for 10 s or longer o Hops; may be able to skip o Can do a somersault o Uses a fork and spoon and sometimes a table knife o Can use the toilet on her own o Swings and climbs	o Does not show a wide range of emotions o Shows extreme behavior (unusually fearful, aggressive, shy, or sad) o Unusually withdrawn and not active o is easily distracted, has trouble focusing on one activity for more than 5 min o Does not respond to people or responds only superficially o Cannot tell what is real and what i's make-believe o Does not play a variety of games and activities o Cannot give first and last name o Does not use plurals or past tense properly o Does not talk about daily activities or experiences o Does not draw pictures o Cannot brush teeth, wash and dry hands, or get undressed without help o Loses skills he once had

Developmental Milestones and Red Flags Checklist

The table above is adapted from material developed by the United States Centers for Disease Control and Prevention (https://www.cdc.gov/ncbddd/actearly/milestones/index.html). It provides information on key developmental milestones and red flags for concerns at particular ages. The website also includes a rich video library showing real-life examples (https://www.cdc.gov/ncbddd/actearly/milestones/milestones-in-action.html).

This table was developed for general guidance in the United States and is not an evidence-based screening tool. The milestones should not be interpreted rigidly and should not be used in a checklist fashion (expecting yes/no answers) to determine if a child is delayed or not. Instead, it is recommended that such a list be used as guidance on trajectories of development. This places more responsibility on the professional assessing the child to interpret findings in the context of the child and family's circumstance. Please see the section on *Taking a Developmental-Behavioral History* for additional suggestions on communicating with families and assessing children's development and behavior.

Appendix 2

Behavioral Challenges and Basic Behavioral Management Strategies

The strategies described below are the purpose of general introduction and do not replace professional advice suited to the particular clinical situation.

Parents often complain about their child's behaviors. Examples of negative behaviors include temper tantrums, damaging objects (e.g., throwing objects), hurting others, or hurting oneself (e.g., biting oneself or hitting head against objects) Some behaviors may be developmentally appropriate (e.g., temper tantrums are normal in toddlers).

The first step in providing support is to clarify to parents that behaviors are the child's way of communication. Usually, negative behaviors are related to an unmet need, distress, or frustration. This is common in children with developmental delays who may have difficulty communicating their needs, frustrations, or understanding expectations. They may also be frustrated by difficulties keeping up with others their age.

Preventing Behavioral Challenges

Positive parenting is a term commonly used to describe parenting strategies that encourage "positive" behaviors (e.g., getting to know your child and what may trigger them, setting a good example, teaching them right from wrong, and being clear about expectations and consequences). The healthychildren.org website provides valuable advice on managing children's behavior and appropriate discipline strategies [23].

Common Behavior Management Strategies

ABC Approach: *An often effective strategy to address behavioral challenges is the* ABC (Antecedent, Behavior, and Consequences).

For example, Mustafa is 4 years old and has minimal spoken language. His mother complains that he often bites his younger brother. Applying the ABC method, his mother was able to observe that Mustafa is usually making noises to get her attention. However, as she is quite busy with household chores, she cannot give him immediate attention. Then Mustafa goes to bite his brother who starts crying which immediately gets the mother's attention. When analyzing this behavior, his mother concludes the following:

Antecedent: feeling ignored.

Behavior: biting brother.

Consequence: getting attention.

By identifying such an Antecedent, Mustafa's mother acknowledges his need for attention by bringing him close to her and getting him to help her with her chores. He is thus getting the attention he needs and is not biting his brother as much. Other options are to have a neighbor or older child support her with housework (or a referral to the camp social worker to consider other support options).

Ignoring: A caregiver's attention is a strong motivator for most children and can be used to manage certain behaviors. One of the best behavior management strategies is ignoring negative behaviors. If there are no safety concerns, caregivers can try to ignore unwanted behaviors and praise behaviors they want to encourage.

Time Out: Time out allows the child to take a break to calm down when frustrated or engaging in negative behaviors. Time out can be used when children begin to understand the cause and effect and consequences of their actions (18–24 months). Use time out as follows:

For example, a child is frustrated and hitting the parent.

1. Warn the child "if you don't stop, you will go into time out."
2. Clearly identify the unwanted behavior (e.g., "no hitting").
3. Start a timer (as a rule of thumb give 1 min of time out for age in years, e.g., a 2-year old will get 2 min of time out).
4. Guide the child to a quiet and safe area where there are no toys or fun activities.
5. If they leave the area restart the timer.

Make sure the child is always safe in time out (e.g., do not place in time in an area with household chemicals, electric equipment, or windows that can be easily opened).

Positive Reinforcement: When a child engages in appropriate behavior, caregivers can give them words of encouragement. For example, if Mustafa does not hit his brother when frustrated, his mother can say "good boy for not hitting." With time this will emphasize the desirable behavior.

Punishment: Many caregivers utilize punishment as the main strategy to manage their child's behavior. Punishment can take a variety of forms (e.g., taking away privileges or more extreme forms of physical punishment).

Physical punishment is discouraged as it can lead to long-term physical and emotional damage in children. It is now also illegal in many countries and there may be legal requirements for professionals to report caregivers who engage in physical punishment to social services or legal authorities. Encourage parents to engage more in promoting positive behavior and avoiding situations that lead to negative behaviors.

For additional information on behavioral management see:

https://www.healthychildren.org/ (American Academy of Pediatrics).

https://www.unicef.org/parenting/child-care/how-discipline-your-child-smart-and-healthy-way (UNICEF).

Recognize Internalizing Symptoms

Be aware, that children who are withdrawn, passive and not being disruptive may also be in need of support. Such "internalizing" behaviors may be signs of grief, adjustment difficulties, anxiety, depression, and post-traumatic stress.

Interventions for Children with Autism Spectrum Disorder

Many resources (often online) are available to support professionals and families caring for children with autism spectrum disorders and social communication difficulties. These include Autism Speaks in the US, which also provides an excellent tool-kit addressing challenging behaviors (https://www.autismspeaks.org/tool-kit/challenging-behaviors-tool-kit) and feeding difficulties (https://www.autismspeaks.org/tool-kit/atnair-p-guide-exploring-feeding-behavior-autism), and the National Autistic Society in the UK (http://autism.org.uk/).

The use of social stories: Social stories are a tool to support children with social communication difficulties learn and anticipate new situations. For example, if there is a plan to change housing, a picture or written story can be created describing the different steps of this change and can be rehearsed with the child before the event. See, for example, https://www.autism.org.uk/advice-and-guidance/topics/communication/communication-tools/social-stories-and-comic-strip-coversations.

References

1. WHO. mhGAP intervention guide version 2.0 [internet]. Geneva: World Health Organization; 2016. p. 1–164. https://www.who.int/publications/i/item/mhgap-intervention-guide%2D%2D-version-2.0
2. Organization WH. mhGAP Humanitarian Intervention Guide (mhGAP-HIG): Clinical management of Mental, Neurological and Substance Use Conditions in Humanitarian Emergencies: 2015; https://www.who.int/mental_health/publications/mhgap_hig/en/
3. Werner D. Disabled village children [internet]. Berkeley, CA: Hesperian Health Guides. https://hesperian.org/books-and-resources/
4. Eapen V, Philip Graham SS. Where there is no child psychiatrist: a mental healthcare manual. London: Royal College of Psychiatrists; 2012.
5. Article 1 - Purpose | United Nations Enable [Internet]. [cited 2020 Jun 21]. https://www.un.org/development/desa/disabilities/convention-on-the-rights-of-persons-with-disabilities/article-1-purpose.html.
6. Kroening ALH, Moore JA, Welch TR, Halterman JS, Hyman SL. Developmental screening of refugees: a qualitative study. Pediatrics. 2016;138:3.

7. Minhas RS, Graham H, Jegathesan T, Huber J, Young E, Barozzino T. Supporting the developmental health of refugee children and youth. Paediatr Child Health. 2017;22(2):68–71.
8. Marlow M, Servili C, Tomlinson M. A review of screening tools for the identification of autism spectrum disorders and developmental delay in infants and young children: recommendations for use in low- and middle-income countries. Autism Res. 2019;12(2):176–99. [Internet] [cited 2020 Sep 6] http://doi.wiley.com/10.1002/aur.2033
9. Wilkinson CL, Wilkinson MJ, Lucarelli J, Fogler JM, Becker RE, Huntington N. Quantitative evaluation of content and age concordance across developmental milestone checklists. J Dev Behav Pediatr. 2019;40(7):511–8. [Internet] [cited 2020 Sep 6]; https://pubmed.ncbi.nlm.nih.gov/31169653/
10. Graham HR, Minhas RS, Paxton G. Learning problems in children of refugee background: a systematic review. Pediatrics. 2016;137:6.
11. Saint-Surin T. Assessing developmental delay in refugee children [Internet]. https://med.virginia.edu/family-medicine/clinics/international-family-medicine-clinic/international-and-refugee-medicine-research/disease-management-and-practice-guidelines/
12. Mishori R. The use of age assessment in the context of child migration: imprecise, inaccurate, inconclusive and endangers children's rights. Children. 2019;6(7):85. [Internet] [cited 2020 Aug 16] /pmc/articles/PMC6678520/?report=abstract
13. Jennifer Aites J, Schonwald A. Developmental-behavioral surveillance and screening in primary care. UpToDate, Post, TW (Ed). Waltham, MA: UpToDate; 2020.
14. Walker SP, Wachs TD, Meeks Gardner J, Lozoff B, Wasserman GA, Pollitt E, et al. Child development: risk factors for adverse outcomes in developing countries [internet]. Lancet. 2007;369:145–57. [cited 2020 Aug 16]. https://pubmed.ncbi.nlm.nih.gov/17223478/
15. Brickell C, Munir K, Brickell B. Grief and its complications in individuals with intellectual disability. Harv Rev Psychiatry. 2008;16(1):1–12.
16. WHO | Training parents to transform children's lives [Internet]. [cited 2020 Sep 27]. https://www.who.int/mental_health/maternal-child/PST/en/
17. WHO | Training in the community for people with disabilities (1989) [Internet]. [cited 2020 Sep 27]. https://www.who.int/disabilities/publications/cbr/training/en/
18. World Health Organization, United Nations Children's Fund WBG. Nurturing care for early childhood development: a framework for helping children survive and thrive to transform health and human potential. Geneva: World Health Organization; 2018.
19. Olusanya BO, Ogunlesi TA, Slusher TM. Why is kernicterus still a major cause of death and disability in low-income and middle-income countries? Arch Dis Child Educ Pract Ed. 2014;99(12):1117–21. [cited 2020 Jun 21] https://adc.bmj.com/content/99/12/1117
20. Gladstone M. A review of the incidence and prevalence, types and aetiology of childhood cerebral palsy in resource-poor settings. Ann Trop Paediatr. 2010;30(3):181–96. [cited 2020 Jun 21] https://www.researchgate.net/publication/46190540
21. Biban BG, Lichiardopol C. Iodine deficiency, still a global problem? Curr Health Sci J. 2017;43(2):103–11. [cited 2020 Jun 21] /pmc/articles/PMC6284174/?report=abstract
22. Abu-Ouf NM, Jan MM. The impact of maternal iron deficiency and iron deficiency anemia on child's health. Saudi Med J. 2015;36(2):146–9. /pmc/articles/PMC4375689/?report=abstract
23. What's the Best Way to Discipline My Child? - HealthyChildren.org [Internet]. [cited 2020 Sep 27]. https://www.healthychildren.org/English/family-life/family-dynamics/communication-discipline/Pages/Disciplining-Your-Child.aspx

Ramzi Nasir, MD, MPH is a Developmental-Behavioral pediatrician who has practiced in the US, Europe, and the Middle East. He currently practices in London, UK (Royal Free London NHS Foundation Trust and The Portland Hospital). He has led and participated in various international collaborations to advance the well-being of children with developmental concerns in underserved and humanitarian settings. These include collaborations with organizations such as Medecins Sans Frontieres/Doctors Without Borders, Society for Developmental-Behavioral Pediatrics, International Society for Developmental Pediatrics, Autism Speaks, International Society for

Autism Research, and Medical Aid for Palestinians. He is also the author of several peer-reviewed publications and book chapters; and developed the first Arabic language Massive Open Online Course (MOOC) on Autism in collaboration with Edraak/the Queen Rania Foundation. He has also provided advice on medical topics to governments in Europe and the pharmaceutical industry. Dr. Nasir completed his medical school and residency training at Indiana University, a fellowship in Developmental-Behavioral Pediatrics at Boston Children's Hospital and received a Master of Public Health degree from the Harvard School of Public Health.

Child Health Promotion for Refugees and Other Vulnerable Populations

14

M. Leila Srour

Introduction

Child health promotion for vulnerable children, including refugees, migrants, asylum seekers, and children living in poverty and difficult circumstances, is the subject of this chapter. These children's precarious lives are often impoverished, exposed to exploitation, social exclusion, and violence. Article 24 of the Child Rights Convention (CRC) recognizes "the right of the child to the enjoyment of the highest attainable standard of health and facilities for the treatment of illness and rehabilitation of health," irrespective of nationality or immigration status.

In 2011, UNHCR estimated over 12 million child refugees who may spend their childhoods displaced. Their childhood experiences have profound and life-lasting effects. Children are resilient, cope, and look to the future despite hardship and suffering. They draw strength from their families and joy in friendships. These children can teach us so much, especially those who have unjustly suffered. Children's participation and capacity building for their protection, with a particular focus on children with special concerns, is one of UNHCR's goals. Parents, teachers, and health care workers can work with children to empower them to advocate for their rights and protection. In school, activities, sports, and creative participatory projects can allow children to explore their talents and use their skills to become active community members. Quality education for child refugees is a big challenge, but there are good examples of innovative programs to improve children's lives [1].

Three levels of disease prevention are addressed in health promotion activities to influence human behavior and improve the health of the community: Primary prevention is measured to avoid illness, such as immunizations and breastfeeding promotion. Secondary prevention is actions leading to early diagnosis and treatment to prevent severe disease, such as education about disease warning signs, how to

M. L. Srour (✉)
Health Frontiers, Vientiane, Laos
e-mail: leila@butterflychildren.org

© Springer Nature Switzerland AG 2021
C. Harkensee et al. (eds.), *Child Refugee and Migrant Health*,
https://doi.org/10.1007/978-3-030-74906-4_14

171

Table 14.1 Disease Prevention Table

Health promotion and prevention	Definition	Examples of health promotion activities for prevention
Primary prevention	Actions to avoid and prevent disease	• Immunizations • Healthy diet • Hand washing • Accident prevention education
Secondary prevention	Actions leading to early diagnosis and treatment to avoid severe disease	• Training of disease warning signs • Use of Oral Rehydration Solution (ORS) • Emergency management knowledge • Improving access to health care
Tertiary prevention	Actions to rehabilitate, recovery after illness, and manage chronic diseases	• Education about use of medications • Community management of disabilities • Education to prevent stigma and allow community integration and support • Psychological rehabilitation from trauma

manage in an emergency, and improved access to health care. Tertiary prevention aims to educate, rehabilitate after a significant illness, and teach management of chronic diseases, including education about medications, community management of disabilities, prevention of stigma, and recovery from traumatic events (Table 14.1).

The Convention on the Rights of the Child (Article 39) [2] requires all appropriate measures to promote physical and psychological recovery and social integration of child victims of neglect, exploitation, abuse, violence, and other degrading experiences. Recovery requires an environment that fosters health and self-respect. Children, especially those lacking a supportive family environment, and unaccompanied minors, need information about safety, child rights, and intervention strategies to prevent abuse and exploitation.

There are many different approaches for child health promotion: teaching children, training teachers, supporting volunteer health care workers, parent support programs, and Child-to-Child. Children share what they learn with other children, their families, and the communities with the support of teachers and health care workers. Creative and innovative examples inspire adults and allow children to use their imagination to support health behavior change [3].

Child Health Promotion to Reduce Epilepsy Stigma

Epilepsy is a highly stigmatizing disease in many African countries. In Gulu, Uganda, an intervention focusing on children as health promoters to educate their community about epilepsy, reduce stigma, improve patients' adherence with medications, and provide first aid for seizures was successful in destigmatizing epilepsy, advancing proper treatment, and overcoming the belief that epilepsy is contagious. In primary schools, health clubs are formed where children, wearing health promotional T-shirts, are trained to teach others using role-plays and creative entertainment to promote awareness and destigmatize epilepsy. Children enthusiastically demonstrated reaching out to people affected by epilepsy, and eagerly reported what they learned to friends and families. Children with epilepsy were encouraged to stay in school, take their medicines, and were successfully integrated into their classrooms. In the community, children and adults with epilepsy were encouraged to seek and receive health care. This program is an example of child health promotion for a very vulnerable population, with the recruitment and training of children as health care behavior change agents [4].

School-based health promotion is a crucial way to improve the knowledge, attitudes, and behavior of children and their families. Schools play a critical role in protecting and promoting the health of children, especially migrants and refugees, including the promotion of good child mental health. The provision of psychological support is the most pressing health care need for migrant children. Involving children in participatory activities in schools improves their self-esteem and control over their own lives.

Child Rights Participatory Approach

Hearing All Voices (UK) Child to Child, London (2013–2016) is a Child-to-Child program to enhance social inclusion, engagement in education, and social participation of vulnerable youth. The young people receive training in the English language, communication, and teamwork. Their teachers and teaching assistants are trained in methods to support young people's participation without being directive. This program uses a Child Rights participatory approach with students aged 16–18 years. The students identify a social problem that they want to address, investigate, design an intervention, implement, evaluate, and plan the next steps to solve the problem. The groups developed projects on a wide range of issues: street safety, crime, homelessness, bullying, and the care of orphans. The students reported improved self-confidence and enhanced ability to communicate with adults. Hearing All Voices illustrates the potential for educational interventions to promote the physical and psychological well-being of vulnerable young people [5].

Case Study: Butterfly Children's Development Center
In Ban Nong Boua, Muang Sing, Luang Namtha province, Laos, children from a dozen different ethnic minorities attend the same primary school. Most started school without a common language, so they needed to learn the Lao language to communicate with each other. Although most families are poor, there is a hierarchy of poverty, with a clear separation of children from distinctly poorer parts of the village. During the school day, the children socialized primarily with children from their ethnic group or similar social strata. The school is located in the center of the village, between the financially more advantaged and less advantaged areas. An after-school program, the Butterfly Children's Development Center, attracted children from both sides, their parents and teachers. The activities focused on inclusion and respect for each other. Cleaning the schoolyard to prepare the area for activities preceded other activities. Creative and enjoyable educational activities developed based on the children's interests and volunteers' skills and experience. Singing, dancing, and cultural events were celebrated daily. A small library of books in the

Lao language, many from Big Brother Mouse books, a program to publish children's books in Lao language, written and illustrated by young Lao authors and illustrators, were used daily both for reading out loud and individually (www.bigbrothermouse.com). The stories in these books creatively illustrate the importance of good hygiene, the use of toilets or latrines instead of open defecation, healthy eating habits, dental hygiene, accessing health care, and nutrition for pregnant women, mothers, and young children. Art projects used available materials, such as recycled paper and crayons. Hand washing after cleaning the school grounds and before other activities was emphasized, using a bucket of water and soap. Marginalized children, including those not attending school and children with disabilities, were all encouraged to participate.

A young blind boy spent 1 year at the school, learning to speak the Lao language until he decided that he liked school and wanted to learn to read and write. At that point, he was sent to the capital city to attend the school for the blind and eventual integration into the local public school. The teachers and students took great pride in the progress of this one child, who first entered the school without Lao language, crying and terrified of the new environment. When he boarded the bus for a longer than 24-h trip to the capital city to start learning Braille, everyone was impressed with how much children can learn.

A computer lab was developed using refurbished donated laptops. With educational software, children learned to add, subtract, multiply, and divide (www.butterflychildren.org). Other games encouraged thinking skills and concentration. Hand washing before the use of the computer lab was required for the safety of the children and computers. The equipment was installed each day with the help of children who were identified as responsible for this job.

Physical activities were encouraged in a simple outdoor play area, an outside covered area with protection from the sun, and use of the kindergarten room with mats on the floor. This program meets the #1 Goal of the UNHCR Framework of Child Protection to provide safe places for children to learn, play, gather, and socialize [1].

The Butterfly Children's development center was a safe place for children to gather when they were not attending school, on weekends, and during school holidays. Their teachers often had received limited education, training, or payment, and their salaries were frequently in arrears for months. For some children, the after-school program was their informal education. Most parents of the children in this village had no educational experience and could not imagine the importance of education or a different future for their children. The after-school program taught the children that learning is fun, productive, and contributed to their future and breaking the cycle of poverty.

Successful health promotion and educational activities require time and consistency. Health behavior change is a long process and best starts in childhood as part of primary and secondary school education. Children need successful role models, promoting health behavior change. Teachers and health care workers can encourage health behavior change, including hygiene, sanitation, healthy food choices, exercise, avoidance of harmful substances, including tobacco, alcohol, and illicit substances, and avoidance of disease vectors.

Substance Abuse Prevention

Alcohol abuse in Laos is a neglected and serious problem. Children are often exposed from an early age to the inebriation of their parents, teachers on school property, health workers at hospitals, older siblings, and even other children. Every party, wedding, and celebration in Laos is an excuse for many to get drunk. A common saying is: "It's not a party if you don't get drunk." Underage children purchase alcohol and young women serve alcohol, making it difficult to resist. Driving while drunk, although illegal, is accepted, along with many tragic accidents, especially of young men. Beer Lao is the most popular drink with extensive advertising and distribution throughout the country. Without health promotion activities, the only message the children receive is that drunkenness is acceptable and pleasurable.

To begin addressing this problem, a poster was developed showing the effects of alcohol on all parts of the body. This inexpensive poster was printed by Save the Children and distributed to hospitals, clinics, and schools around the country. For many young people and health care workers, this was the first education about alcohol's dangerous effects. Organizing alcohol-free celebrations with children sharing the simple pleasures of singing, dancing, and enjoying life allow them to see that alcohol is not required to have fun together.

The promotion of tobacco to children in Lao is forbidden, but often not enforced. Young people may not consider the risk of nicotine addiction or the adverse effects of second-hand smoke. Children's development centers, tobacco-free, are an excellent example for all children and their caregivers. Promotions of tobacco, including the distribution of single cigarettes, should be reported to the Ministry or Department of Health.

Child-to-Child approach to Health Promotion

Traditional didactic health education with passive advice to children often fails. The Child-to-Child approach to health promotion focuses on child-centered participation. Children and adults learn best with active involvement, addressing the communities' concerns and interests. When health education belongs to the children, they can portray the messages in culturally and developmentally appropriate ways to all age groups. Useful health information from an early age and in a practical manner can improve and protect their lives, giving them a sense of personal responsibility and community involvement. Practical knowledge, skills, attitude, and values are needed for children to acquire healthy lifestyle habits for their entire lifetime. Health education should be taught in a way that leads to direct application at home, school, and community. Child-to-Child has many wonderful examples of children's health promotional activities conducted in low resource countries throughout the world. These activities build young people's confidence in themselves, self-esteem, and leadership skills, beyond the health care message alone (Fig. 14.1) [6]. With the cooperation of health and education sectors, Child-to-Child approaches can be used in schools, health centers, youth groups, preschool, nonformal settings, and integrated with existing programs.

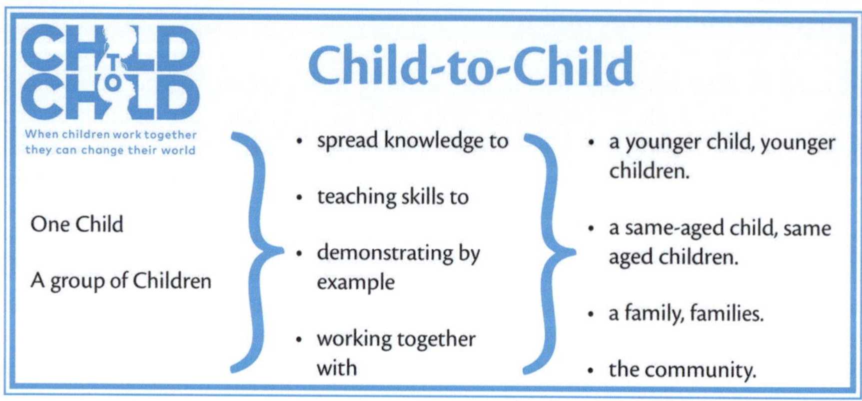

Fig. 14.1 The Child to Child approach - the flow of learning

Begun by David Morley in 1978 to honor the International Year of the Child, 1979, the program is built on the well-known situation of an older child being responsible for a younger sibling, while the mother is busy elsewhere. The older child, sometimes only 4 years old, may not understand the severity of unaddressed problems such as malnutrition, diarrhea, injury prevention, hygiene, and safety. The Child-to-Child program aims to put the older child in a better position to deal with these and other vital issues for all children.

Child-to-Child is free, with all materials available online with no copyright, translated into multiple languages, and easy to translate into other languages as most of the materials are visual and created by children. Child-to-Child activities are low-cost, sustainable interventions, which can reduce the need for outside interventions, allow for local management, and improve the quality of children's lives. Child-to-Child Trust, Institute of Education, 20 Bedford Place, London WC1H 0AL, UK. Tel: (+44) 2076126648, or by email at: ccenquiries@ioe.ac.uk [7].

Close and active working partnerships with project workers, government, agencies, and the community are required to coordinate health promotion. As parents may not be ready to accept health messages from their children, children can create dramas for the community to share their knowledge about health messages. With the support of other sectors, health care messages can be spread more widely by local news and social media.

There are many inspiring examples of Child-to-Child activities. In India, boys made a puppet show to teach about oral hygiene. In Zambia, children put on a play about HIV/AIDS. In another creative activity, a young girl gives ORS to a younger sibling and shows her mother how to prepare and administer oral rehydration [6].

Case Study: Bhutan Refugee Camps in Nepal

In Bhutanese refugee camps in Nepal, 50% of the refugees were less than 16 years old, with high child morbidity and mortality. Once health services were established, the focus was on long-term primary health care with specific prevention programs.

First, children were asked to draw pictures showing: "What makes me healthy?" These drawings helped to show what children understand and remember from the health education they received. "What makes me happy and unhappy" drawings revealed the simple things making them happy: clothes, toys, friends, food and unhappy: shouting, beatings, and other abuses. During the Child-to-Child training workshop, a survey of priority health topics was conducted, revealing the need for early childhood education, support for special needs children, and coping with refugee life. After the survey, discussions and activities were planned using puppets, drama, and games with the children and young people [6].

In Laos, a small hospital scene was created with roles assigned for the receptionist at the hospital, doctor, nurse, patient, family members in a variety of health care emergencies. Children took turns participating in various roles. Learning objectives were how to recognize an emergency, what to do, who to call, where to go, how to help, and how to care for the patient and family. They used props such as pretend "medical equipment" and homemade face masks. The drama can be performed for the parents and community, rehearsing how to respond and support in a medical emergency. There is always laughter, but moments of seriousness and discussion of how realistic the drama mirrors their own life experiences. Children shared stories of health care emergencies they had witnessed without knowing how to help.

Children's participation is valuable in decision-making for program activities. Specific health care concerns change based on the different ages of children and the problems to be addressed. Children between 3 and 6 years may suffer from excessive discipline, poor hygiene, and not attending school. Children of 7–10 years may be involved in child labor, child trafficking, lack clean drinking water, face discrimination, lack health care, and suffer from abuse by drunken adults. Issues for older children are early marriage, unplanned pregnancies, alcohol and drug abuse, violence, and lack of extra-curricular activities. These are examples, but there are many more health and life issues to be discussed, with all health campaigns beginning with cleaning up the environment and hygiene promotion.

Inspiring accounts of Child-to-Child successes in delivering and implementing public health messages are found in challenging locations such as the West Bank, Gaza, Romania, Yemen, Somali refugee camps, Zaire, and in Goma with Rwandan refugees. Children in extremely challenging circumstances can promote public health messages and reach out to the community. In Yemen, for example, a land mine awareness and accident prevention program with Child-to-Child included reaching out to disabled children [6].

Community Surveys and Action

With guidance and support, children and young people can conduct community surveys, diagnose problems, and make plans to address concerns raised by the survey. There are six recommended steps in the Child-to-Child methodology to address a health care problem: identify the problem, study, discussion, plan actions, act, and evaluate. Simple questions with yes and no questions can be developed. Children can collect the information and display results on charts to show the

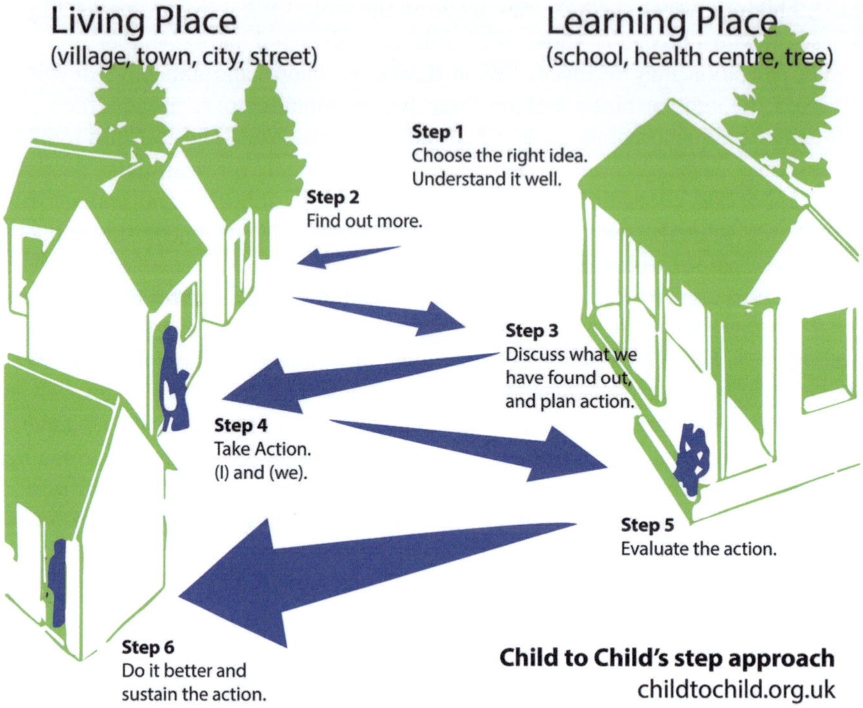

Fig. 14.2 The Child to Child approach - stepwise activities

results. Making the community diagnosis raises the children's awareness of the problem and is the first step to finding solutions. Then, conclusions can be drawn, and a plan developed (Fig. 14.2) [8].

The Child-to-Child approach to health promotion can be incorporated into a wide variety of programs in school, out-of-school, and curriculums. Active learning methods using art, drama, role-plays can be blended with other subjects. By strengthening children's participation and integration in the curriculum, the importance of health is strengthened. The most effective programs involve children in the decision-making [9].

Child-to-Child and Children Living in Camps

Children living in camps have experienced and continue to experience difficult circumstances. Recognizing and building on children's natural abilities to share, learn, and play together encourages them to put into practice what they are learning to help each other. Fun, happy, and busy children improve everyone's morale and spread health messages in the community [10].

Sanitation can be improved, even when latrines are not available or not appropriate for young children, to prevent diarrheal disease and parasites. The importance of immunizations and the diseases they prevent can be shared with children. Child-to-Child health messages about diseases are simplified, so children can understand and share the information with each other and their families. Each message has activities for the children to promote responsibility. Kids enjoy dramatic performances, role-playing, puppets made from a bag, a potato, or just a finger with a face drawn on it, which can advance to filming and video. Children enjoy acting out how to help a sick person with comfort, water, food, good hygiene, entertainment with stories, songs, and games. Diarrhea is a topic children enjoy discussing, as all topics about defecation are humorous for children, and as most have experienced diarrhea.

Adult organizers of children's activities need to be sensitive to everyone's needs. All necessary approvals from the authorities should be obtained. Willingness to fit in with overall plans and with other educational activities is mandatory. Planning committees should include children and their parents.

Children with disabilities are essential participants and may need additional support and integration. Most children know about disabled children who are hidden or excluded. Visits to excluded children will allow relationships to develop, and playing together can foster inclusiveness. Recognizing the strengths of these children can encourage them to help themselves with the support of other children for their disability. Deaf children are often identified as children who cannot talk. With a few words in sign language, children can begin to communicate with deaf children and welcome them to school.

Helping children with disabilities allows children to integrate with heart-warming and inspiring lessons. A young Lao boy, born missing a lower leg, was unable to attend school, learn the local language, and have friends. His family lived in extreme poverty, and his mother *was caring for other children, so she was unable to help him. He showed his frustration with destructive and dangerous behaviors. When he was integrated with the support of the other children, and supplied with a prosthetic leg, he became an excellent student, empathetic, and now aims to continue his studies to help others with disabilities.

Promotion of Healthy Nutrition and Lifestyle

The International Code on the Advertising of Breastmilk Substitutes

Exclusive breastfeeding for the first 6 months and continuing breastfeeding with complementary foods until 2 years old saves infants lives [11]. The advertising of formula products unfairly competes with limited public health promotion of breastfeeding. The International Code on Marketing of Breastmilk Substitutes is designed to protect breastfeeding from promotions by the formula industry. Violations of the Code should be reported to the Ministry of Health and International Babyfood

Action Network (IBFAN, https://www.ibfan.org). Each year, there are many violations of the Code, especially promotions offering incentives to health care workers. This is particularly serious where health care workers' salaries are low. The enforcement of the Code depends on observers to report violations.

In Laos, advertising campaigns of formula products to the public promoted breastmilk substitutes as the best food for infants' health and development. The Nestle formula logo, of a mother bear holding a baby bear in the breastfeeding position, was on cans of coffee creamer, leading poor parents to believe it was good food for babies. Infants fed coffee creamer developed severe malnutrition, and some died. Research and publication of the findings led to the end of the advertising campaign, and the removal of the logo from coffee creamer. The formula logo was changed with the removal of the baby bear. Stronger legislation was implemented to control formula promotions in Laos and elsewhere [12]. International support is often needed to protect breastfeeding, as formula representatives may have strong connections with national health care professionals.

Nutrition Promotion

Gardening can improve nutrition by planting and harvesting vegetables, fruits, and beans, in school gardens and at home. Children can be encouraged to make better food choices and to carefully spend limited financial resources on nutritious foods, rather than wasting on ubiquitously available junk food.

In the Guatemalan highlands, children are at high risk of malnutrition, with some departments reporting 70% childhood malnutrition. Wuqu' Kawoq (the Mayan Health Alliance) (http://www.wuqukawoq.org/) has a nutrition program aiming to improve children's diets. The mountain hillsides are covered with cornfields, limiting dietary diversity. Children's diets are deficient in protein and vitamins A, C, and folic acid. Water is scarce, and community water supplies are forbidden for agriculture. Most families use chemicals, pesticides, and fertilizers, which harm the environment and deplete financial resources. Traditionally, fields are burned after the harvest, depleting soil nutrients. To address these issues, Wuqu' Kawoq's Guatemalan nutritionists and agronomists teach the families to produce home-grown chemical-free vegetables, based on their preferences and rich in missing nutrients. The square-foot gardening technique with raised beds can yield an abundant harvest in a small area, conserving water, but requires good quality soil. Soil health is improved with worm compost and dry leaves. Natural pesticides are made with soap, chilies, and other local ingredients. Filters for recycled laundry water allow families to conserve their limited water supply. Fertilizers are produced organically with food and garden wastes. Response from the families has been positive. Surveys conducted before, during, and after follow the children's nutritional status and dietary improvements.

Growing Health began in Butare, Rwanda, at a hospital, to provide food for patients, as hospitals do not provide food for patients, many of whom are malnourished and extremely poor. The local organizers consulted with the mothers of malnourished children, teaching and promoting nutritious foods, good hygiene, and the value of kitchen gardens. Vegetables are grown near the hospital and used to feed nutritious meals to the patients. The program has grown to be a large farm with farmers, agronomists, managers, educators, cooks and is supported by donations and volunteers. Beans, sweet potatoes, kale, sorghum, bananas, avocados, passion fruit, and more are grown and consumed in the hospital. An outreach program provides teaching and training in target villages. The program is a model for Rwandan health care facilities (https://kuzamuraubuzima.rw).

The Promotion of Complementary Food to Children over 6 Months

Photos of varieties of foods grown locally and inexpensive in local markets promote the use of tofu, soft fruits, and vegetables, eggs, rice or noodle soups with vegetables, meats, oil added to improve the nutritional content and peanut sauce. In each location, what is available should be evaluated for the best nutritional value for effort and price. A Lao Language book, titled "Good Nutrition for Mother and Baby," is published by Big Brother Mouse (http://www.bigbrothermouse.com/books/goodnut-book.html).

Remote floating villages on Tonle Sap Lake, Cambodia, have diets limited to rice and fish, of dwindling supply due to climate changes, dams, and overfishing. A Cambodian nurse, working with The Lake Clinic, promotes the building of floating gardens to grow vegetables to improve childhood nutrition. The promotion of the gardens includes nutrition education for the families and training the children to build and care for the gardens (https://www.lakeclinic.org).

In Laos, papaya salad is a healthy food choice with ingredients from the community with no cooking required. The preparation is shredding the papaya, adding ingredients to the mortar, taking turns pounding with the pestle, test tasting, and adding seasonings. Papaya salad making contests are fun and nutritional activities, requiring minimum organization and local resources. First, a list of ingredients is prepared. Children are asked to bring what they can find: papaya, chili peppers, peanuts, mortar and pestle, knife, wildflowers for decoration, banana leaves for plates, sticky rice, tomatoes, lemons, and water bucket for hand washing. The children are divided into groups with two older kids in each group. The ingredients are divided between the groups. Judging is based on everyone's involvement, good hygiene, a song or chant, creativity, environmentally friendly (no plastic), and taste. A book written by a Vietnamese social worker, Xuygen Dangers, Tammakhung Forever, has the recipe and poems and chants in Lao and English. Peanut sauce is another example of a nutrition-dense and inexpensive culturally correct choice. After the judging, everyone gets a reward, fruit, boiled egg, or another healthy item, and to eat the salad or peanut sauce with sticky rice. Teachers and parents are the judges, and everyone has a healthy snack. Photos, drawings, and posters can be made to document the event and remind everyone about available healthy foods that children can prepare. Further discussions include food choices on a minimal budget, and growing papaya, chilies, and tomatoes in home gardens.

Conclusion

Child health promotion is essential to protect and improve the lives of vulnerable children, refugees, asylum seekers, and children living in poverty worldwide. Children and young people enjoy promoting healthy living to their friends and families. For over 30 years, the Child-to-Child participatory model has modeled children helping others to evaluate health problems, search for solutions, and implement health behavior changes. With the essential support of the local community, national approvals, and cooperation with local and international groups, children can learn, teach, and implement health behavior change in their communities and improve their own lives. Child health promotion should be child-centered, imaginative, and fun for children to result in successful health behavior change that reaches even the most vulnerable children and their families.

References

1. A framework for the protection of children [internet]. UNHCR; 2012 [cited 2020 May 18] p. 36. www.unhcr.org
2. Convention on the rights of the child [internet]. UN Commission on Human Rights (46th sess. : 1990 : Geneva); 1990 Jul [cited 2020 May 21]. Report No.: E/CN.4/RES/1990/74. https://www.unicef.org/child-rights-convention/convention-text
3. Hjern A. Health of refugee and migrant children Technical guidance The Migration and Health programme Health of refugee and migrant children Technical guidance [Internet]. World Health Organization; 2018 [cited 2020 May 18]. http://www.euro.who.int/__data/assets/pdf_file/0011/388361/tc-health-children-eng.pdf?ua=1
4. American Academy of Pediatrics. ICATCH Grants Website [Internet]. Community/AAP Sections/Section on Global Health (SOGH)/ICATCH/ICATCH Grants. 2020 [cited 2020 Jul 16]. https://services.aap.org/en/community/aap-sections/international-child-health/icatch/icatch-grants/
5. Conway C, Bonati G, Arif-Fear L, Young T. Hearing all voices—transforming the lives of vulnerable youth: the power of participation. Learning for Wellbeing Magazine [Internet]. 2017 Mar 15 [cited 2020 May 22];(3):12. https://www.l4wb-magazine.org/mag03-art03
6. Harman P, Scotchmer C, editors. Rebuilding young lives: using the child to child approach with children in difficult circumstances [internet]. Child to Child Institute of Education 20 Bedford Way London WC1H 0AL United Kingdom 0044 (0)207 612 6649; 1997 [cited 2020 May 18]. http://www.childtochild.org.uk/wp-content/uploads/2014/10/Rebuilding_Young_Lives-Using_the_C2C_Approach.pdf
7. Child to Child. Child to child website [internet]. Child to Child. 2020 [cited 2020 Jul 16]. www.child-to-child.org
8. Bonati G. Child to child training manual [internet]. Child to Child Institute of Education 20 Bedford Way London WC1H 0AL United Kingdom 0044 (0)207 612 6649; [cited 2020 May 18]. 111 p. http://www.childtochild.org.uk/wp-content/uploads/2014/10/Child_to_Child-Training_Manual.pdf
9. Early years children promote health case studies on child-to-child and early childhood development [internet]. The Child-to-Child Trust; 2004 [cited 2020 Jun 7] p. 141. www.childtochild.org.uk/wp-content/uploads/2014/10/Child_to_Child-Early_Years_Promoting_Health.pdf
10. Hanbury C, Gifford D. Child-to-child and children living in camps [internet]. London: Child-to-Child Trust; 1993. [cited 2020 May 18]. http://www.childtochild.org.uk/wp-content/uploads/2014/10/Child-to-Child-and-Children-Living-in-Camps.pdf

11. Zhao M, Wu H, Liang Y, Liu F, Bovet P, Xi B. Breastfeeding and mortality under 2 years of age in Sub-Saharan Africa. Pediatrics. 2020;145(5):e20192209. [cited 2020 May 18] [Internet]. http://pediatrics.aappublications.org/lookup/doi/10.1542/peds.2019-2209
12. Barennes H, Andriatahina T, Latthaphasavang V, Anderson M, Srour LM. Misperceptions and misuse of bear brand coffee creamer as infant food: national cross sectional survey of consumers and paediatricians in Laos. BMJ. 2008;337:a1379.

M. Leila Srour, MD, FAAP, MPH, DTM&H is an international volunteer, supporting the training of pediatricians in developing countries. From 2002 to 2013, Leila volunteered with Health Frontiers supporting the training of Lao pediatricians and the continuing medical education of the graduates. With her husband, Bryan, they supported the Butterfly Children's Development Center, an after-school program in their village in Luang Namtha, northern Laos. Leila volunteers with Health Volunteers Overseas, supporting pediatric training programs in Indonesia, Bhutan, Cambodia, Nepal, and Laos. She is the chair of the pediatric steering committee for Health Volunteers Overseas, and a member of the SNIS noma research group. Leila graduated with an MPH from Loma Linda University in 2001. Leila worked as a general pediatrician in Santa Barbara 1984–2001. She is a CHLA pediatric residency graduate in 1983, after graduating from Loma Linda Medical School in 1978.

Part IV

Editor's Introduction: Field Guide

At the time of this manual's writing, the coronavirus pandemic has spawned unique challenges for healthcare providers around the globe. Even in highly resourced settings, we are faced with shortages of hospital beds, ventilators, doctors and nurses, even gloves and masks—all at a time when numbers of the sick and dying continue to increase daily. Such overwhelming demand paired with scarcity of resources is not new to many parts of the world, where providers must find creative solutions for clinically complex and ethically challenging situations, constantly. Pandemic or not, these challenges and complexities are often daily realities in the field—which are now even more trying as refugee settings globally grapple with COVID-19.

When we meet a refugee or migrant child in the field, at any given juncture along his or her path of flight, we must address the health needs they bring to us—bearing in mind their particular psychosocial, cultural, and historical context. This Field Guide is intended to help you do just that—address the range of problems that may be brought to your exam table—using culturally appropriate, holistic, evidence-based, practical approaches. This section is not intended to provide an exhaustive academic review of all pediatric conditions; rather it aims to provide you with a toolkit of clinical pearls from a panel of seasoned humanitarian workers. We have abstracted their guidance on the most common pediatric presentations in these settings, collected their most salient tricks of the trade, and have complied a vetted list of references and appendices following each chapter for those wanting further knowledge.

This section walks you through how to prepare for a field experience, both personally and materially; how to set up data management systems and field pharmacies even in rugged conditions; how to conduct nutritional surveys and develop infectious disease surveillance systems; and how to protect the delicate health of a newly born refugee in a resource-poor setting. We cover common respiratory, gastrointestinal, reproductive, and adolescent conditions, and address the difficult questions and considerations that arise at the end of a child's life. We discuss the general management of chronic conditions, burns, bites, and other common presentations, and explore how interpreters can help you understand much more than spoken languages.

We hope this Field Guide will equip you with the tools you need, be it during a pandemic, prolonged armed conflict, or other natural or human-made disaster—wherever and whenever you may find yourself along a particular child's path of flight.

Further Reading

- Blundell H, Milligan R, Norris SL, Garner P. WHO guidance for refugees in camps: systematic review. BMJ Open. 2019;9(9):e027094.
- Denno D. Global child health. Pediatr Rev. 2011;32(2):e25.
- Esmaili BE. Caravans and containers: children on the move, immobilized. Pediatrics. 2018;142(3):e20181470.

Preparation and Well-being for Humanitarian Workers

Christian Harkensee and Sarah Walpole

Introduction

Even with a lot of experience, working in a humanitarian setting can be challenging, unsettling, and confusing. This chapter aims to help you as a humanitarian worker to prepare for deployment and to support you to look after your own and your team members' physical and mental health. Having clarity about your motivation, expectations, and goals is the first step towards preparedness for the unexpected that you are likely to encounter. Such awareness can help you to prepare, including recognizing what stressors you might experience, and which approaches to self-care may help you.

Why Work in Humanitarian Settings?

You may already have thought about whether and why working with refugees could be for you. Many humanitarian workers are driven by a desire to help others and a belief that they can have more impact in a low resource setting (altruism)—their motivation can be "charged" with idealism and the desire to live to high moral values [1]. Such values may be philosophical, political, or religious. Speaking to others, their reasons are more personal in nature, such as experience working in a different setting for own personal development, to learn more about their own

C. Harkensee (✉)
Queen Elizabeth Hospital, Gateshead, UK

S. Walpole
Health Education England North East, Newcastle, UK

Newcastle University, Newcastle, UK

Infectious Diseases Department, Newcastle Hospitals, RVI, Newcastle, UK
e-mail: sarah.walpole@doctors.org.uk

© Springer Nature Switzerland AG 2021
C. Harkensee et al. (eds.), *Child Refugee and Migrant Health*,
https://doi.org/10.1007/978-3-030-74906-4_15

abilities and how to cope with change and challenges, or to learn more about different people, places, cultures, and situations. Some are attracted to this type of work with a spirit for adventure, testing their mental and physical limits. Others have specific goals for career development. You may wish to gain or practice skills by working in a different setting, for example, to practice clinical skills in a low resource setting, communication skills in a highly challenging situation, or language skills in a different country; to gain experience that you can present to potential future employers or collaborators, i.e., to "build your CV" to develop a career in the humanitarian or development sector [2]; or to fill a career break or gap between jobs. Some people embark on placements in humanitarian settings to mark or provoke a change in work or personal circumstances. Most commonly, it is a combination of several of these drivers that motivate people to do humanitarian work.

This chapter does not advocate that any motivation is more or less valid than another, rather than whatever your motivations are, it is worth spending time to recognize them before embarking on placement and to consider whether working in refugee health is the best way to achieve what you hope to achieve. Most people will be motivated by more than one factor and some motivations might require more caution and consideration than others. If what you really need is a break from your current situation (especially consider this if you have just ended a job, a relationship, or another significant life change), then there may be other ways to recalibrate before, or instead of, going to work in a refugee setting. Volunteering and working in refugee settings may appear to offer a break, but it is usually fraught with physical, mental, social, and emotional demands, and not an easy or healthy way to take space to review your priorities, heal trauma, or find a new direction.

It is worth considering how realistic your expectations are and what you can put in place or do before, during, and after your placement to maximize the benefit of your placement to you, your colleagues, and the population you serve. You may also want to consider the impacts on and perspectives of colleagues at home, your family and friends, and your employers (current and/or future).

What Might It Feel Like to Work in Child and Family Refugee Health?

Migration rarely takes place over a short timeframe; refugees often spend months traveling. When working in refugee health settings, your experience will vary greatly depending on the population that you are serving and the location of your work. Your own background and perspective and the perspectives of those with whom you work will also have a significant influence.

Whether your relationships with colleagues are good, tolerable, or difficult can be the difference between having a positive or negative experience. You are likely to work with a diverse group of colleagues, often of a range of ages, backgrounds, and experience. Adaptability and transferable skills may be more relevant to lead, plan, and manage than experience or seniority. Members of the community that you serve may often be among your colleagues, whether they are acting as translators, trained health professionals (from nurses, to doctors, to outreach workers/health promoters), or receptionists, cleaners, administrators, or other support workers for a clinic or service.

It is also important to remember that work in humanitarian settings and other refugee settings often involves long hours, intense work schedules, and frequent professional and social contact with a small group of colleagues. In many settings, security issues require that a curfew is in place and you may not be allowed to go out after work. Movement restrictions may be such that you are only allowed to visit certain streets or locations, or only allowed to go out when accompanied. Particularly if your placement is short (weeks or months), if your language skills are limited, and depending on the type of setting that you work in, it may not be possible to socialize with anyone other than your immediate colleagues. You may well live in a compound, apartment block, house, or tents with your colleagues and have little of your own private space. In some projects, volunteers share a bedroom. Conversely, in some projects, you may have very limited contact with colleagues or opportunity to socialize at all, for example, if you have a small team and an early curfew. One author's personal experience included living in a compound with the eight expat colleagues where some people shared rooms and the arrangement did not provide any possibility to speak in privacy. There was a 6 pm curfew, so any socializing was between the same eight colleagues, which provided creativity and fun much of the time, but also tensions and the need to find ways to "take time out." As well as sharing experiences with and learning from great colleagues, the author wrote to friends at home, read, and took up yoga. In another placement abroad, the author was one of two expats. They lived in an apartment building and had a curfew which allowed for little time to go out after work. Again, ensuring healthy habits such as eating properly, sleeping well, drawing boundaries around work time, individual pursuits, and contentment with time alone were key to maintaining balance, health, and successful placement.

Case Study: Reflections on Volunteering in Greek Refugee Camps
A group of volunteers shares lunch around a table in Northern Greece. Meanwhile, the population that they have come to work with eats inside tents in a large industrial building. The setting and physical circumstances are different, but perhaps an even greater divide exists between the sense of control and the future possibilities that these two groups hold.

The volunteers come from Australia, Belgium, Norway, Spain, Syria, the UK, and the USA. What unites them is their decision to go out into the world to provide healthcare to people living in refugee camps. Yet their backgrounds and the factors that motivate them vary. Some came here because they wanted to do something to respond to the "migrant crisis" that they have seen reported on the news; some are motivated by religion; perhaps others are looking for a sense of purpose or a setting where they can see immediate positive effects of their work. Some are staying for 3 weeks, some for 3 months or more.

Those living in the camps have lost their livelihoods and are also prohibited from creating new livelihoods due to the instability and lack of control over their lives, the burden of not being able to plan their future, and the anxiety that they have about their children's future. Many of those living in the camp do not like labeling themselves as "refugees", as the term is associated with either positive or negative connotations. These refugees told us that they want to be seen as the individuals they are, rather than as a group.

There is a weighty psychological impact from the challenges that those living in the camps face day-to-day. After weeks, months, or years of life in a tent, it is not only important to address the psychological trauma that refugees have been through previously, but also along the arduous journey that they have taken.

Refugees with whom we spoke who were living in a "temporary" refugee camp and waiting for an opportunity to continue their journey, said that many of their expectations are not met. The ability to meet these expectations may be limited by the resources available, yet it may be possible to go further towards meeting their expectations and wishes even working within existing resource constraints.

Recognizing and addressing the ways in which expectations are not or cannot be met may help. For example, what refugees find with regard to medical care may be very different from what they were accustomed to at home. They may think care is not good because they are used to being able to buy antibiotics over the counter at the pharmacy and do not like antibiotics being restricted. People from many countries, including Syria, expect earlier referral to specialist care, as they are not familiar with the role of general or family practice [3]. Asking patients about their expectations and explaining when and why they can and cannot be met may help them to accept the services as they are.

Psychological trauma is often present and perceivable, but both providers and recipients of healthcare may be reluctant to initiate a conversation about it. Patients from many cultures feel they should defer to the physician and wait to be asked, while doctors may not feel comfortable asking and may not be prepared mentally and emotionally to hear the stories [4].

Volunteers sometimes struggle to know where to begin to address such deep-rooted and extensive trauma, especially if their knowledge of the political, economic, social, and cultural context is limited. Adding to this the time pressures that are often faced in emergency or post-emergency setting, the challenge further increases.

Volunteers may expect gratefulness from the people that they have gone to help, and then feel disheartened that many of the patients they see present with conditions that are largely psychologically mediated and for which they cannot provide any certain or quick solutions. Their sacrifice of time and effort may even be countered with dissatisfaction and disappointment from refugees whose priorities and desires are not met.

The experience of working in a camp has made us feel humble—about our own expectations. There is little we can do to alleviate the situation the people in the camps suffer—especially the uncertainty that prevents them from concluding the past and facing the future. However, there is much we can do by consciously and truly listening and trying to understand [5, 6]. As volunteers, we may have some influence on the lives of others, but we may not be aware of all of the different types of influence that we have [7]. *One of the most rewarding experiences as a volunteer is bearing witness to the astonishing level of resilience and resourcefulness that many refugee families pertain, which helps them to bear difficult circumstances and master their future. At the same time, our senses and awareness sharpen for the often hidden vulnerabilities, for which we can become strong advocates.*

Exploring Approaches to Working in a Humanitarian Setting

The previous section has explored different motivations that you might have for choosing to work in a humanitarian setting. The next few pages are dedicated to reflection on and ideas about preparing to work with refugees in humanitarian settings, while looking after yourself when in the field and thereafter.

This section explores the more practical tasks of preparing for a humanitarian deployment: Recognizing your own skillset and considering what you wish to offer, looking for and planning a placement/assignment, and preparing for the physical, social, and psychological aspects of working in a humanitarian setting.

What Knowledge, Skills, Experience, and Abilities Will You Bring to the Field?

When thinking about what you can and cannot bring to the field, you can think beyond clinical and health promotion skills. Just as important as your skills and experience as a clinician, manager, public health expert, or other health professional, will be your ability to adapt to different environments, think innovatively to address challenges with limited resources and confined working arrangements, collaborate with colleagues from different fields, different backgrounds, and organizations, and do all this and look after yourself in circumstances of frequent change and uncertainty. Although well-organized programs may offer appropriate predeparture training and briefing, this does not always happen. A tolerance for uncertainty and changing roles is essential, especially in the early weeks of a humanitarian emergency.

Bearing in mind your goals for the placement and the types of skills that you have to offer should help you to decide about the positions you will seek. Examples of the kind of work that health professionals often plan to do include: supported clinical roles; clinical lead for a clinic or a program; health advisor or other management roles at different levels; roles in health promotion; roles related to research be that data collection, data analysis or other aspects of design or delivery; and teaching roles.

Many organizations, but by no means all, will have a process of clinical supervision and/or progress review, depending on the length of your placement. Whether or not there is a process like this to engage with, you may want to consider keeping a record of your expectations, goals, and progress, and trying to recognize how these are evolving.

Finding and Planning a Placement

Having considered why you want to go and work in refugee health and what kind of role you would like to work in, you may want to pay attention to certain practicalities so that you know what you want before you start to look for a placement.

- Are there any situations or scenarios that you are more or less drawn to, for example, due to having connections to a particular cause, or due to having studied the context? (Bear in mind that having a personal connection to a context *may* be an important reason not to work there as it may reduce your ability to be objective, or might increase the emotional strain that working in the context puts you under. Equally, sometimes, a connection to a context may be a positive motivation for you to work there.)
- What levels of insecurity and risk are you willing to accept and maintain your own well-being and ability to work well within—e.g., conflict zone, infectious diseases outbreak?
- How important is it to you to have free time and your own private space? It may be important to check on the accommodation arrangements.
- How "remote" are you willing and able to be? Is internet access important to you? Do you find it important to be able to visit shops or a bar?
- Do you have any access requirements, health issues, or other needs to take into account?
- How long do you want to go for? Of course, this might vary depending on the above factors—if you are in a less stable, more remote, and more challenging placement, you are likely to experience more strain on your ability to feel comfortable.

Considering this in advance will give you a good starting point from which to identify what you are looking for and explore the kinds of placements available. Much of the above information may not be available at the stage of applying, but it should be possible to find out more by contacting the organization or talking to someone who has worked for them (someone known to you or the organization could put you in touch with someone who has previously worked in a similar role).

In terms of where to look:

- Employment websites, e.g., humanitarian jobs.
- Websites of and bulletins from humanitarian organizations, e.g., MSF, Doctors Worldwide.
- Updates from humanitarian and health and social justice organizations, e.g., People's Health Movement.
- Updates from professional bodies and local networks for health professionals interested in global health, e.g., the Royal College of Physicians and Health Professionals for Global Health in the UK or the American Academy of Pediatrics Section on Global Health in the US.
- Talking to friends and colleagues.

- Finding out from those who you meet who have worked away, where they have worked.

Many people find it difficult to first enter into this sector of work, and it would be beyond the scope of this chapter to give specific recommendations [8]. In general terms, volunteering experience, however short, is beneficial as it will build confidence and help workers develop a reputation and network that opens up further opportunities. The sector is highly fluctuant, and although formal education and training (e.g., undergraduate/postgraduate training in a relevant profession) are essential, education alone will not secure a position. What many organizations value highly is practical experience with evidence of defined outcomes (e.g., having managed a project with evaluation, written a report, published a research paper, delivered teaching/capacity building, etc.), and evidence of use of transferable skills.

Stress and Stress Responses of Humanitarian Workers

Unique stressors have unique effects. In addition to the physical dangers, relief workers are at risk for behavioral and emotional readjustment problems following traumatic exposures on deployment [9, 10]. It is only natural to be physically and emotionally affected by such experiences, although the long-term impact will depend on your physical and emotional health when you depart for your post, previous traumatic experiences, the degree of awareness and self-care, the degree and quality of planning and preparation, and the amount of support provided in the field and afterwards. Humanitarian workers are often driven to this type of work for its potential to promote personal growth, develop awareness, compassion, self-discovery, testing one's limits, and opportunity for building deep friendships and comradery. For most people, this personal growth outweighs and counteracts the distress that is experienced with traumatic events. Nevertheless, a significant proportion of humanitarian workers in crisis situations (up to one-third) do experience more severe stress symptoms, and some may need psychological support for symptoms of Posttraumatic Stress Disorder (PTSD) or depression [11]. It is important to recognize such symptoms and to seek or offer support early.

Stress reaction symptoms can be broadly categorized into four domains: emotional, cognitive, physical, and interpersonal. In the early stages, or if symptoms are relatively mild, you may notice the following in yourself and others [12, 13]:

- *Emotional symptoms*—Feelings of shock, fear, grief, anger in the acute situation, resentment and guilt (survivor's guilt), feeling ashamed, overwhelmed, helpless, feeling numb, and detached.
- *Cognitive symptoms*—disruption of normal logical thinking, feeling confused, disoriented, indecisive, worried, problems with memory, attention span and concentration, unwanted memories, self-blame.
- *Physical reactions*—feelings of tension, restlessness, edginess, sleeping difficulties or excessive fatigue, lack of energy but unable to rest and recover. Physical

symptoms such as achiness, headaches, backaches, panic attacks, change in appetite, being easily startled.
- *Interpersonal reactions*—Feelings of distrust, wanting to isolate and withdraw, or feeling irritable, aggressive, seeking conflict. Feeling rejected, abundant, distant. Leaders may become over-controlling, judgemental.

If you notice a colleague is beginning to display these symptoms, it is important to be there, listen, share, have patience, support the person, giving them space and time for a break. Some people may not be aware of the change in their behavior, and people around them notice these first—it is critical to intervene at this stage.

Once symptoms become more severe, immediate intervention by someone skilled in psychological help, and if needed evacuation out of the situation may be necessary. "Red Flags" for severe psychological distress include: Feeling extremely dissociated and numb, intrusive reexperiencing ("flashbacks"), hyperarousal, severe anxiety, severe depression, extreme memory avoidance (self-medication, drugs, alcohol), and feeling suicidal.

To a degree, it is possible to predict which experiences lead to severe stress symptoms, such as direct experience or witnessing any of the following:

- Life-threatening danger or physical harm
- Danger or harm to children in particular
- Extreme human violence or destruction
- Intense emotional demand of the work
- Extreme fatigue or sleep deprivation
- Extreme loss—mental, spiritual, emotional, physical
- Extended exposure time to danger or loss
- Extended emotional/physical strain

It is important to note that certain medications (e.g., antimalarials such as mefloquine) can trigger or worsen emotional symptoms [14]. The degree to which relief workers can bear these experiences depends very much on their own level of mental and spiritual resilience (which can be prepared) but also their own personal history of exposure to trauma (including previous relief work), chronic physical or mental illness, chronic emotional imbalance, experiences of poverty and discrimination, recent major life events, stressors, or emotional strain. While such experiences cannot be reversed, processing the experiences and developing coping strategies can build resilience in the run-up to a deployment.

What Organizations Can Do

The onus for preparation and support must not be on the relief workers alone; humanitarian organizations that deploy employees and volunteers have a duty and responsibility to keep staff and volunteers safe and supported [15]. This is increasingly being recognized, and while many organizations have developed very good programs, the psychological support for relief workers often remains inadequate. It is on the organizations, but also their partners, governments, multi-national bodies (e.g., UN, WHO), and workers themselves to push for better support. Organizations can work on many levels to prepare and support workers:

Preparation:

- Clearly define the purpose, expectations, and goals of any field position, and communicate this effectively.
- Maintain an effective management and leadership structure.
- Provide comprehensive health and accident insurance, repatriation support if needed, and appropriate risk management.
- Pre-deployment training and briefing information (in verbal and written formats).

In the field:

- Ensure that all new volunteer arrivals are given an induction, including orientation to all safety protocols, who to inform should any concerns arise and the location of key locations and supplies to ensure safety and well-being.
- Provide all the necessary tools and equipment to do the work safely and efficiently.
- Establish robust communication pathways.
- Ensure consistent and adequate supplies in the field, both to run the project and ensure staff well-being.
- Nurture a culture of support, including a humanistic approach to staff management.
- Early recognition of stress and contingency planning in place for all levels.
- Clearly defined roles and functions with supervision and support.
- Defined shifts, briefings and debriefings, breaks, and time away.
- Buddy systems and experience sharing sessions to allow team members to "check-in" and raise any issues affecting their well-being or others, allowing for monitoring of well-being.
- Availability of immediate psychological support and evacuation if necessary.
- Focus on staff development of skills, knowledge, and experience.

After completion of deployment:

- Exit Plan: Debriefing, opportunity for bilateral feedback, formal recognition.
- Aftercare: Ensure well-being, proactive counseling and support, retention.

Preparation: The "Grab-Bag Concept"

The "Grab-Bag Concept" is a framework for humanitarian workers to prepare for their deployment to a disaster or crisis. A grab bag is a bag that contains the items a worker needs to be self-sufficient for a short period of time, which they carry with them at all times and "grab" in the case of an emergency evacuation.

The content of a grab bag depends on two main factors: The environment where the worker deploys to (e.g., climate, local resources and facilities, culture, level of hostility, duration) and their own experience and preferences. Less experienced workers tend to put more items into their bag, whereas more experienced ones often become more "minimalistic," having developed experience, skills, and resilience.

To understand this concept better, it is helpful to look at examples from expedition and survival training. Italian mountaineer Reinhold Messner revolutionized climbing in the Himalayas by moving from traditional "Expedition Style" (a large number of climbers and Sherpas with an enormous amount of material equipment would "besiege" a mountain for a long period of time) to "Alpine Style" (a small number, or even a solo climber, would ascend a mountain fast and with minimal equipment). As Messner himself described this, the difference that made such a bold approach possible was not in the equipment or physical constitution, but in the mind—trained instinct, experience, and confidence; although to an outsider his climbs appeared outrageously risky, for his own risk assessment they were perfectly within his safe abilities and comfort zone [16]. Likewise, German survivalist and humanitarian activist Rüdiger Nehberg pushed the art of survival to the extreme—on one of his trips he entered the Amazon rainforest essentially naked, only to find and develop everything he needed, surviving on his experience, skills, and mental resilience [17].

The Grab-Bag Concept looks at someone's needs in four categories: The mental and spiritual needs and capabilities; experience, knowledge, skills; the environment; and physical needs and capabilities.

Mental and Spiritual Needs, Capabilities, and Preparation

Your mental preparation and motivation is the most complex, but also the most important part of your preparation, as mentioned above. All other preparation follows on from this initial process.

- *Expectations*—imagine you come back from the deployment—what do you expect to have experienced? What may have changed for you? How do you cope if your expectations are not met by your work?
- *Working and living with a team*—You may have to take a step back from your deepest convictions and beliefs for becoming pragmatic, for the "greater good" of the community you want to serve and the team you work with. You may be working and living closely with people you do not know or like for a prolonged period of time—have a strategy in mind how you deal and cope with this. Feeling

safe and secure—What level of risk are you willing to take? Imagine the worst-case scenario, and ask if you and your loved ones would cope with it.

- *Stress and resilience*—You may have to work and live well outside your comfort zone for a prolonged period of time. Work may be demanding, and you may experience a lack of basic facilities and privacy. What are your normal stress busters? Would they work in a different environment? If not, consider learning a new strategy that does not rely on any equipment or technology (e.g., meditation, mindfulness, or religious practice). It is important that you have these techniques well established before you go—e.g., if you want mindfulness practice to be effective when you are under stress, start practicing and make it a habit weeks or months before you actually go. Consider your support network—how can you keep in touch to access this support? What if you have no internet access?

Experience, Knowledge, Skills, and Preparation

Once you have some clarity about why you do this work, what your expectations are, and what level of challenge you are prepared to accept, the next step is about more specific preparation for your work.

- *Gain confidence*—This can be done through training and experience. If you plan to go to a challenging environment (e.g., conflict zones), consider training (e.g., HELP, HEAT, survival courses) but also plenty of practice to gain experience (e.g., survival weekends in your nearest forest, wild camping, practice bushcraft skills, or foraging).
- *Being part of a team*—Have a good understanding of your own personality and what you can and cannot bring to a team. Undertaking psychometric testing with qualified feedback (e.g., Belbin, Meyers-Briggs) can give you great insights in how you function, what your preferences, strengths, and weaknesses are. Have some simple activities and games in mind that could strengthen team spirit without needing much material (e.g., pocket chess set and set of playing cards). Consider developing skills that are useful for working and living with other people—e.g., psychological first aid, counseling, coaching/mentoring, communication skills training.
- *Choose specific courses and workshops that are relevant for your area of work*—Practice that knowledge where you live to gain experience—e.g., seek voluntary roles in the city where you live to gain experience working with vulnerable people and to build a support network. You are likely to find a lot of like-minded people you are working with, e.g., those working with homeless people or refugees in your home town who will understand your motivation and experiences.
- *Have an escape plan*—Think through all possible scenarios that would make your position in the field unbearable or untenable, and think through how you can get out if needed (which should include, e.g., diplomatic and repatriation routes and options). Be as detailed as possible, and do your research. Share this with your organization and your loved ones.

- *Study carefully your organization's policies and provisions*—you can often recognize a reputable organization by the level of care and support they provide to their employees and volunteers.

The Environment

The place where you go will help to determine how you need to prepare mentally and spiritually, and what skills and experiences you need to bring. This section focuses more specifically on environmental factors that need to be considered in your preparation.

- *What is happening now in the place where you are going?* Obtain the most current information from reputable news outlets and from the organization that is deploying you. Ensure with your organization that you clearly understand the aims, objectives, and terms of your deployment.
- *Learn and read as much as you can about the country/area where you are going.* Ensure you obtain reliable information (see Resources section at the end of this chapter). Try to understand as much as possible about politics, culture, and religion. Find someone from the country/region living in your home city to ask questions and make connections.
- *Learn some of the language.* If you have the time, try to learn the language or at least learn some simple expressions—this will go a long way in breaking the ice and building trust and respect.
- *Geography and climate.* Study maps, weather, and climate reports to gain a good understanding of the conditions and challenges.
- *Personal safety.* Understand what the risks are, and how to mitigate these. Have knowledge about how and where to seek help in the country, and how reliable this is. Understand well what to do and what not to do in case you find your safety is threatened. There are several online and face-to-face courses for safety on deployment (see Resources section).

Physical Needs, Capabilities, and Preparation

Going through mental and spiritual preparation, reflecting on experience, knowledge, and skills, and the environment eventually leads to the physical preparation of the actual grab bag.

There are really only two ground rules about the grab bag: It must be light, clearly weighing less than 10 kg including all contents, and everything must fit into a small backpack of no more than 20 liters. The actual content is very much determined by your personal needs. Start by collating all the things you think should go in, put them on a scale, and check if they would fit into a bag of that size. If your things exceed weight or volume, there are two approaches to solve this: Firstly, go back to mental and spiritual needs, skills, knowledge, and experience, and examine carefully what your needs really are, or if by achieving a new skill, knowledge or experience you could spare some of the items altogether. The other approach looks at the chosen items to see if they could be replaced by something smaller or lighter. Think through the following aspects:

- *The grab bag itself*—Choose a simple, light bag made from robust material (e.g., a "day pack" rucksack). Try it on to ensure it is comfortable. Be prepared to carry this for extended periods of time—train for it before you deploy by filling it with 10 kg (e.g., water bottles) and carry it around on a daily basis. For more comfort, you could consider cutting off the carrying system (such as shoulder straps) and replacing it with a carrying system designed for a larger backpack (such as better padded shoulder straps or a hip belt). You do not need a rain cover—use a strong 50 liters plastic trash bag to line your grab bag from the inside, and close this with a plastic clamp to make it waterproof. For some deployments, a grab bag may be all you are allowed to bring. Think in categories of your grab bag that will make you completely self-sufficient. Do not bring anything that you cannot afford to lose, such as items of high physical and emotional value.
- *Your physical health and well-being*—Get a health check with your doctor and dentist well in advance (2–3 months) in case you need any vaccinations or any treatments. If you are on prescription medicine bring at least 2–3 times the supply that you need and carry it in your hand luggage. Check any legal restrictions in the country where you go, and inquire in advance with the country's consulate how you can bring prescriptions legally (you may need to bring a letter from your doctor and a formal permit). If you are not a healthcare professional, do a First Aid training course. Prepare a personal first aid kit (an example kit list is in the Appendix) and bring a spare amount of any first aid supplies that you could share with team members if needed. Check the country's health information (links in Resources section) to learn what you may need to bring, e.g., repellents, ITN bed nets, malaria prophylaxis. Find out what items can be bought locally. Bring personal hygiene items—best in small plastic bottles, lightweight.
- *Physical fitness*—The required level of physical fitness depends on the type of deployment and environment. Going into a well-developed established setting for a short period may be less physically demanding than going into a disaster area. As a general principle, any deployment into an area that is politically unstable, a disaster zone, or has an extreme climate is more demanding on the body and a basic level of physical fitness should be considered. Nevertheless, the situation may change rapidly even in presumed stable areas.
- *Clothing*—Choose lightweight, comfortable clothing according to expected temperature and climate. Fast-drying synthetics are preferred. If temperatures fluctuate, use a "layer" principle—rather than one very warm and one very light piece of clothing choose a small number of light-mid insulating clothes that you can combine for warmth. Avoid anything that looks military. You may only be able to bring one set of clothes to change—for clothing care consider bringing a mini sewing kit for repairs, a small plastic brush, a small bar of soap, and a clothes line. These items are multi-functional, but consider buying them in the country.

- *Shelter*—You may be provided with accommodation, but consider bringing at least an emergency blanket, sleeping mat, and/or bivouac bag. Further need for shelter equipment may be determined by the environment and security of shelter—you may consider bringing a sleeping bag and mat, lightweight tarpaulin (3 × 4 m), or even a tent. Look at equipment for endurance runners or lightweight backpackers [18, 19]—there is now a great choice of very lightweight equipment available. Experiment with building simple survival shelters with materials only that you find in the environment [20].

- *Food and water*—Think 2–3 days emergency supply for a grab bag. Choose some emergency food that is energy-dense, lightweight, and tasty (e.g., nuts, protein bars). The amount of water (use a simple plastic bottle, or thermos flask for cold temperatures) depends on the availability of water in the environment—the drier, the more you should bring (and this would be the only excuse to exceed 10 kg weight!). Consider bringing a small filtration device (e.g., life straw) and water disinfection tablets. If you think you need to prepare food yourself, consider bringing a fire-resistant metal cup and a multi-cutlery (spoon and fork in one, plastic). A small amount of coffee/tea/sugar/sweetener could provide a great physical as well as mental health boost. In case that your organization tells you that you need to bring a cooking system, consider a lightweight gas cooker or a high-efficiency system such as a Jetboil. Study food that you can potentially forage in the environment where you are going—but ensure with information from local people what is edible and what is not. Ensure you prepare your food in a hygienic way.

- *Navigation and communication*—Plan for all possible navigation and communication scenarios that you may encounter. With regards to communication, explore what facilities are available—e.g., reliability of local phone networks. Install useful apps (see Resources section) for communication and navigation on your phone, install a fresh battery, bring a solar phone charger, and plug adapter. Consider learning how to use a simple radio, a satellite phone, and the Morse code depending on the approaches used by your organization. When the network is poor, or if electricity or safety is a problem consider bringing a simple old phone which has a long battery life and works with 3G networks.

Your requirement for navigation skills depends on the type of deployment, the environment, and how likely you may find yourself having to find your own way back. Map reading can be a very useful skill and allow you to learn about the area that you are living and working in. If you can find one, get a local topographic map in 1:25,000. Even if it is not the most up-to-date, you may find important landmarks that can help you orient, and train yourself [21, 22]. Or, attend a navigation course to learn how to use a map and compass rather than relying on GPS. For some environments (e.g., sea, feature-less desert) a GPS navigation device is essential unless you know how to use an old-fashioned sextant!

- *Laptop/IT*—Bring a small, cheap, low energy consumption, lightweight laptop or tablet which you only use for your humanitarian deployments. The chance that it will get screened at border crossings, or lost, is high. Put only the essential software and data on it, and reset it after each deployment. Use up-to-date security software and password protection. Do not store sensitive data on the device. If you cannot avoid bringing sensitive data (i.e., with patient information), store them on a secure cloud platform or put them on an encrypted micro SD card which you could discard inconspicuously if necessary. Consider downloading textbooks and guidelines to inform questions and decisions, and bringing a simple outdoor medicine pocket book [23]. Bring a power adapter, surge protector, card adapter, and Ethernet cable. Consider bringing a solar charger with an adapter or spare power adapter ("brick").
- *Money and documents*—Most theft or mugging is opportunistic, and perpetrators are often satisfied with grabbing some easily accessible valuables and running off. Have some small change and a few banknotes in your pocket at all times. Key is to split any cash, credit cards, and important documents, keep them in different places/pockets, the most important ones in hidden places. Be inventive with stitching additional inside pockets, hides in belts, shoes, underwear, hats, and bags. Keep a record of all valuables in a safe place. Use several credit cards and keep them in different places. Make use of travel money cards with little money on them in case you get forced to disclose a pin. Use travel apps to store electronic copies of important documents such as passports, flight tickets or insurance certificates and details. Nominate a person at home to manage your affairs, and leave them with document copies and detailed instructions on what you want them to do, under which circumstances.
- *Simple tools*—There are several useful tools and items that are highly functional: a small multi-tool or pocket knife (make sure you store that in check-in luggage), high-quality torch or headlight (with solar charger), gaffer tape (fixes almost anything from holes in your pockets to broken bones), superglue, and a small notebook with a pencil in a waterproof zip-lock bag. You may also bring a couple of survival tins for smaller items that you can select according to need, e.g., a fishing line, wire saw, fire starter, etc.
- *Medical kit*—Bring a small medical kit with some basic diagnostic tools and medicines, to treat patients but also team members should they fall ill. Spend some time to think about possible training you require, in particular, emergency and life support training.
- *Your personal mental health*—Bring yourself a simple treat—e.g., a music playlist on a simple music player, a mindfulness/meditation/biofeedback phone app, a favorite movie on a tablet, a book, or some sweets.

Summary

Having a resilient mindset and having done the right physical and mental preparation is essential not only to make yourself useful to the people you want to help, your team, and your organization; but also to make your volunteering a rewarding and enjoyable experience. While the grab-bag concept helps you to best prepare for the more challenging environments, it is also a very useful framework to use for any kind of trip, even your next holiday.

Appendix: Resources for Preparation for Humanitarian Work

Courses:
- HELP: https://www.icrc.org/en/document/helpcourse
- HEAT: Offered by several organizations in several countries, an example: https://www.separinternational.com/heat-training/
- International Federation of the Red Cross learning platform (various courses): https://ifrc.csod.com/client/ifrc/default.aspx
- Disaster Ready (various online courses): https://www.disasterready.org/
- UN field security online courses: https://training.dss.un.org/
- RedR courses: https://www.redr.org.uk/
- Global Health Learning Center: https://www.globalhealthlearning.org/
- Relief Web: https://reliefweb.int/
- Centre for Excellence in Disaster Management: https://www.cfe-dmha.org/
- How to use a two-way radio: https://www.csudh.edu/Assets/csudh-sites/dhpd/emergency-preparedness/two%20way%20radio%20protocol.pdf

Travel Medicine Links:
- Centers for Disease Control (US): https://wwwnc.cdc.gov/travel
- National Health Travel Network and Centre (UK): https://nathnac.net/
- MD health: https://redplanet.travel/mdtravelhealth/destinations/
- Check travel advice for your destination in your country of residence, and check with your country of destination consulate's website for any advice. Be aware of any legal vaccination requirements (e.g., yellow fever).

Destination Research:
- Do a google search on the country/place of your destination, identify reliable sources of information
- Check local and international reliable news outlets about most up-to-date information
- Visit your countries foreign ministry website for country-specific information, e.g., https://travel.state.gov/content/travel.html (US), https://www.gov.uk/government/organisations/foreign-commonwealth-office (UK)

- Country information on the CIA World Factbook: https://www.cia.gov/library/publications/the-world-factbook/
- Travel risk map: https://www.travelriskmap.com/#/planner/map/security
- Road Travel Safety: https://www.asirt.org/
- Travel Safety in general: http://globaled.us/safeti/, http://globaled.us/plato/
- Global weather: https://weather.com/, https://www.metoffice.gov.uk/, check national/local weather forecasts, depending on environment check specific weather forecasts, e.g., mountain, coast/sea

Mental Health and Well-Being Links:
- The Center for Mind Body Medicine: https://cmbm.org/self-care/
- Disaster Rescue and Response Workers 2017 https://www.ptsd.va.gov/professional/treatment/early/disaster-rescue-response.asp
- A movie about the experience of humanitarian workers deployed to the Haiti earthquake: http://amybrathwaite.com/portfolio_page/kick-at-the-darkness

Generic Links:
- Global Health Quick Medical Reference: https://sites.google.com/view/hswtllc/global-health-quick-medical-reference
- AAP Pediatric Disaster Topic Collection: https://www.aap.org/en-us/advocacy-and-policy/aap-health-initiatives/Children-and-Disasters/Pages/Pediatric-Terrorism-And-Disaster-Preparedness-Resource.aspx

Phone Apps:[1]

- Travel documents and preparation: https://www.tripit.com/web
- Survival/Bushcraft: Survival Guide, SAS Survival Guide, Wild Plant Survival Guide, Bushcraft
- Maps/Navigation: Waypoint, View Ranger, Karta, Avenza
- Communication: Google translate
- Medical tools: Medline/Pubmed, Medscape, Up to Date, resuscitation apps, medical calculators, Drug reference apps
- Safety/Security: Life 360, phone tracker
- Humanitarian General: HSP (Humanitarian Standards Partnership), OCHA humanitarian kiosk, UNHCR Emergency Handbook, CBM humanitarian hands-on tool
- Mental Health: Mindfulness, Head Space, Meditation, Zazen, Buddhify, Inner Balance

---

[1] Please note: This is a random selection representing some experience by the author who has no stake in any of these apps.

First Aid Kit List

Diagnostics/tools	Injury/wounds	Medical care
Gloves, facemasks, hand sanitizer	Selection of plasters and dressings	Small number of syringes, injection needles, venflons/butterflies, alcohol wipes
Thermometer	Burns dressing	Pain killers: ibuprofen, paracetamol. Consider ketamine or opiod analgesic (e.g., fentanyl, tramadol, codeine)[a]
Pulse oximeter	Hemostatic dressings	Antibiotics: ceftriaxone (for emergency), oral amoxicillin, clarithromycin, ciprofloxacin, co-amoxiclav
Blood pressure cuff and manometer	Gauze, bandages	Strong antihistamine, IV/oral steroids
Scissors, pincers, tick remover	Stitches, Steri-strips, wound glue, scalpel	Anti-emetic (ondansetron), omeprazole, racecadotril
Tourniquet	Antiseptic fluid and cream	
Mini otoscope/ophthalmoscope	Eyewash (0.9% saline)	
Gaffer tape	Tranexamic acid tablets	
Pocket emergency mask, Guedel/nasopharyngeal tube	Dental repair kit	

[a]Be aware of legal restrictions in many countries

A Simple Mindfulness Exercise

This is a simple exercise to become aware of your thoughts and feelings, putting these into a wider context of reality, letting go and relax. You can do this for as long as you like (minimum 5–10 min) and this works best if you make this kind of exercise a regular habit before you go on your deployment

- Find a quiet space where you can be undisturbed.
- Find a comfortable sitting position, on the floor or on a chair, with your upper body and head upright and self-supporting. Rest your hands in your lap or on your thighs. Roll your head in a circle a couple of times in each direction to relax your neck and back muscles.
- You can close your eyes (or keep them half open, focusing on some imaginary point in the distance).
- Gently sway your upper body from side to side and back and front with ever smaller movements, until you feel you are sitting well balanced. Then remain as motionless as possible for the rest of the meditation.
- Take 2–3 deep breaths, and then allow your breathing to settle into a normal, comfortable rhythm.

- Observe your breath (without altering it in any way), feel the cool air entering your nostrils, flowing down your throat, entering your chest, pushing out your abdomen. Feel it leaving your body the same way. Stay with the breath; if it helps you can quietly count your breaths on breathing out.
- It is absolutely normal that thoughts and feelings will very quickly distract you from observing your breaths. When you notice this, give the thought or feeling a simple short label (e.g., "thinking about my daughter" or "feeling happy"; or simply: "thinkng" or "feeling") without elaborating on it, and return simply to observe your breathing.
- Thoughts and feelings are like floating clouds in the sky of life. They come and go, the sky remains. We have a choice if we feed our thoughts and feelings with our energy, or allow them to simply pass by.

Do this exercise on a regular basis—regardless of how you feel or what your thoughts are. If you make this routine, you may find that you can more easily activate this state of mind by taking 2–3 breaths and close your eyes for a moment, for example, in a stressful situation.

References

1. Asgary R, Lawrence K. Characteristics, determinants and perspectives of experienced medical humanitarians: a qualitative approach. BMJ Open. 2014;4(12):e006460.
2. Ripoll Gallardo A, Djalali A, Foletti M, Ragazzoni L, Della Corte F, Lupescu O, et al. Core competencies in disaster management and humanitarian assistance: a systematic review. Disaster Med Public Health Prep. 2015;9(4):430–9.
3. Burnett A, Peel M. Health needs of asylum seekers and refugees. BMJ. 2001;322:544–7.
4. Shannon P, O'Dougherty M, Mehta E. Study: communicating torture and war experiences with primary care providers. Ment Health Fam Med. 2012;9(1):47–55.
5. Shannon PJ. Refugees' advice to physicians: How to ask about mental health. Fam Pract. 2014;31(4):462–6.
6. Sheikh A, Gatrad R, Dhami S. Consultations for people from minority groups. BMJ. 2008;337(1):a273.
7. Huschke S. Performing deservingness. Humanitarian health care provision for migrants in Germany. Soc Sci Med. 2014;120:352–9.
8. Gedde M. Working in international development and humanitarian assistance. 1st ed. London: Routledge; 2015.
9. Britt TW, Adler AB. Stress and health during medical humanitarian assistance missions. Mil Med. 1999;164(4):275–9.
10. Rizkalla N, Segal SP. Trauma during humanitarian work: the effects on intimacy, wellbeing and PTSD-symptoms. Eur J Psychotraumatol. 2019;10(1):1679065.
11. Lopes Cardozo B, Gotway Crawford C, Eriksson C, Zhu J, Sabin M, Ager A, et al. Psychological distress, depression, anxiety, and burnout among international humanitarian aid workers: a longitudinal study. PLoS One. 2012;7(9):e44948.
12. Smith EC, Holmes L, Burkle FM. The physical and mental health challenges experienced by 9/11 first responders and recovery workers: a review of the literature. Prehosp Disaster Med. 2019;34(6):625–31.
13. Young T, Pakenham KI. Risk and protective factors for aid worker mental health: the effects of job context, Working conditions and demographics. Disasters. 1 May 2020.

14. Nevin RL. A serious nightmare: psychiatric and neurologic adverse reactions to mefloquine are serious adverse reactions. Pharmacol Res Perspect. 2017;5(4):e00328.
15. Salmani I, Seyedin H, Ardalan A, Farajkhoda T. Conceptual model of managing health care volunteers in disasters: a mixed method study. BMC Health Serv Res. 2019;19(1):241.
16. Messner R. My life at the limit. 1st ed. Seattle, WA: Mountaineers Books; 2014.
17. Nehberg R. Wikipedia. 2020 [cited 2020 May 4]. Available from: https://en.wikipedia.org/w/index.php?title=R%C3%BCdiger_Nehberg&oldid=950211713.
18. Ladigan D. Lighten up! A complete handbook for light and ultralight backpacking. 1st ed. Guilford: Falcon Guides; 2005.
19. Clelland M. Ultralight backpackin' tips. 1st ed. Guilford: Falcon Guides; 2011.
20. Wiseman JL. SAS survival handbook. London: Harper Collins; 2003.
21. Wilson N. The SAS tracking & navigation handbook. 1st ed. Guilford: Lyons Press; 2002.
22. Cliff P. Mountain navigation. 6th ed. Crayke, York: P. Cliff; 2006.
23. Duff J, Gormly P. Pocket first aid and wilderness medicine. 11th ed. Milnthorpe: Cicerone; 2012.

Further Reading

Johnson C, Anderson SR, Dallimore J. Oxford handbook of expedition and wilderness medicine. 2nd ed. New York: Oxford University Press; 2015.
Lindemann H. Alone at sea. New York: Random House; 1958.

Christian Harkensee, MD, PhD, MSc, DLSHTM, DiMM, MAcadMEd, MFPHC (RCSEd), FHEA, FRCPCH made his first humanitarian experience in Central America in 1987. Since, he became a doctor (Humboldt University Berlin, Germany, 1997), pediatrician and pediatric infectious diseases and immunology specialist (the UK, 2012), researcher (PhD in immunogenetics, the UK, 2012), medical educator (2003), and mountain- and expedition doctor (2017). He has done humanitarian disaster relief, development, and capacity building work in many countries ever since; and is currently leading a health service for refugee children and families in the North East of England.

Sarah Walpole, BSc Int Health, MBChB Med, MSc(Res) Med Educ, MRCP is an Infectious Diseases registrar in Newcastle, the UK. She has worked in various medical and pediatric specialties, completed an Academic Clinical Fellowship in medical education with cardiology, and worked as a Medical Activities Manager and Medical Educator for MSF in DRC, SAMS in Greece, Doctors Worldwide in Bangladesh, and Health in Harmony in Indonesia. She continues to provide telemedicine consultations to junior doctors in Bangladesh. She champions planetary health, including the Association of Medical Education in Europe and the Centre for Sustainable Healthcare. She cofounded the UK's Climate and Health Council and IFMSA's "Healthy Planet" during her studies of International Health at University College London and medicine at Leeds University. She is committed to protecting access to healthcare, including by maintaining the UK's NHS as a publicly funded and publicly provided service, and has undertaken research on privatization with the Centre for Health in the Public Interest.

Environment of Care: Initial Assessment

16

Philip Bruce Murray

Introduction

Finding themselves in a foreign, often unattractive setting, refugee and migrant children face stressful challenges daily that include overcrowding, the loss of privacy and personal space, and a multitude of potential health threats. The need to feel safe is an undeniably important and universal human need that can only be met by the provision of adequate security, along with shelter, clean water, adequate nutrition, and timely and compassionate health care. These common challenges and needs cut across all displaced populations, regardless of location or context. A broad humanitarian response must recognize these needs and, in a coordinated effort with other national and international groups, begin to provide the necessary services in the midst of a chaotic, ever-changing, and at times, hostile environment.

No two refugee settings are the same. They may differ depending on their physical environment, location, the cause of the displacement, and whether the displaced population is relatively homogeneous or whether it is comprised of various ethnic groups with multiple languages, styles of dress, customs, and food. The routine and rhythm of a child's life is suddenly disrupted. Settings for refugee settlement may also vary from extremely rural areas of open land to preexisting refugee camps, or increasingly now, to urban areas.

Refugee camps, as well as integrated urban settings, differ not only in their geographic location but in other important ways that affect the environment of care for both the refugees as well as for the health worker. An important factor to consider across settings initially is the stage of development or phase of the humanitarian response.

P. B. Murray (✉)
Josephine County Public Health Department, Grants Pass, OR, USA

Medical Teams International, Portland, OR, USA

© Springer Nature Switzerland AG 2021
C. Harkensee et al. (eds.), *Child Refugee and Migrant Health*,
https://doi.org/10.1007/978-3-030-74906-4_16

Emergency Phase

The initial awareness and response to a crisis may occur during the migration of an affected group to a new physical setting as they flee a natural catastrophe, armed conflict, persecution, or other threats. Initially, the population may move into an urban or rural setting, into a preexisting refugee setting, or even into an unoccupied field or forest. An example of a refugee settlement arising where there was no prior human habitation was seen in August 2017 when upwards of 700,000 Rohingya began their migration into Bangladesh to the site of an elephant forest reserve adjacent to a preexisting refugee camp to escape the genocide in Myanmar. Here, almost all services available locally needed to be greatly expanded, relocated, and rapidly developed. In rural settings such as this, the initial priority may be constructing primitive tarp and stick tent clinics within the camp in order to provide IV hydration, to distribute ORS and nutrition supplements as needed, and to diagnose and treat lower respiratory infections and diarrheal illnesses. In this early emergency phase, in addition to quickly establishing essential public health services (provision of water, sanitation, shelter, and hygiene) as well as emergency health care, a chief concern is to address the basic needs of the pediatric population. In most refugee settings children usually account for more than half of the total population.

Another chief concern in the emergency phase is to quickly disseminate information in the camp that the medical team being assembled is prioritizing care for children with loose stools, cough, and fever in order to identify children at greatest risk from diarrhea and pneumonia. This highlights the importance of reaching out to refugee community leaders. These local partners can then help disseminate key public health directives and can help develop lasting and vital partnerships between the relief effort and the refugee community at large, with the formation of a community health worker (CHW) program. This is a crucial step in creating a system to share vital information around vaccination, hygiene practices in the home, and when to seek medical attention. A capable CHW program also provides the care team with valuable information about the culture and health care practices and beliefs of the population they are serving, and it may begin earning the trust of the refugee population. These initial relationships between humanitarian workers and the refugee community may grow into mutually beneficial partnerships that should continue to develop over years to come.

In urban settings, the challenges of addressing refugees' needs are equally complex. If the population move was abrupt and unplanned, the refugees may disperse widely throughout a city, usually into lower income or tenement areas. This may make it difficult to track or follow them, much less try to provide for their essential needs. Inadequate shelter, water, and sanitation may present barriers to addressing safety, hygiene, and health needs. Humanitarian response teams may need to employ mobile medical units to travel from site to site to do initial assessments of pediatric populations and address vaccinations and primary care needs. The existing infrastructure in urban settings may be fragile and rapidly overwhelmed due to the number of displaced persons arriving in a short period of time.

In the emergency phase of a humanitarian crisis, the correct selection of the volunteer health workers with respect to their training and background in pediatric care is crucial. The "first-in teams" of health workers and responders need to be experienced, adaptable, self-reliant, and possess leadership skills to mobilize cooperation. Cultural awareness and sensitivity help them to forge relationships with the refugee community and with other NGOs, host country organizations, and UN agencies to meet the myriad initial needs.

Evolution of the Humanitarian Response

Eventually, over the ensuing weeks to months after the onset of a humanitarian crisis, the refugee crisis will evolve. Basic needs of the population will be met more successfully, and more substantial health care facilities will appear. Field outposts for care within the camp may still be needed for primary care but referral facilities and hospital capacity will have developed and matured. The range of services offered to the pediatric population will also have expanded to include broader nutritional care for the moderate and severely malnourished, a more complete menu of vaccinations, improved and expanded pharmacy services, and established referral networks to better address subspecialty needs. The range of skills and experience levels of health workers brought into this environment will correspondingly expand.

The detection and treatment of infectious diseases is one of the highest priorities in the early stages of a humanitarian crisis. However, food insecurity in children especially, manifesting as wasting, stunting, and acute severe malnutrition, also ranks high among the leading early health concerns. In protracted disaster settings, the specter of malnutrition remains throughout the duration of living in a refugee environment and poses an ongoing threat to child welfare. Undernutrition may lead to devastating long-term effects on growth, cognitive development, immunity, and disease susceptibility. Malnutrition is felt to be the single greatest noncommunicable risk for morbidity and mortality of children in these populations. In Chaps. 11 and 22, the effects of malnutrition, its manifestation, detection, and treatment will be covered in greater detail.

The context of refugee settings may differ widely depending on the nature, scale, and location of the humanitarian crisis. Accordingly, health workers may encounter a broad range of attitudes, perceptions, and expectations of healthcare. Genocides, wars, natural disasters may provoke sudden and unexpected migration without warning and rarely discriminate by social strata or economic status. Often those who now find that they are homeless may well be previously well-educated professionals from all walks of life. They may continue to expect high-quality medical care even in this new, unfamiliar refugee setting. They may anticipate that their children will be seen for primary care needs by only experienced pediatricians or subspecialists when those services may not be available. These dilemmas require patience and understanding by the health care worker, in order to earn the trust that is so necessary, and to work effectively within the boundaries of care that a refugee setting imposes.

In addition to these challenges, refugee migration may be a protracted ordeal taking many months to years. The difficult journey may result in multiple international border crossings while experiencing cultural and language differences, discrimination, and overt hostility. Eventually, the arduous trip does end, but all too often prematurely and far short of the original goal, with expectations of a better life often shattered. The living conditions where they are ultimately halted are usually overcrowded and squalid refugee settlements or urban tenements where adequate protection, shelter, nutrition, and healthcare are lacking. Children are especially vulnerable physically and emotionally, at each stage of the journey. Repeated efforts of migrants to legally achieve asylum and to leave the refugee settings are met with prolonged bureaucratic obstruction that may last for years, often masking blatant discrimination due to xenophobia, racism, and the perceived economic insecurity of the destination country. The following sections are designed to cover specific pediatric health care priorities in the first phase of humanitarian response. This is intended to be a broad overview and review of the concerns in the early stages of a crisis, and as such is not intended to be comprehensive.

In assessing communicable disease threats, public health measures are crucial in recognizing vulnerable populations, performing disease surveillance in new arrivals, and in tracking disease contacts. Early in a humanitarian crisis, identifying diseases that have the greatest potential to develop, spread, and cause severe disability and mortality is crucial. Risk assessments done early on are designed to target those diseases at the highest likelihood to develop and spread. In the early phase of response, infection control and disease prevention mean targeting the major communicable disease threats to children.

Communicable Diseases

Measles and Other Communicable Disease Detection and Prevention

At the top of health priorities is assessment of the risk of measles, especially if the camp population is from an area of low immunization rates. Of the four major killers of children under 5 years old (including lower respiratory tract infections, diarrhea, and malaria) measles remains as the most important risk to prioritize initially. Spread by both person-to-person contact and the airborne respiratory route, the impact of measles on a community is influenced by overcrowded conditions, poor sanitation, lack of health care resources, and malnutrition, which are all factors commonly found in refugee settings. In an unvaccinated cohort, measles may be the most infectious communicable disease known [1].

Measles vaccine has been a significant public health advance since its introduction in the 1960s. Despite a significant decline in measles-related deaths over the last 60 years due to vaccination and better management of complications, the disease may still be lethal in a vulnerable population. To prevent widespread dissemination of the virus and large outbreaks of the disease, vaccination efforts must be started early (within the first week of humanitarian response is optimal), achieve a goal of >94% coverage to reach "herd immunity" levels, and provide two doses separated by at least 28 days. Age groups to vaccinate should include 9-month olds to 14-years old, but extending vaccinations up to age 29 has been necessary in some large camp outbreaks [2]. In most settings in the world, the MMR (measles, mumps, rubella combination) is the vaccine of choice because of its simplicity, effectiveness, and safety. The disadvantage of both MMR and monovalent measles vaccines is that they require a cold chain (refrigeration), which presents a great challenge in the early days of a humanitarian crisis.

Despite the best public health efforts, measles outbreaks still occur in refugee settings. It is crucial that health care workers be able to identify, isolate, and treat cases as effectively as possible. Measles is transmitted by coughing and sneezing with subsequent entry into the lungs followed by widespread dissemination leading to systemic infection. The incubation period is 7–21 days and it is important to realize that the prodromal symptoms (fever >38 °C, coryza, and/or conjunctivitis) occur 4 days prior to the rash. Koplik spots (multiple small white plaques on the buccal mucosa) may also appear 1–2 days prior to the rash. They may be seen in ~70% of cases and are important to look for as they are pathognomonic for measles [3]. The typical measles rash starts on the face and spreads peripherally, lasting 3–7 days. The disease can cause severe pneumonia, as well as otitis media, diarrhea, and sometimes fatal encephalitis. A state of immune suppression may develop that can last for 2 months or more. Malnutrition (especially vitamin A deficiency) is a significant contributor to life-threatening complications. Early case detection, treatment, and isolation are paramount, as are community efforts to begin contact identifications and infection control measures.

Treatment of measles is supportive, including close fluid management, nutrition support, vitamin A supplementation, and antibiotics for clinical pneumonia as bacterial superinfection is possible. There is no effective antiviral therapy. Vitamin A administration (100,000 units for ages 6–11 months, 200,000 units for 12–59 months) is vitally important as it appears to reduce complications, severity of the disease, and mortality.

Prevention of Diarrheal Illnesses Including Cholera

Fecal oral transmission is the common mode of transmission of all infectious diarrheal illnesses. Therefore, key to prevention is assuring that clean water is available in public settings as well as in the homes, adequate and accessible toileting and sanitation facilities are in place, and hygiene measures are taught and practiced (see Fig. 16.1). Broad public health initiatives with widespread community participation on topics such as hand washing, and safe food preparation and serving are critical. Having CHWs disseminate culturally oriented hygiene information as well as soap, basins, and clean water to individual residences may have a significant influence on the reduction of diarrheal illnesses.

Fig. 16.1 Hand drawn poster on the wall of the diarrhea treatment unit, October 2017, Kutapalong Refugee Camp, Cox's Bazar, Bangladesh. (Author's photo)

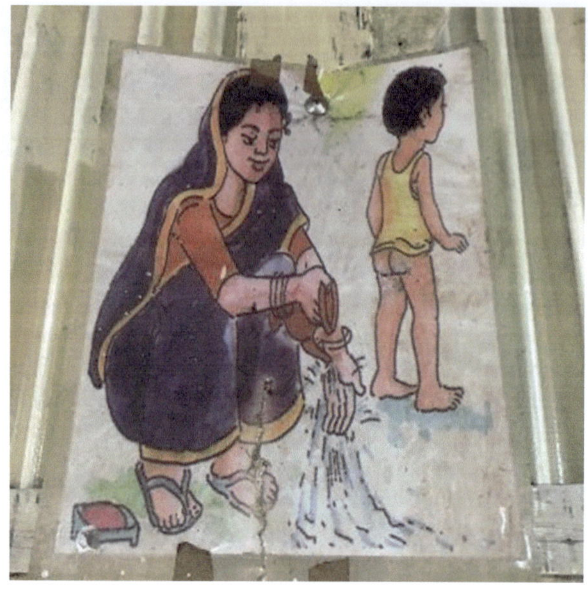

Cholera, which will be covered more in Part 4, Chap. 24, "Gastrointestinal Issues in Refugee Settings" section, is the most dangerous form of acute watery diarrhea. All of the infection control measures noted above assume even a greater sense of purpose during a cholera outbreak. Urgent treatment requires aggressive oral, and at times intravenous, rehydration of affected children. Special inpatient diarrhea treatment units may need to be created to consolidate the treatment required.

Water, Sanitation, and Hygiene

Pivotal to the prevention of diarrhea in a refugee setting are instituting measures to establish clean water sources, to provide adequate means for disposal of human waste, and to promote effective hygiene methods. In accordance with standards promoted by the Sphere Project it is estimated that a minimum of 15 liters a day per person, regardless of age, are needed to meet the requirements for drinking water, cooking purposes, and hygiene, and that the aim should be to provide 30–40 l/person if possible [5]. Assessing the water availability is done by measuring the output of a water source over 1 min multiplied by the time in minutes that the source actually runs per day. Dividing the total volume of water from a source daily by the number of people it supplies will generate the number of l/day/person. Furthermore, access to the water source should be no more than 500 yards away from the household, with no more than 30 min of waiting in a line. These are important parameters for unaccompanied children especially, as they are often assigned the task of water collection for the family and are at heightened risk for gender-based violence and abduction at water collection sites and toileting facilities. Additional water capacity may be needed for the demands of institutions, clinics, schools, places of worship, and governmental and NGO camp facilities. These goals may be extremely difficult to meet in the early chaotic days of establishing the infrastructure of a new refugee settlement. In the earliest stages of a disaster, the quantity of water provided trumps quality as thirst and severe dehydration are major causes of early morbidity and mortality, especially in children. Clean or sterilized water is then the very next priority to meet once possible.

The key questions regarding initial water supply are: what are the sources of the water currently being used and are they safe? The answers may depend on multiple factors: the physical location of the refugee settlement, presence of preexisting water sources and intact plumbing, feasibility of drilling wells, presence of surface, ground, or river water that will require purification, capture of rainfall, or even logistical capacity to truck in freshwater. After water filtration, dry or liquid chlorine for purification for personal use requires accurate and careful measurement for drinking as well as for disinfection purposes but may be a useful adjunct to obtaining clean, potable water (see Gastrointestinal Issues in Refugee Settings, Chap. 24 for chlorination recommendations). Point of use water treatment in the homes may employ microfiltration devices, ultraviolet or solar disinfection methods. Natural UV light (sunlight) exposure for 8 hours is an effective way of water disinfection for small volumes, but the water must be free of visible matter and the container must be clean and transparent.) Boiling clear and filtered water for 1 min (3 min if above 2000 m) is another option but requires a continuous source of fuel such as wood, charcoal, or rarely available propane gas fueled stoves. Boiled and filtered water may quickly become contaminated again if adequate clean and covered water storage containers are not available.

Sanitation measures should start as soon as humanitarian relief arrives. First, specific areas or open spaces should be designated for defecation, separated, and screened off by gender, while pit latrines (or optimally, pour-flush latrines) are being dug. Both practices should be placed away from the clean water access points and away from lakes and streams where children may play (see Fig. 16.2). Access and use of toilets must be safe and protected, especially for women and children, at any time of the day-night.

The goal is that no more than 20 people or 4 households share one latrine [5]. Individual household latrines may be more culturally acceptable and more hygienic but usually are limited by available space and resources. Secure, gender-specific latrines are optimal when feasible. Public health measures of providing soap and water stations for hand washing and education on proper hygiene techniques for toileting are essential and are again a key motivation for utilizing refugee CHWs as soon as they may be identified and trained.

Promoting public education on hygiene techniques is crucial to prevention of water-based disease outbreaks. However, introducing new practices in a culturally acceptable manner is key and involves close coordination with refugee representatives who are respected within their communities. Priorities of a capable WASH program therefore include: safe water transport and storage, proper maintenance of latrines, education on the importance of hand washing after defecation particularly,

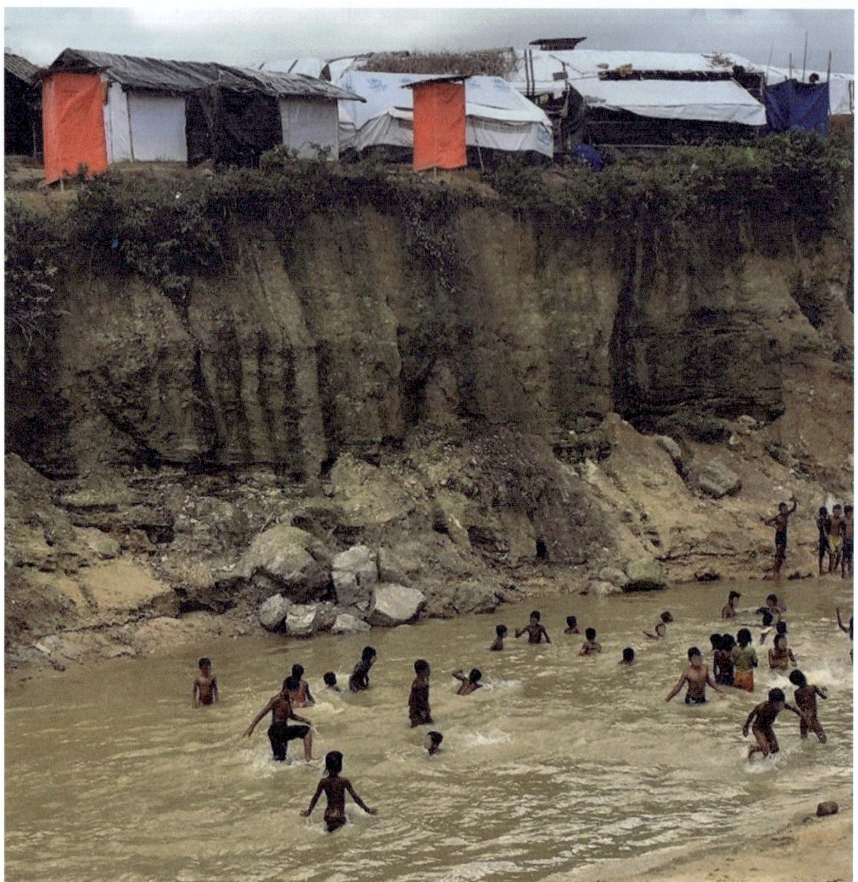

Fig. 16.2 Orange latrines sit above the contaminated stream flowing through Kutupalong Refugee Camp, Bangladesh, October 2017. (Author's personal photograph)

proper food storage and preparation, and appropriate care of those affected with diarrhea within the household.

Shelter and Clinic Settings

In an ideal world, displaced children would come in an orderly fashion to a location that was already well organized and designed with sufficient security, community space, adequate family shelters, and appropriate infrastructure for water, sewage, health care, and food procurement. Refugees certainly do not live in that world. When they flee the disaster in their homeland it is often collectively, under chaotic and dangerous conditions, bringing only the clothes that they wear and possessions that they carry. Once they reach a zone of perceived safety, sometimes across an international border, further trauma, fatigue, hunger, and thirst become the main concerns. Their highest priority is safety for themselves and for their family members. Often they will cease their journey out of sheer exhaustion and claim a very small parcel of open or available space that may scarcely be large enough for the family to lie down upon. Their first nights may be spent on bare ground before even primitive shelters are erected from sticks and thin plastic sheeting. When available, tents may provide more substantial yet still temporary housing. As thousands and thousands more arrive, often many days before there is a coordinated national or international response to the crisis, a new refugee settlement is born.

Unfortunately, the overcrowding and lack of adequate shelter and basic services that are common in hastily assembled refugee settlements provide a fertile environment for the diseases and malnutrition that soon come to characterize them. The direct link between shelter and health in these settings is well known. By necessity, the initial humanitarian health response may be a similarly primitive tarp lean-to or tent set up to treat those affected by diarrhea and respiratory problems. Access to antibiotics (especially pediatric formulations) and other essential drugs, oral rehydration fluids, and IV fluids is especially important at this early stage. Alternately, if roads and vehicles are available, use of mobile medical units may be an effective way to access the sick in remote reaches of a new settlement or urban setting, especially for those too weak to travel to established clinics or hospitals.

Safety

In Maslow's paradigm of human needs first published in 1943 [6], the importance of safety, particularly in regard to the needs of children, is the second most important foundational block of his hierarchical pyramid of human motivation. It rests just above the basic physiologic needs such as thirst and hunger. There is no better illustration of this than in a refugee setting where populations often escape from an area of extreme danger only to land in a setting of chaos and inconsistency. Children will likely be very sensitive to the insecurity of their new setting. Where they need reassurance and rhythm, they more often encounter unpredictability and lack of structure resulting in further emotional and physical harm. Early in the formation of a new camp, child-safe zones for play, learning, self-expression, and blanket feeding programs should be established in the community to address these needs.

In 1994 the UNHCR published "Refugee Children, Guidelines on Protection and Care" [7], recognizing the unique vulnerability of refugee children facing multiple threats to their physical, emotional and spiritual security, and their developmental well-being. This report is periodically updated and summarizes international consensus on the minimal standards for expected care. It promotes the concept that we should all be advocates for children especially in the refugee setting where disease, undernutrition, and physical injury are common. It covers many aspects of child refugee risk including threats to the rights of a child under international law, the importance of their native culture, the prevention of abuse and exploitation, and the unique challenge of unaccompanied minors.

Safety also means that children, in particular, must be physically protected in their new and foreign environment. Security, both armed and unarmed, is usually provided by the host country army or state police force. In addition, establishing or reinforcing community watch and supervision programs is critical. These can develop spontaneously, especially if the overall population is relatively homogenous in regard to language and culture. If not, systems must be put into place to protect children and especially unaccompanied children as they are easy targets of conflict and abuse between dissimilar groups and even within their own culture.

Humanitarian Work in the Setting of Scarce Resources

One of the greatest adjustments for new humanitarian aid workers is that care, as we know it in our developed world, is difficult if not impossible to emulate in the stark reality of a refugee setting. When even basic necessities such as water, food, shelter, and security are in short supply, providing high-quality medical services to a diverse displaced population presents a tall challenge. There are certainly published guidelines by UNHCR for essential medication lists and for what comprises basic health care services that should be available and considered even in the early days of the catastrophe [8, 9]. However, there are often great challenges to meeting these standards—pulling together the necessary pediatric medications, IV fluids, administration sets, bandages and dressings, minor surgical sets, splints, water supply, purification means, nutritional support, latrines, waste disposal, adequate physical clinic structure, necessary human resources, and the list continues. One must come prepared to face these challenges with creativity and adaptability. Success depends on the ability to handle shortcomings, inefficiencies, omissions, and frustrations as calmly and as productively as possible. Creative and collaborative problem-solving can be an effective way to work through the frustrations seen daily. Especially in the early phase of a humanitarian response where essential supplies and meds are still in the process of being mobilized, it is vital to remember that your very presence, your calmness, and your compassion are important therapeutic tools in themselves.

The Importance of Collaboration and Partnership

The complex history of how a coordinated multifaceted international response to humanitarian disasters developed is not within the province of this book. Going back as far as the founding of the International Committee of the Red Cross (ICRC) in 1859, there have since been many humanitarian calamities around the world that have shaped the subsequent policies of international response. The genocide in Rwanda in 1994, the Darfur conflict and famine of 2004, and the earthquake disaster in Haiti in 2010 are just some of the more recent sentinel events that have helped shape a code of humanitarian conduct, improved leadership, a more coordinated international response, and ultimately, more accountability. Does that mean that modern disaster response is now a well-oiled model of efficiency and cooperation?

No, unfortunately not. However, the humanitarian response has evolved and become significantly more successful through improved interagency communication, coordination between key players with different priorities and constituencies, and more transparency in how responsibility is delegated.

In the setting of a new rapidly developing disaster the host country must decide if it is capable of handling the needs within its borders or whether it needs international support. If outside assistance is requested it is usually under the auspices of the UN Office for the Coordination of Humanitarian Affairs (OCHA), which helps to mold the international response across UN, governmental, and non-governmental lines of command and communication (see Fig. 16.3). The host nation's response and ongoing participation in the crisis is absolutely critical and their active participation and consent is vital to the long-term success of the project and ultimately the recovery and reconstruction phases. Figure 16.3 illustrates the interrelationship of the different actors in disaster response and the importance of cooperation between agencies [10].

Once a disaster response is underway, the various actors must work collaboratively to manage the four major sectors of immediate concern: WASH, shelter, nutrition, and health. No one sector reacts in isolation as there are multiple layers of shared responsibilities. Each sector has its own area of focus, but none function independently of the other (see Fig. 16.4).

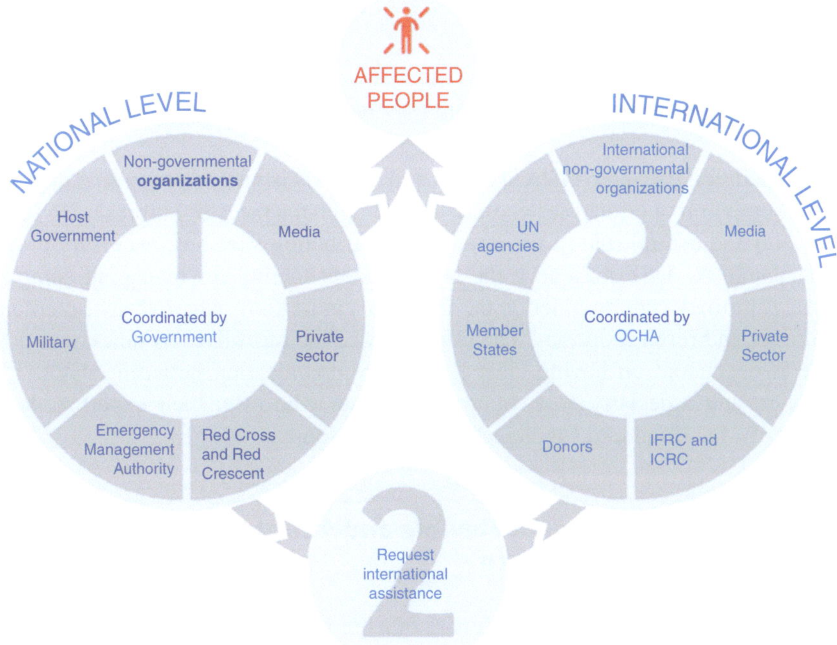

Fig. 16.3 Graphic(s) provided courtesy of the UN Office of Humanitarian Affairs

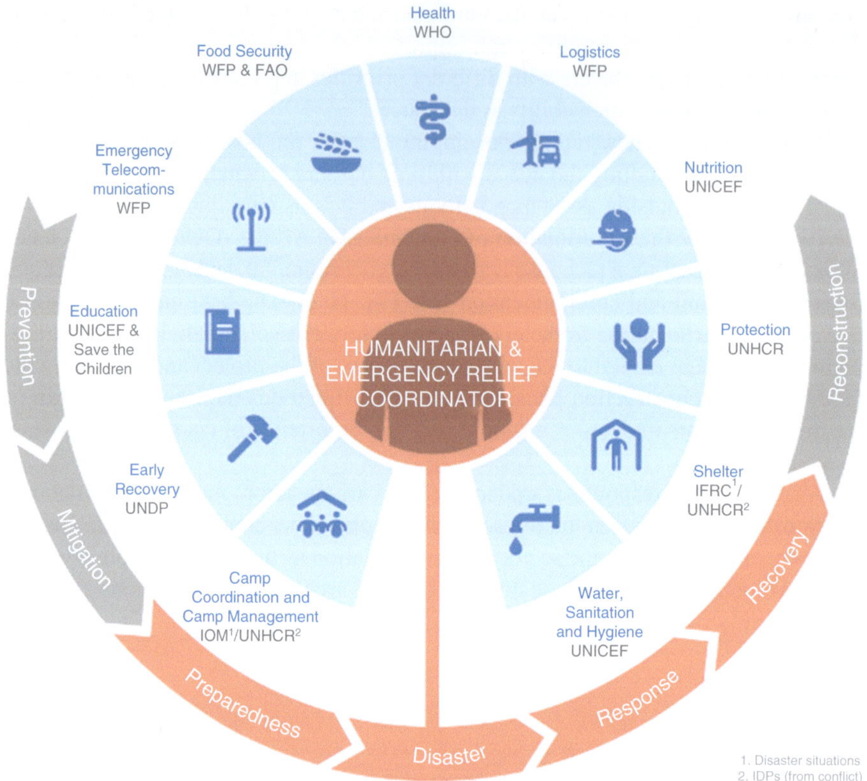

Fig. 16.4 Graphic(s) provided courtesy of the UN Office of Humanitarian Affairs

Cooperation between different actors and agencies is vital to preventing duplication or omission of critical services. In the example of a measles outbreak, UNICEF may play the central role in procuring and distributing vaccines, necessary drugs, and vitamin A. MSF may have the best inpatient facility for managing complex cases. A primary care provider on the front lines must know where to access crucial resources and referral options. The effort to save the most lives as quickly as possible is dependent on having clear lines of communication between NGOs, UN agencies, and especially host country authorities who offer their expertise, local familiarity, facilities, and supplemental human resources.

Importance of Remaining Flexible and Adaptable in a Changing Circumstance

Especially early on in the response phase of a humanitarian disaster, health workers will find themselves in a uniquely different environment of care than they are accustomed to. They may find themselves to be "displaced" as well and coping with new challenges each day. Even if they know in advance the specific role that is expected of them, they should not be surprised to encounter difficulties with their new environment on several levels:

1. Instead of a well-equipped clinic or hospital setting, they may find themselves improvising in crude handmade structures (e.g., tarps, tents, lean-tos) or in an overcrowded tenement located in a vast inner city. Electricity, plumbing, and clean water may be unreliable or unavailable. Climate may be harsh and unfamiliar. A health worker should anticipate noise, lack of adequate space, confusion, and rarely enough time to do a thorough evaluation of the child.
2. Communication with host country staff and patients will require interpreters, who may be unpaid volunteers. Much can be "lost in translation" as one navigates an oral history with an ill, frightened child through a distraught parent, via an inexperienced interpreter.
3. The displaced population may be of an entirely different culture with alternative perspectives on health care. Parents may not initially trust someone foreign to them to see, much less touch, their children. Parent and caregiver understandings of basic health concepts may fall far from usual expectations.
4. Those that are displaced may not yet feel safe in their new homes and may be processing fresh emotional and physical traumas. You will likely need to find clever and creative ways to entertain or at least distract frightened children in what may be an unusually spartan or unattractive setting. Trauma-informed care is paramount.

In short, both the health worker and the population served are displaced and are functioning in new environments of care. It is important not to forget that the workers as well as refugees may be processing great changes, although on wholly different scales. Sharing experiences with coworkers and having protected personal time may shed new light and perspectives on these experiences and the role one plays therein.

Do not be daunted by the enormity of the world's grief.

Do justly, now.

Love mercy, now.

Walk humbly, now.

You are not obligated to complete the work.

But neither are you free to abandon it.

(The Talmud, Micah Chapter 6, verse 8)

References

1. Durrheim D. Measles-the epidemiology of elimination. Vaccine. 2014;32:6880–3.
2. Lam E. Measles. In: Townes D, editor. Health in humanitarian emergencies. Cambridge: Cambridge Press; 2018. p. 386–99.

3. Lefebvre N, Camuset G, Bui E, et al. Koplik spots: a clinical sign with epidemiological implications for measles control. Dermatology. 2010;220:280–1.
4. Measles photo from Mayo Clinic website: patient care and health information. Measles symptoms and causes. Mayoclinic.org/diseases-conditions/measles/symptoms/syc-20374857.
5. Water supply, sanitation, and hygiene promotion. In: The sphere handbook 2018. Rugby: Practical Action Publishing; 2018. p. 89–156.
6. Maslow AH. A theory of motivation. Psychol Rev. 1943;50:370–96. Republished online by Green, CD. Classics in the history of psychology. Toronto. ISSN: 1492-3713, http://psychclassics.yorku.ca/Maslow/motivation.htm.
7. UN High Commissioner for Refugees (UNHCR). Refugee children: guidelines on protection and care. 1994. Available at: https://www.refworld.org/docid/3ae6b3470.html.
8. UNHCR's essential medicines and medical supplies policy and guidance. 2013. Geneva. https://www.unhcr.org/protection/health/527baab09/unhcrs-essential-medicines-medical-supplies.
9. UNHCR. Emergency handbook, primary health care staffing standard, version 1.7. Geneva: UNHCR. https://emergency.unhcr.org/entry/93522/primary-health-care-staffing-standard.
10. OHCA. This is OHCA, coordination. Geneva. 2015. Available at: https://www.unocha.org/sites/dms/Documents/this_is_ocha_2015.pdf
11. OCHA Services Humanitarian Response. What is the cluster approach? Geneva. Available at: https://www.humanitarianresponse.info/en/about-clusters/what-is-the-cluster-approach.

Philip Bruce Murray, MD, DTM&H was trained as a general internist at the University of California, San Francisco. He has practiced in academic settings, on a Native American reservation, and in private practice in rural communities California and Oregon. Since 2006 he has done volunteer work in multiple low resource settings including refugee camps in Uganda, Greece, and Bangladesh. He has written clinical protocols for both acute and noncommunicable chronic diseases for different international NGOs. He assisted in the Rohingya humanitarian disaster in Bangladesh in 2017, helping to develop early field clinics and opening a 24-bed field hospital for acute diarrheal illness. He was involved in the capacity building of Bangladeshi physicians teaching refugee medicine, tropical disease, and epidemic management on two subsequent trips in 2018. He now works for Josephine County, Oregon, as COVID-19 medical liaison and contact tracing coordinator.

Data Collection, Surveillance, and Response to Epidemics and Pandemics in Refugee Settings

17

Ramin Asgary

Introduction: A Surveillance System for Infectious Diseases

Through gathering information and data on health indicators on a regular basis, public health surveillance functions as a "test" to assess the community-level health status. Surveillance will help monitor and understand the population health over time, investigate disease distribution, devise prevention strategies, prioritize health actions, ultimately estimate and plan for adequate response and treatment and maintain routine health activities. Just as a complete blood count test for a patient could help identify early signs of an underlying or imminent infection, the constant disease surveillance at the community-level provides an important window into current disease trends or an impeding infectious disease outbreak.

The surveillance information will help health personnel in early detection of a significant health issue with a high risk of transmission to the population, and better prepare them in addressing the prevention and management of specific infectious or noninfectious diseases such as Cholera, Shigella, SARS, or a chemical and environmental exposure. For example, diarrhea occurs in refugee settings on a regular basis and at some baseline level, especially among children. But if we observe that a significant number of adults present with diarrheal symptoms or with a specific presentation such as bloody or voluminous watery diarrhea, this will be an indication of an important public health issue. Similarly, if diarrhea is accompanied by fever and occurs in a vicinity or around a specific well or water point in a refugee settlement, or within other subgroups of the refugee population, it could indicate an impending epidemic.

R. Asgary (✉)
Department of Global Health, Milken Institute School of Public Health and Elliott School of International Affairs, George Washington University, Washington, DC, USA

Department of Medicine, Weill Cornell Medical College, Cornell University, New York, NY, USA
e-mail: ga263@columbia.edu

C. Harkensee et al. (eds.), *Child Refugee and Migrant Health*,
https://doi.org/10.1007/978-3-030-74906-4_17

In a refugee setting, one of the first public health strategies should be to set up a well-functioning, reliable, and reproducible public health surveillance system [1–3]. This largely happens through syndromic surveillance, meaning that the data is largely collected via observation or questioning of the population, as there is often limited avilability of patient-level laboratory tests. However, most of the broader control strategies will involve some form of testing such as assessing the presence of coliform pathogens at water sources or regular or intermittent malaria testing. The basic concept is to assure a wide set of health indicators are regularly collected so that we can observe and assess trends and predict an outbreak.

It is important to have a set of criteria for the detection of an impending epidemic. Multiple different types of thresholds have been used for different diseases [1, 3]. These may have to be adjusted depending on the size of the population or characteristics of that specific disease. For example, studies have shown that a rate of 15 or more cases of meningococcal meningitis per 100,000 persons per week, or higher than a baseline or usual average rate in a specific population, over two or more consecutive weeks were sensitive and specific with a high likelihood (predictive value) for an impending meningitis epidemic. If the population size is small, then doubling of meningitis cases from 1 week to the next over a 3-week period should increase the suspicion of an impending outbreak. A significant increase in the admission of children/patients 5 years and above also suggests the likelihood of an outbreak.

Surveillance definition: It is an ongoing, systematic collection, analysis and interpretation of health data essential to the planning, implementation, and evaluation of public health practices that is closely integrated with timely dissemination to those who need to know and use it [1, 2]. Surveys are complementary to surveillance. They supplement rapid health assessment strategies and ongoing surveillance. They could be used intermittently with focused assessments that collect population-based health data. General types of surveys include; convenience (non-random), simple random in which a randomly selected group of responders or observation occurs, cluster surveys in which random selection of respondents or observations happens in geographic clusters, or exhaustive sampling through widespread random selection in a large population [1–4].

The practical steps in surveillance could be categorized in the following phase responses: Immediate actions, long-term actions, setting up systems, and protection. These include identification of cases, case definitions, community mobilizations and communication strategy, generic or specific targeted action plans, human resource needs and training, coordination among actors, isolation and protection of the vulnerable population, therapeutic and or treatment modalities, and external resources [1, 2, 5].

Key aspects of an effective surveillance system: Simplicity, timelines, accuracy, and regular feedback to the people who collect data and indicators. The simplest monitoring procedure is weekly tabulation of admissions and consultations by diagnosis in health centers and regular household visits and data collection. Frequent feedback of the results to local clinics or field hospital personnel will increase reporting as well as allowing the institution of preventive measures.

Devising an Epidemic Response: The Basics

Strengthening Surveillance

Local literate non-health or health workers can be trained quickly to collect information in regards to clinical case definitions, admissions to hospitals, or diagnoses made in ambulatory sites, and complete weekly reports (see Appendix 1 for an example). Simple software such as EpiInfo and Excel could be used. Data needs to include sociodemographic information such as age or date of birth, sex, date of consultation or diagnosis, actual diagnoses, current residence in the camp, social characteristics such as customs and norms, new arrivals, particular ethnic group, and time lived in the camp [1, 2, 5]. Cases of disease or death could be presented and tabulated in numbers per 1,000, 10,000 or 100,000 per week [1–3]. The Epidemic Response includes plans for immunization, including necessary equipment, medication distribution to patients, and informing the public about plans.

Case Detection

Epidemics require case definitions that include clinical data. For example, in case of bacterial meningitis it could be "an illness with sudden onset of fever above 38.5°C with one or more of the following: neck stiffness, altered mental status, and petechial or purpuric rash" [4]. Ideally, laboratory diagnosis, if available, should be performed early in the epidemic to confirm the source pathogen. In case of meningitis, this could be via a positive CSF antigen or a positive culture. Case definition could be a *suspect case* when the patient meets only the clinical definition or a *probable case* when the patient meets clinical case definition plus some of positive tests (for example, a turbid/purulent CSF or positive gram stain) or be part of an epidemic and linked to another case [4, 5]. *Confirmed cases* will be a probable case plus lab confirmation. Each clinical case definition will have some sensitivity (likelihood to detect all genuine cases) and specificity (likelihood that a negative test exclude the disease in all genuine negative cases) in itself. Generally speaking, we choose a high sensitivity case definition when the disease is highly communicable, has a high case-fatality rate, or we do not care to identify many who do not have the disease. We prefer clinical case definitions with higher specificity when we try to identify the genuine cases, do not want to treat people without disease (because of risk of resistance to medications such as in TB or HIV) or when the disease has a relatively low case-fatality rate. Table 17.1 in Appendix 2 presents some case definitions. Detailed examples of case definitions are presented in Chap. 16.

Prevention and Epidemic Control

Epidemics create high fears, could be very fatal, and could cause rapid influx of many patients to health facilities and disrupt health systems. Rapid assessment of suspected cases and identification of high-risk groups are the key. Priority should be given to early collection of specimens or samples to confirm the causative agent and to determine serogroup as well as antibiotics or treatment resistance patterns [1–4]. An epidemic committee needs to be assembled to coordinate public health efforts, gather information from different parts of the refugee settlement, plot the course of epidemic, coordinate intervention efforts, and promote the community knowledge and skills on control measures such as prevention and protection, vaccination, and to overcome unreasonable fears and rumors. Coordination to get medical supplies and medications, personnel, and equipment is urgently needed because most epidemics will evolve quickly, intensify, and then fade away within the first 12–18 weeks [1–6].

Phases of an Epidemic Response

The course of an epidemic depends on the specific type of the pathogen and its propensity to spread (reproductive rate). However, for most of the highly contagious infectious agents you could follow this simple timeline [1, 3, 4]:

Weeks 1–2 should focus on rapid assessment: case definition, lab confirmation, defining outbreak (person, place, and time).

Weeks 3–4 should focus on response planning such as setting up committees, establishing and strengthening surveillance, preparing for and implementing population- and individual-level prevention and protection strategies, communication, planning vaccination if plausible, and mobilizing supplies.

Weeks 4–8 should focus on containment strategies including vaccination campaigns if needed, isolations and treatment or supportive health facilities, medical treatment such as standard protocols, case-finding, and follow-up visits, and continuing surveillance.

In some specific diseases, such as meningitis, chemoprophylaxis for close contacts could be considered and planned during the early weeks of the epidemic. In many such cases, vaccination of contact is easier and cheaper than chemoprophylaxis, but this does not treat carrier state and will not prevent transmission to other susceptible patients. In rapidly spreading diseases, the attack rate (the proportion of at-risk individuals who contract the disease after the exposure in a given time period) can exceed 1% very soon. Therefore, a large population can be regarded as close contact. In general, despite recent studies suggesting some impacts, mass antibiotic prophylaxis is ineffective because of reinfection of asymptomatic persons, and it also diverts resources from higher priorities. The important aspects to remember is emphasizing prevention, having available and ready health teams to react immediately through a contingency plan, and that every outbreak requires a specific response.

Prevention of Sporadic Cases

In the refugee setting, it might be difficult to differentiate between sporadic and epidemic cases. Therefore, it is important to collect baseline data outside an outbreak to understand the frequency of sporadic and endemic cases. If there are many sporadic cases in one section of the camp or settlement, try to address potential epidemics with appropriate responses to contain, or vaccinate the entire population at risk if there is a vaccine. Due to overcrowding and unsanitary living conditions, refugees are at higher risk of epidemics and data from hospital or clinic admissions can help detect the epidemic appropriately and timely [1, 3, 6]. A delayed response can quickly lead to high mortality and morbidity.

General Approach to Data Collection for Surveillance and Outbreak Management

There are six *key principles*:

(a) Only collect data which are useful and can be acted upon in the field.
(b) All health agencies and facilities should be involved.
(c) Create simple and standardized forms to be completed weekly or every 4 weeks.
(d) Devise simple case definitions.
(e) Use a mix of passive and active data collection (clinic-based morbidity and mortality is passive and surveys and home visits are active).
(f) Engage staff early in the process and seek and provide timely feedback.

Critical issues in rapid assessment of epidemics include linking the assessment results to the program decision-making to determine priorities that are coordinated by a lead agency or group and integrated with other assessments. It requires planning, authority, and credibility. Nevertheless, essential programs should not wait for findings from the assessments and should continue until findings are available.

Importance of Health Information System (HIS)

The main objectives are to monitor trends (such as vaccine-preventable diseases or nutrition status), redirect public health programs, detect epidemics, and evaluate health care interventions. Therefore, establishing a Health Information System is important in refugee settings. Data collection in itself has limited value if it is not well-thought-out. There is a need to balance methodology with concerns over security, resources, and time. In refugee settings, the quality of the data itself and the process of its collection, or their analysis including historical trends, meaning, or characteristics may be limited and biased. Common issues include incomplete data in places where access is limited, biased secondary data from other agencies or government, under-reporting due to sociopolitical concerns or lack of training or support, low sensitivity of data (too specific or too broad), and non-population-based information or unclear denominators. More information on data management systems is provided in Chap. 18.

General Approach to Collecting Morbidity and Mortality Data in Refugee Settings

There are considerations on top of routine data collection from the population in the camps and health centers. Please see Table 17.2.

General Ways to Collect Data

Methods could include; rapid health assessment (RHA), targeted surveys, regular surveys, and ongoing surveillance. RHA helps determine the magnitude of emergency, health and food needs, availability of local resources, needs for external resources, and developing a plan of action. Establishing surveillance and HIS comes next [1, 4, 6]. See Appendix 3 for a sample targeted survey.

General Types of Data

For RHA collect the following [1, 4, 6]:

1. Background information including
   (a) social, economic, political (from any sources such as UNHCR, UNICEF, governments, NGOs, other agencies or people in the field)
   (b) population size from registration data, food distribution or refugee registry or from community leaders (start collecting these early)
   (c) survey (convenient or cluster sampling)
   (d) visual inspection and aerial photos (has a risk for overestimation)
2. Demographics:
   (a) sex ratio, age groups (especially under 5)

Table 17.2 General approach to collecting morbidity and mortality data in refuges settings [1–6]

- Set up screening posts to screen newcomers at the entry points
- Emphasize on proportional morbidity and mortality (number of cases per 10,000 population or number of deaths per 1000 or 10,000 population in a given time period) in the acute phase
- Collect age and sex-specific incidence of diseases for infectious, hazardous, and trauma/violence-related conditions
- Pay particular attention to cases of diseases that were not previously reported or observed in that setting
- Calculate attack rate for diseases with public health importance and a propensity for epidemic or high mortality such as:
  - Diarrheal diseases (bloody or watery, cholera, shigella, etc.)
  - Malaria, skin diseases such as scabies, meningitis, measles, mumps, diphtheria (other vaccine-preventable diseases)
  - Lower respiratory tract infections
  - Other important environmental conditions such as toxins and or exposures to irritants

(b) rates of new arrivals and departures, an estimate of denominator, size, and conditions of vulnerable groups (single-headed households, unaccompanied minors, pregnant, elderly, minorities, disabled, adolescents, etc.)

3. Vital health data which includes: background health problems or vaccination rates, source of health care, impacts of disruption of services, mortality and morbidity data, nutritional status, and environmental risks and health conditions.

How to Collect Data During RHA

Interviews with key informants, direct observation of the environment in refugee settlements, limited surveys, and local community and refugee settlement health services (health facilities, government, NGO, or camp staff), their conditions and size, personnel, supplies, and infrastructures. These should be coupled with ongoing morbidity and mortality reports from surveillance and from the health or non-health facilities. There needs to be an assessment of the potential or current impact on health systems such as loss of medical staff (in a previously well-functioning health system), destruction of infrastructures, and discontinuation of public health services in war-affected areas or natural disasters (i.e., disruption of expanded program of child immunization or vector control measures) [1, 4].

Broader Prevention and Control Strategies

The most important task should be assuring access to water and shelters. Lack of access to water causes dehydration, contributes to poor hygiene and diarrhea or skin diseases such as lice (typhus), scabies, and conjunctivitis/trachoma. Supply enough water and its accessibility first, then assure water quality by treating water and testing it, regularly. Simultaneously, create a system for sanitation and waste management. Water quality measurement forms usually include data on the specific water points, conductivity (mS), pH, and number of fecal coliform per 100 ml in the sample water [1, 6].

- *Sanitation and hygiene*: There needs to be a system for excreta control within 2–3 days of arrivals of refugees. Focus on identifying and establishing defecation areas, shallow trench latrines, or collective latrines. Generally, one latrine per trench per 50–100 people is a good start. Trench latrines are often not well accepted, even though they are the only option in acute phases of an emergency, and people best accept household or small group latrines. Access to latrines needs to be safe particularly for women and children at any given time. Latrines should be maintained on a regular basis using local community members with a scheduled approach. Consider soil composition and plan for one latrine per 20 persons or per family, and distribute soap [1].
- *Wastes control is important*: Run-off rainwater is usually safe. Soakaway pits at water points and roadside collecting systems should be accordingly planned. Waste collected from the washing areas or health facilities should be evacuated. The waste disposal should be at least 2 m from underground water sources. For

solid waste, cleaning teams with trucks or even donkey cars need to be organized, and there should be planning for some form of landfill system. The trench or individual pits should be covered daily. To help families with cleaning wastes, distribute tools, and assemble volunteer teams. Medical wastes are an equally important source of infectious diseases outbreak. Set a system to dispose of dead bodies and always protect corpses from animals that is acceptable to the population. Most burial places are assembled in good soil and on the outskirts. If the mortality rate is high, communal graves could be used in an urgent phase with the possibility to relocate later. In cholera, disinfection of the body should be considered before burial. The body should not be returned to the family in circumstances where disease transmission is very likely [1–3, 7].

- *Site cleaning*: Refugee sites have to be appropriately and regularly cleaned to prevent intermediate carriers such as vectors from spreading the disease or limit exposures. All health facilities and feeding centers need to follow the sanitation and hygiene rules as well. Linking sanitation with the surveillance system and monitoring mortality and morbidity is important to identify weak points of the sanitation system [1].

Shelter and Environmental Factors

Proper shelter is an important part of protection against diseases. Cold weather or extreme heat is detrimental to the health of children or elderly and expose them to a wide range of illnesses. For example, acute respiratory infections in children are more prevalent or will be more severe when adequate shelter or warming equipment is not available. Similarly, environmental exposures to smoke or indoor cooking without appropriate ventilation systems contribute to respiratory infectious diseases or asthma-like attacks in children or worsening of COPD in the elderly. Location of the refugee settlement and soil composition of the camp area are important considerations considering easy access to water, farming opportunities, proximity and safe distances to domesticated animals or herds, and burial places or cemeteries [1].

Logistical Considerations

Supply Chain and Maintenance of Critical Activities
During an epidemic assuring that basic supply chains are available and that the transport system and market activities are functioning are enormously important. Supply chains for field hospitals and health facilities including storage and stocking of medical supplies and medications and laboratory tests, and their safety and maintenance requirements, must be ensured.

Transport and Referral Systems
Some critical or advanced care activities or procedures may need transferring patients outside the camp/settlement for further care. A reliable referral system through prior assessment of and coordination with outside health facilities should

be planned. Volunteers will be needed to accompany patients as well as cars and drivers to function as ambulances. Liability issues should be addressed.

Capacity Building and Staff Training

Build some capacity and train staff to effectively detect and respond to an epidemic and set up a functioning surveillance system. This is often difficult to assure in the camp because most trained or experienced people have opportunities to leave the situation or look for jobs outside the settlement. Involve community leaders to identify and train potential educated camp residents who can read and write. Teachers and younger adults are often good sources for targeted and advanced trainings in diverse topical areas not only related to the health but also social issues or the basics of psychosocial support or assessment, food and nutritional assessments, water or sanitation, supply chain, advocacy and health promotion, infection control and hospital/health facility sanitation, camp organization and coordination. They could also help with maintaining or building physical structures of health facilities or renovation when needed or with sectoring the camp, assessing new arrivals, contact tracing, and collecting morbidity and mortality data. This will nevertheless help build local capacity for the community [1].

Internal and External Sources of Support

It is important to identify all sources of potential support locally, funding or human resources, and externally from the surrounding or international community (either volunteered or paid staff or in kind donations). Assure that you regularly communicate the status of the refugees and their needs through international channels and local and regional entities so that the potential sources of funding, extra support for areas that are not your areas of expertise, or complementary services could potentially be provided by others. UNCHR, WFP, WHO regional offices, Ministry of Health, OCHA, and a wide range of international non-governmental organizations are often part of a cluster response or at the national level of the host or affected country that could provide additional resources.

Infection Control Strategies

There are important steps to implement and follow for infection control as described below. For more detailed information regarding each step, please see Appendices 4 and 5.

Isolation Needs

During the epidemic, it might be necessary to create isolation units within the field hospital or other health facilities. This will help avoid spread of the disease to other patients or community members during the most infectious phase of the disease.

Personal Protective Equipment

Aside from routine standard infection control equipment, the need for different or complementary protective equipment depends on the specific agent that caused the epidemic. Plan for and discuss with your team why they need PPE, the type of PPE they need, who needs it, and when they need it [8]. Assure that your staff understands their activities and responsibilities and knows about transmission routes. Droplet transmission is from coughing, sneezing, and respiratory exposures and contact transmission is from the pathogens that live on the surfaces. Airborne pathogens could be transmitted via breathing with the infected case in the same room or through talking. Surgical masks are generally recommended when working in isolation units. Vaccination of staff, if available, should be prioritized. Advise staff and support them to look out for their colleagues and take their time in caring for isolated patients. Use posters to help staff get reminders and establish a practice of buddy system to reinforce appropriate practices and provide support.

Contact Tracing

Establishing a well-functioning contact tracing system is essential to help identify all potential susceptible individuals who came in contact with an infected person. Use a simple form that could include the location and address of the infected person and all household or close contacts since the start of incubation period or symptomatic period for that specific disease [1, 4, 5].

Mapping Resources

This is an important part of epidemic response as many health and social resources are vital to provide an appropriate and effective response. It is also important to identify weakness, exposures, or risks for epidemic in different localities within the refugee settlements and assess or provide opportunities for protective measures such as sectoring or quarantine or screening of the new arrivals.

Management Pillars of Epidemic Response for Major Communicable Diseases

There are many infectious diseases that predispose the refugee population to epidemics including diarrheal diseases, malaria or other vector-borne diseases, acute respiratory tract infections, and vaccine-preventable diseases such as measles [4–7]. Skin diseases and other environmental conditions or exposures such as lead poisoning are also important. Please see Appendix 6 for specific information regarding diarrheal, vector-borne, and respiratory diseases.

Crisis Management in Epidemics, Pandemics, and Other Health Emergencies

The major components of crisis management include rapid assessment, establishing surveillance and data collection, critical thinking, crisis center and committees, action plans, organization and communication strategies, training of staff, and coordination with actors and across sectors. Effective leadership with team approaches across disciplines, availability and access to external resources, environmental assessment and control, and capacity building are equally important [1, 7–10].

Leadership, Incident Plans, Team Management, Collaboration, and Coordination Across a Spectrum of Services

Being well-prepared beforehand is critical during health emergencies. This needs a leadership plan to identify people who can coordinate the response among all stakeholders, and bring people together around a common goal. Community leaders and other community assets need to be involved early in any planning and response with a clear and agreed-upon chain of command and process of decision-making that is open to revisions and when more information is available. Often a central location within a settlement needs to be identified, that is accessible to all, as a command center to maintain lines of communication, access, and collaboration across different sectors. People involved in the leadership team need to be from all important social and health sectors and subsectors.

Critical Thinking and Systems- and Practice-Based Learning

Critical thinking is vital in preventing and or responding to many population health emergencies. Many of emerging diseases with propensity for epidemic or pandemic are zoonosis in origin meaning that they originate from animals, mostly wild animals. Diseases that have been successfully controlled in the past are reemerging despite availability and access to vaccines, and new infections such as SARS 1&2, H5N1, West Nile, and Lassa Fever have emerged. In understanding all these infections, there are some main characteristics to consider: source of infection, reservoir for pathogen, immunogenicity, pathogenicity and virulence, ease of transmission, contagiousness or infectivity, disease-specific morbidity, case-fatality, and mortality, and the degree of impact on the society (impact on public health or social disruption). Understanding potential transmission routes are important as some of these diseases are transmitted through aerosol or breathing air and droplets, others via vectors such as mosquitos, fleas, lice, or ticks, or via food, water, objects, or physical items. In general, routes of transmission are fecal-oral, aerogenous, direct or indirect contact, and blood. It is also important to understand the basic reproductive rate for each disease or pathogen which means the average number of persons infected by each patient in a totally susceptible population. There are periods during the illness when the infectious agent can be transmitted (see Fig. 17.1) [9].

Fig. 17.1 Transmissibility period in infectious diseases [9]. (Courtesy of Nurses on the Frontline; George Washington University)

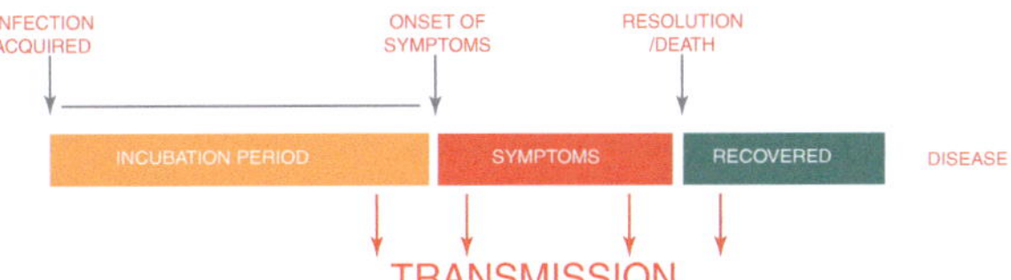

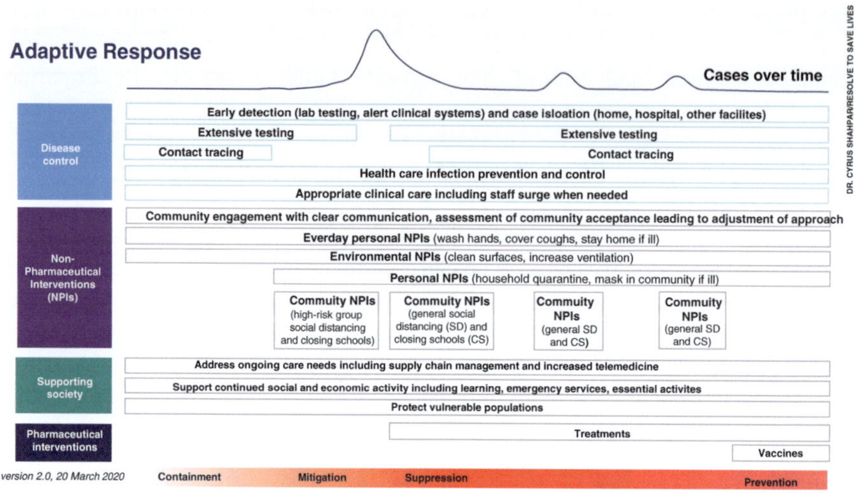

Fig. 17.2 Adaptive response to epidemic and pandemics [10]

Shedding of an infectious agent by an infected but otherwise asymptomatic patient could be important in exponential transmission of a newly emerging disease (e.g., SARS-Cov-2) either directly or through vectors [11, 12]. Social isolation or quarantine may help delay or dampen the quick spread until appropriate treatment or vaccines are developed. Maximum time of the incubation period determines the duration of quarantine or isolation following the exposure. Transmission can occur during an asymptomatic period up until early recovery. For example, in SARS-CoV-2 this quarantine period was first established as 14 days [12, 13]. An epidemic or pandemic will present with a very high number of initial cases when the transmission is at the community-level, rapidly increase within 3–6 weeks, and then subside over a longer period of time and when most susceptible people are infected, isolated, died, vaccinated, or otherwise protected by other measures. Figure 17.2 presents general strategies to address pandemic or epidemic at different levels [10].

During large-scale epidemics or pandemics when the health system is overwhelmed, there are many fatalities, and restrictions or quarantines are often implemented. Therefore, collect and record information from the patients or the deceased [9]. For emerging or reemerging infection, the immunity level might not be known, present, protective, or long-lasting. Therefore, prepare for a second or third wave of the disease until a vaccine or effective treatment is available and widely used [14]. Please see Appendix 7 for Table 17.3, which presents critical thinking steps when encountering a potential epidemic of an unknown infection or other mass health emergencies [9].

Preparation and Planning for Health Emergencies

Professional preparedness plans for large health emergencies (including infectious/ biological, chemical, nuclear, and or explosive emergencies) are needed for the health personnel and community. Keep health personnel up-to-date on data and information and perform regular drills. Develop basic support plans for healthcare providers and essential workers, and their families, and people with special needs (orphans, elderly, disabled, mentally ill, pregnant, etc.) in case of shortages or lock-downs. Please review detailed information and instructions regarding these plans at the individual, facility, school, and community-levels presented in Appendix 8 [9]. Learning from experience and current practices, and understanding how local health and social systems work are of prime importance. Not all guidelines or recommendations are going to be applicable to all populations, universally. Nuances are important and the effectiveness of all scientific approaches rests on local capacities, possibilities, and resources.

Communication Strategies, Awareness Campaigns, Health Promotion and Education

It is vital to help disseminate accurate information and encourage the community to use well-established social venues or legitimate supporting platforms to obtain up-to-date and proper information regarding their risks and receive updates [1, 9, 15]. Providing accurate and timely information and encouraging individuals to avoid exposure to negative or distorted news could be vital to effectively and efficiently use limited resources in refugee settings. Set up community-level communication strategies and use local volunteers to communicate proper information regularly with the population. Use positive and forward-looking language and attitude to communicate and encourage your community or individuals to focus on positive contributions, strengthen the response to the epidemic, and provide recognition and or rewards, accordingly [9]. Have an open line of communication at all times to address misinformation or rumors. Stay vigilant, monitor social media, talk on the camp corners, and listen to what is said in the community and household level. Accurately describe uncertainty as well as certainties and comment on the accuracy of information coming from outside and clarify whenever needed. Seek help from the population and community itself and accordingly change the format and delivery methods to improve communications [1, 9, 15]. Develop informational posters, radio talks, and or social media activities, speakers, and utilize community health workers. In health promotional activities, focus on available resources, use short messages (customized to the local norms), avoid jargons, focus on only messages that could change risky behaviors, and avoid excessive information about the disease. Excessive information may contribute to more questions than answers and distract from learning. It is better to focus on behaviors that you want to change, be realistic of possible changes, and provide less risky behaviour alternatives.

Social and Community Mobilization and Engagement, Resilience, and Recovery

Always have a plan for social mobilization and get as many as community members as possible involved in the planning and provision of services. When people are engaged they better understand limitations and constraints and feel and accept more responsibilities and accountability. Try to involve people from each and all sectors, ethnic backgrounds, age ranges, gender, and other sociodemographic characteristics as much as possible [1]. Always keep an eye on community resilience and be realistic about and use all community-level coping strategies that are available. Epidemics take a huge toll on the community and could create fears and anger and psychosocial stresses and could disrupt community cohesiveness and its governance [9, 15]. Plan for a quick recovery period even if it is not at sight or possible at the whole settlement level. Plan ahead about the next steps if cases go down or some people get better and usual activities could restart or usual needs become more prominent again. Plan for psychological support and recovery, aid the families who lost the head of household or person who generated their income, and plan for and encourage neighborhood-level support and contribute in any way possible [9]. Provide moral support and encourage togetherness and bring different sectors together.

Internal and External Resources

Utilizing an inclusive approach, explore and understand the regional- or national-level emergency response plans including the related agencies and their resources. Identify professional societies and or individual experts that could help refine local responses, share lessons, and provide a unified approach.

The Covid-19/SARS-CoV-2 Pandemic and Refugees

At the time of this book's publication, a full understanding of all aspects of SARS-CoV-2/Covid-19 has not yet been reached; however, many of basic principles of epidemics and outbreak management apply to this particular pandemic. SARS-CoV-2 has a presymptomatic infectious period, high transmissibility, and relatively high case-fatality rate for vulnerable groups (such as elderly, HIV positive, weak immune system, malnutrition, etc.), many of which are represented in refugee populations [11–17]. It is important to have a plan to keep essential healthcare and medicine for patients especially those with chronic needs such as hypertension, HIV, diabetes, and TB [15]. Most patients at risk of dying due to SARS-Cov-2 need critical care services which are not available in refugee settings. Although rapid testing and isolation may be available in some situations, admission and isolation of cases may not be practical or helpful and could even infect healthcare personnel and add more risks to other patients. General prevention at the population level such as social distancing or mask distribution to curb the transmission may also not be much feasible in the refugee settings [15]. Considering resources, the main strategy could be protecting the most vulnerable population from getting the disease and having severe outcomes [14, 15, 18]. Modeling studies suggest that during both low and high transmission phases, sectoring the camps into smaller sections, if possible, could be an effective approach to dampen or flatten the epidemic curve especially if implemented early [19].

Practical Approach to Protect the Most Vulnerable Groups

Without a vaccine or treatment, ideally those most vulnerable should be separated from their families and close community contacts until the transmission rate falls below a reasonable threshold or when the net reproductive rate (or the number of individuals that are infected by one person with the diseases) falls below 1. This type of isolation is often not practical as some vulnerable people depend on family caregivers; alternatively the entire family could then be isolated from the community [15, 18].

At-Risk People

There is some data on subgroups with higher risks for the worst outcomes. There are also strategies to protect them at family/household, neighborhood, or larger camp levels [12–16]. Each poses opportunities and challenges. Please see Table 17.4 for detailed information. Irrespectively, infection prevention at any type of gatherings of vulnerable people is ineffective without good standard infection control, and could pose more risk of infection in a short time period. They could also be impractical because of family structures, lack of broader support systems, or psychologically challenging to the families and community. A clinical case definition could be satisfactory; however, many cases are asymptomatic in early stages or have vague mild symptoms. Therefore, establishing good surveillance and outbreak control in such gathering facilities is extremely important. In the end, house-level protection and semi-isolation may be more practical for vulnerable people.

Case Management at the Household and Health Facility Levels

At each health facility, temperature should be checked for all patients and a sign should instruct patients to inform greeting staff about any flu or Covid-like symptoms (i.e., new onset of either subjective or measured fever of >100.4 °F (>38 °C), or cough, or shortness of breath, or sore throat, or loss of smell or taste). Patients with symptoms should be given a mask and isolated in a designated screening area, ideally in a separate room away from other staff or patients. If these patients deem to be infected then they should be given masks and isolated from the rest and a contact tracing be initiated [20]. General supportive care is the mainstay of treatment both at the facility and household level. Mild symptoms could be managed at home [21]. Moderate to severe

Table 17.4 High-risk groups and strategies to protect them [12–16]

At-risk people for more severe outcomes	General considerations

• Age 50 or above (higher in >70).
• Hypertension, Diabetes, cancer, or other chronic diseases.
• Immunosuppression or HIV, TB, or malnourished adults, and severe other medical conditions that increase the risk.
• Multi-organ autoimmune disease in children.
  – Children do not appear to be at higher risk of serious infections
• Children are unlikely to be super-spreaders:
  – However, they could facilitate the spread of disease as they are more likely to be asymptomatic and therefore continue in the public or have contacts with others.
	• They should be ideally protected through:
	  – Avoiding going outside, limiting family visits, avoiding extended family visits, resting and living in places with adequate ventilation and air circulation, avoiding sharing sanitation or hygiene tools, and separating eating or conversation areas as much as possible.
	• Providing masks or face shields will provide more protection when in close proximity or contact with other household members.
	• The household members should also avoid:
	  – Mass gathering (weddings, large family gatherings) or close contacts with others, so they are less likely to be infected and infect household high-risk persons in return.
	• If possible, a separate room or area in the household could help protect the most vulnerable.
	  – Then one caregiver could be identified to live with and help them.
	  – A caregiver already recovered from Covid-19, within months postinfection, would be a better choice.
	• Other forms of protection at the neighborhoods or extended family levels, or larger and camp level could include:
	  – A specific house or shelter prepared for a group of vulnerable people isolated from the rest, or isolation or quarantine areas in camps' periphery, which would need good infection control procedures, social distancing, good ventilation, caregiving measures, clean food and supplies, masks or cloth masks, and cleaning materials such as disinfectants, soap, and water.
	  – Generally, any large gatherings of vulnerable people are ineffective without good standard infection control and could pose more risk of infection in a short period of time.
	  – These also could be impractical at times because of family structures, lack of broader support systems, and psychologically challenging to the families and community.
	  – Establish good surveillance and outbreak control in such facilities:
	    Due to asymptomatic cases or with vague mild symptoms, clinical case definition may not be fully effective.
	• In the end, house-level protection and semi-isolation may be more practical for vulnerable people.

symptoms especially worsening shortness of breath should be kept in the health facility. Moderate or severe illness, especially with worsening shortness of breath or other consequences of Covid-19 infection, can be defined as illness due to suspected or confirmed Covid-19 that requires further medical evaluation and should be kept at a health facility. Please see Appendix 9 and other CDC guidelines for some useful tips and instructions for caregivers, self-care at home, or when patients leave the health facility [20, 21].

PPE for Health Personnel, General Public, or Household Contact of an Infected Person

Households or the general public could use any form of protective masks that is sealing the nose and mouth. Eye protection or face shield could be used for very vulnerable persons. You can teach the community to make homemade cloth masks using CDC or WHO recommendations [8, 20]. Household-level isolation requires a single room or closed off area (partition or physical barrier) that allows for at least 6 ft/182 cm distance with others. For health personnel, surgical masks, or even two masks, face shields or goggles will add to protection. In SARS-CoV-2 or Covid-19, small droplets may be carried by dust or suspended in the air for a while and be aerosolized during procedures such as intubation, nebulizers or oxygen therapy. In such situations, and since there will be no negative pressure room, N95 or N99 masks (used in occupational hazard settings and paint or construction workers) should be used if available. All droplet and contact precautions are important at health facility and household levels.

Surveillance, Basics of Infection Control, Isolation, and Quarantine

Surveillance system was discussed previously. Clinical case definition alone in settings where upper respiratory infections are common may not be sufficiently specific and could pose a burden to the family, community, or health care system. They should later be modified when testing available or tailored down when cases trend down. Syndromic surveillance for severe forms of respiratory distress syndrome will help with its early detection. Establish screening, isolation and quarantine, and testing when available. Testing will help better prioritize resources by differentiating suspected, probable, and confirmed cases and assess the impact of prevention measures. Handwashing should be encouraged, and soap and water should be provided to each household. If possible, a single bathroom or toilet per family, and also for isolation or quarantine units are required. Gowns, gloves, and clot masks could be disinfected and reused. Ethyl alcohol above 80% could be reasonably disinfectant (follow WHO recommendations) [7, 8]. Quarantine period should ideally be 14 days but also as low as 7–10 days depending on resources [20]. Visitors could gather using social distancing in meeting areas to see loved ones. Ideally set up mobile health facilities close to quarantine or isolation sections. Trained community volunteers should help high-risk persons without social support.

Community Engagement and Mobilization

Basic approaches have been described previously. Active engagement and communication with all stakeholders, addressing fears and misinformation, providing accurate information and education, and liaising with surrounding communities and within the refugee settlement are the key elements. Communication committees could help devise appropriate health education methods and content and communicate rationale to improve adherence. Action plans and activities should be coordinated and coupled with existing services and emergency responses.

Logistics and Staffing Needs and Training

Community volunteers should be trained for a wide range of logistical support. Covid-19 epidemic could effectively isolate the refugee settlement from the outside and create fears among the surrounding communities or residents. Most businesses could come to a halt due to lack of trade or economic activities in surrounding communities, which will affect basic supply chain in the settlements. Therefore, supplies need to be ordered, delivered, stoked and stored, and rationed if necessary, and early support from external sources should be pursued. International agencies would need to support the delivery of essential goods and public services such as food, fuel, construction materials, infection control and treatments supplies, and trained medical or public health personnel.

Appendix 1: Example of Monthly Surveillance (Morbidity and Mortality) Report

In Patient/Hospital Morbidity and Mortality Year	weeks: 1 to 5 January		
	< 5y	> 5 y	Total
Total inpatients at the beginning of the month:	13	10	23
Total admissions per month:	54	122	176
Total exits per month:	53	112	165
Discharged	49	90	139
Defaulters			0
Transferred	3	20	23
Deaths	1	2	3
Total inpatients at the end of the month:	14	20	34
Average length of stay (days) *			5.9
Bed Occupancy ratio % *			73.5
Hospital mortality ratio (deaths/exitsx100)	1.9	1.8	1.8
% under 5			32.1

Morbidity				%
Diarrhea	2	1	3	2%
Bloody Diarrhea		3	3	2%
Respiratory Infection	20	10	30	18%
Malnutrition	11		11	7%
Malaria (confirmed)	1	1	2	1%
FUO			0	0%
Sepsis			0	0%
Neonatal Sepsis	3		3	2%
Gastritis & Gastric Ulcers		8	8	5%
UTI & Nephrolithiasis		3	3	2%
STD & PID's			0	0%
Skin and SC infections	1	2	3	2%
Domestic trauma and wounds	3	14	17	10%
War trauma & Wounds		1	1	1%
Tetanos			0	0%
TB			0	0%
Meningitis (confirmed)			0	0%
Measles			0	0%
Hepatitis/Jaundice			0	0%
Typhoid Fever (suspected)			0	0%
Leprosis			0	0%
Delivery		20	20	12%
Gyn Obst cases		28	28	17%
Surgical cases	5	5	10	6%
Chronic disease		9	9	5%
Other	7	7	14	8%
TOTAL	53	112	165	100%
Number of transfusions			0	
Nb of parachecks positive			0	
Nb of parachecks done			0	

Mortality				%
Diarrhea			0	0%
Bloody Diarrhea			0	0%

Appendix 2

Table 17.1 Examples of case definitions [1, 4]

Condition	Clinical Case Definition	Laboratory[a]	Others
Acute lower respiratory tract infections	Any case of fever with cough and rapid breathing (>50/min): >60/min for children <2 months >50/min for children 2–11 months >40/min for children 1–5 years >30/min for >5 years **OR** Chest indrawing	Usually none[a]	

Meningitis	• Clinical: an illness with sudden onset of fever above 38.5 °C with one or more of:
	  – Neck stiffness
	  – Altered mental status.
	  – Petechial or purpureal rash
		• Laboratory: positive CSF antigen or positive culture	• Suspect: Meets clinical definition
			• Probable: Meets clinical plus
			  – turbid/ purulent CSF or Positive stain
			  OR
			  – part of an epidemic and linked to other cases
			• Confirmed: A probable case plus lab confirmation

Cholera	• Suspected case: Any patient developing a rapid onset of severe watery diarrhea (usually with vomiting) resulting in severe dehydration.	Rapid dipstick test	

[a]For infectious diseases such as Tuberculosis, HIV, or Malaria there are multiple point-of-care laboratory tests that could help with case definitions but they are often not used in the context of the epidemic

Appendix 3: Sample Targeted Survey

Date: **CAMP:**   **SECTION:**
Number: **CLUSTER #:**
SEX:
1. CAN YOU READ OR WRITE? 1. Y   2.N
2. AGE?   AGE MARRIED?
3. HOW MANY CHILDREN DO YOU HAVE?   #MISCARRIAGE/DEATH?

4. WHAT IS YOUR HOUSEHOLD MONTHLY INCOME?
5. DO YOU WASH HANDS/CHILDREN AFT TOILET/BEFORE MEALS? 1.Y   2.N
6. WHY SHOULD ONE WASH HANDS?

7. DO YOU HAVE SOAP AVAILABLE AT HOME NOW? 1.Y 2. N   HOW LONG?
8. HOW OFTEN HAVE YOU OR YOUR CHILDREN AT HOME HAD DIARRHEA
 OVER PRIOR THREE MONTHS? CIRCLE ALL THAT APPLIES
1. NONE   2. ONCE   3. TWO 4. OR >
1.ONE KID   2.MORE THAN ONE KID   3.MYSELF
9. DO YOU WASH YOUR HAND BEFORE FEEDING INFANT? 1. Y   2. N

10. HOW OFTEN DO YOU EAT FOOD IN A DAY?
1. ONCE   2. TWICE 3. THREE TIMES
 IS IT ENOUGH? (1.Y   2.N)
11. OVER PAST MONTH HAVE YOU EVER EXPERIENCED HUNGR
BECAUSE OF LACK OF FOOD OR LACK OF MONEY TO BUY FOOD? 1. Y   2. N
12. OVER THE LAST MONTH DID YOU/ANY ADULT EVER
CUT SIZE OF MEALS OR SKIP MEALS TO GIVE TO CHILDREN? 1. Y   2. N
13. DO YOU USE CONTRACEPTION (PILLS or INJECTION) NOW? (Y N) EVER (Y N)?
 WHY?
14. HOW MANY WIVES ARE HERE WITH YOU?
15. DO YOU FEEL SAD? (Y   N) EVERY DAY? (Y   N)   HOW LONG?
16. DO YOU HAVE SLEEP PROBLEM (Y   N)? DO YOU CRY OFTEN (Y   N)?
WHY? HOW OFTEN?
17. DO YOU FEEL TIRED EVERYDAY (Y   N) ? PAIN (Y   N)?
18. HAVE YOU EVER HAD PRENATAL CARE? (Y   N)
19. DO YOU HAVE BEDNETS? (Y N) FOR EVERY FAMILY MEMBER (Y N)?
 HOW OFTEN DO YOU USE THEM? AND WHY?
OBSERVATIONS: LOOK FOR;
 INDOOR SMOKING/OVEN? (Y   N)
DOES HE/SHE KNOW WHY IT IS IMPORTANT? ASK TO DESCRIBE
TOILETS (Y N)   BEDNET (Y   N)   VACCINATION CARD (Y   N)
MEASURE AND RECORD MUAC FOR CHILDREN IN AGE RANGE

Appendix 4: Broad Infection Control Strategies [1, 6, 8]

Isolation needs	• Needed for epidemics of some infectious agents such as Measles, Diphtheria or viral Hepatitis, SARS, and TB (specific PPE requirements and ventilation).
	  – Implement appropriate infection control practices, training of healthcare as well as supply or support staff, and monitoring of exposures.
	  – Cholera units are also utilized to improve care and efficiency of case management.
	  – Other viral conditions with high reproductive rates or high case-fatality rates such as SARS and Ebola also need specific isolation and treatment units sealed off from the rest of hospital or health facilities with specific PPE requirements (gown, gloves, face shields or goggles, masks, or bodysuits) and more stringent infection control practices.
	• Create a triage unit based on the characteristics of epidemic agents to identify and isolate suspected cases and reinforce routine practices of handwashing, regular cleaning, and disinfection to prevent spread of the disease to staff or other patients.
	• Establish cleaning services for environmental surfaces using water and detergent and hospital level disinfectants. Current recommendations are chlorine solution of 0.5% concentration for surfaces but ethyl alcohol could also be used.
	• Assure staff wears surgical masks and appropriate PPE when working in isolation areas.
	• It might be necessary to create a quarantine corner for all new arrivals or isolate a section of the camp or settlement to control the spread of an infectious agent.

PPE	• In community settings, masks are not generally recommended for most infectious diseases but they could be recommended depending on the extent of infection, type of agent, and availability of treatment, etc. See section on Covid-19 for specific related information.
	• Mask should be appropriately disposed after usage.
	• Train staff in the proper order of donning and doffing PPE starting with hand washing, gown, mask/respirator (seal check), googles, and gloves when donning and gloves, gown, googles, mask/respirator, and hand hygiene when doffing (see Appendix 6 for donning and doffing).
	  – Gowns protect clothing from droplets and splashes.
	  – Surgical mask is for droplet precautions and decreases the risk of splash to nose/mouth. Respirator (N95) is for high risk activities that are airborne producing such as CPR or suctioning or intubation or oxygen therapy or for airborne diseases such as TB.
	  – Goggles protect eyes from droplets and splashes. Face shield will do the same.
	  – Gloves protect hands from direct contact with pathogens. Without gloves, a pathogen that lives on the surface and is touched could later be transmitted to the mouth, eyes, or nose accidentally. It is important to choose an appropriate size. It does not replace hand washing, however. In some hospitals acquired infections such as *Clostridium difficile* both hand washing and gloves are an important part of infection control. Change gloves when needed and in between patients and wash hands in between.
	• Advise staff to put on PPE before entering the patient's room or isolation. General tips include:
	  – Do not touch your PPE, keep hands away from the face, and avoid touching unnecessary areas in the patient's room.
	• Make sure you disinfect equipment that you use in patient care in between patients (i.e., stethoscope or other equipment).

Contact tracing	• It will help identify other cases who did not yet come to clinics or health facilities and helps map the hot spot in the camp or settlements. • It also helps health authorities identify hot spots and seal off or sector the camp or settlement to prevent epidemic spilling off to other areas in the settlement and to accordingly dedicate resources for vaccination, treatment, or supportive care. • Contact tracers could be local community volunteers with the ability to read and write and should be trained in proper case identification, registration, and tracing. • The close contacts should receive prophylaxis treatment or vaccinated if applicable, or be quarantined for the entire period of the disease incubation period (often a maximum time of an incubation period).
Mapping sources	• Trained community health workers or local volunteers will need to evaluate the camp/settlement for any potential support systems including: – Storages and stoking, transport and roads, fuel and supplies, food distribution points, water points, community gathering areas, vulnerability or strengths of physical and social infrastructures such as characteristics of physical spaces or health facilities, community leadership or leaders, sociocultural assets, livestock, farming, proximity to fuel supplies or firewood or forest or burial areas, etc.

Appendix 5: Images for Donning and Doffing PPE (CDC)

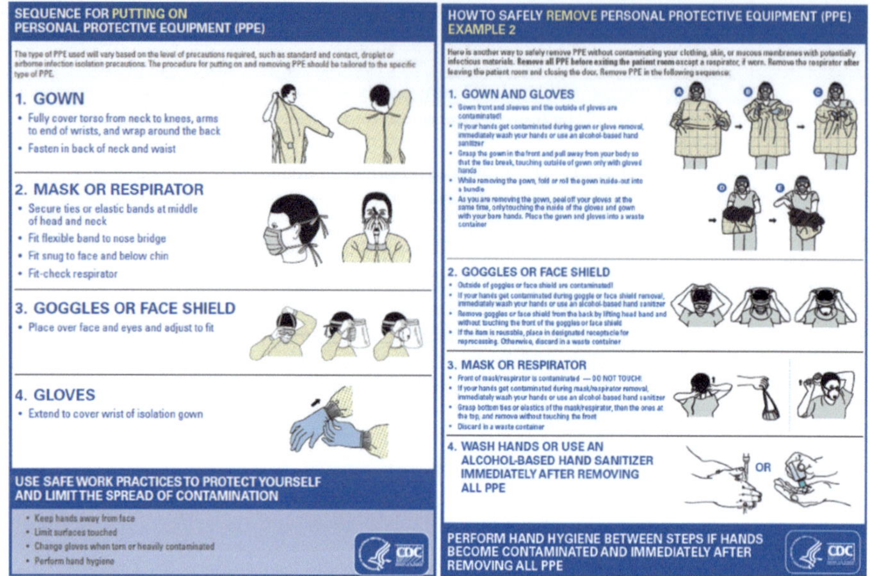

Appendix 6: Pillars of Response to Diarrheal, Vector-Borne, and Respiratory Diseases [1, 6]

Diarrheal diseases	• Focus on prevention by improving accessible water, personal hygiene, and adequate sanitation system. • Provide food ration if needed. • Set up surveillance with protocols and standard simple forms. • Emphasizes warnings signs such as adults with death above 5 per week, increase in bloody diarrheal cases, and a rise in diarrheal case-fatality. Record cases and deaths and perform case-control assessment to detect the source. • Improve case management: early rehydration and oral rehydration therapy (ORT) centers, and continue feeding. • Corpses could present a risk and should be disinfected with chlorine if needed. • Mass chemoprophylaxis is not recommended in diarrheal diseases as it diverts attention and resources from effective measures and could contribute to antimicrobial resistance. • Selective prophylaxis is also not recommended as it may require a large-scale control system. • Stool samples at the end of outbreaks could confirm the disappearance of pathogens such as Cholera.
Vector control for communicable diseases	• Ideally set refugee sites far from potential breeding sites; avoid or eliminate breeding sites. • Larvicides, periodic spraying of houses and shelters with residual insecticide (especially when low prior immunity level) could help. Residual insecticide often lasts 6 months. • Consider distribution of impregnated mosquito in high-risk areas to decrease transmission. Distributed annually or every 3–5 years depending on the materials and potentials.

Respiratory diseases	Prevention measures are often nonspecific. • Address risk factors; low birth weight, malnutrition, poor breastfeeding practices, Vit. A deficiency, indoor air pollution (cooking smokes and or tobacco), overcrowding, chilling in infants (due to poor shelter, distribute blankets), low prior vaccination rates such as for viral or bacterial infections. Vaccination is the most important specific prevention control strategy (DPT, Polio, HiB, PNM, etc.). Establish surveillance systems to collect morbidity and mortality and develop tables and simple case definitions. • For respiratory infections or meningitis surveillance systems should assure monitoring by age to categorize higher risk groups. Management should focus on: early diagnosis and case management to decrease mortality, coupled with immunization (DPT and childhood vaccines), accessible health system, and simple treatment protocols. Case management includes antibiotic at home or health facilities along with supportive measures. • Antibiotics are often oral and the choices should be in accordance with the national policy of the host country. They should be easy to administer and cost effective, and simple supply chain and storage requirements. • Assuring oral hydration, continuing feeding, warming, and antipyretic are recommended. • Case definitions and clinical diagnosis should be tailored as needed and should be consistently applied. • For example, when severe malnutrition, rapid breathing, or chest in-drawing is not sensitive for Pneumonia. • In refugees over 10,000 you can have more than 100 cases daily in meningitis epidemics. • A standard protocol and questionnaire have to be developed for doctors, nurses, and community health workers. • Gather historical, clinical, and demographic data of the cases, create special wards in the health facilities, and shelters should be planned for cases or suspected cases. Isolation: In some specific diseases, isolation may be needed in health facilities or at home. Proper protection needs to be provided to family members caring for the loved ones. Most cases such as meningitis are not transmitted by casual contact or dried fomites. But others are (including Covid-19). Active case finding in refugee camps needs to be set up and carried out by health workers or trained personnel. You can treat non-epidemic cases using usual case treatment. For most epidemics of respiratory infections, limiting mass gathering and increasing space between beds are warranted. Vaccination: • Logistical component of vaccination campaigns is the most important part. • Provide vaccination cards or use general vaccination cards. • Assure and follow the cold chain process. There are 7–10 days cold boxes that could be used. • Order vaccines and assure supply chains. The vials could include 10–50 doses. • Assure specific protocol so each case receives the specific dose and frequency needed. • Train vaccinators in proper hygiene and infection control to avoid the spread of other viral infections such as HIV or hepatitis. • If vaccines are not available for the general population then strategies could initially focus on higher risk groups. • For specific conditions routine vaccination during non-epidemic periods may not be effective because of the short duration of protection in children (e.g., meningitis). • If there is a strong reason (for example, an epidemic in the last season), then preventive vaccination could be justified. • Most vaccines need a specific time period in order for them to mount antibodies. It could be 5–10 days. Therefore, vaccination largely reduces secondary cases. In cases such as meningitis epidemic, since infected individuals can still transmit after immunizations, vaccination of high-risk groups may not stop the epidemic, therefore monitor the disease trend in unvaccinated as well. • Most respiratory infections or other diseases with a tendency for epidemic clusters within specific geographic areas of the refugee settlement or camp. Therefore, identifying those areas through active and passive surveillance and vaccinating population in those areas should be first on your list.

Appendix 7

Table 17.3 Basic critical thinking during an unknown epidemic or mass health emergency [9]

Critical thinking	Action plan
Most infectious diseases are presenting with a flu-like syndrome that is very common. The key is: • To have a high index of suspicion. • Be vigilant. • Look for trends and number of people presenting with the same type of presentation that is considered unusual for that locality or season or is different from usual trends. A well-functioning surveillance system is a key to alert of an impending epidemic.	Basic approach in addressing public health or mass health emergencies (infectious, chemical, or nuclear) include: • Preparation, assessing the situation, taking appropriate personal precautions. • Assessing if multiple cases are presenting or an epidemic is going on. • If multiple cases: – Perform triaging, assessing contacts with the potential pathogen (sometimes decontamination is needed if applicable). – Assessing if the patient is contagious, and isolating the patient and all exposed persons, and finally treating and recovery.
Basic critical thinking approach at the patient level starts with being prepared, using standard precautions (gloves, gowns, mask, eye protection, and handwashing) plus N95 mask. In assessing individuals or groups of patients with the same symptoms or presentation: • Consider protecting staff, other patients, and yourself • Use personal protective gear • Obtain a good history for exposure and timelines • Perform exams and or further studies	If there are many patients presenting like this individual and they are at different stages: • Triage patients based on triaging principles. If there is no other similar case: • Investigate if this patient had any contact with other infected patients with known disease or suspected disease. If there are similar cases: • Isolate (if applies) and provide medical care (supportive or specific). If no similar cases: then assess the patient to see if she/he is contagious. If the patient is contagious: • Isolate the patient and all exposed persons. If not, then continue to assess and diagnose the condition and treat accordingly.

Appendix 8: Preparation and Planning at Different Levels for Crisis Management During Mass Health Emergencies [9]

Health care workers individual level	• Health care workers should be familiarized with their facility-level plan including relevant units that are necessary when responding to a health emergency: – Infection control, engineering and logistics, supplies, security, admission and transfers, pharmacy and storage, etc.
Health facility level	• Identify potential locations such as guest houses or warehouses that could be used as additional makeshift facilities in case of overflow of patients. • It might be necessary to transfer patients to other potential units in the health facility or field hospital that are not usually used for emergency care or admission but in case of epidemics or pandemics could be converted to emergency stations or patient rooms for a sustained period of time. • Ensure that there is a plan for protecting healthcare personnel and nursing staff when they provide care at patients' homes especially in regards to contagious infection agents during epidemics or pandemics. • For clinics, there might be a need to create isolation areas as well. • If possible, establish plans for noncontact patient care in case of epidemics or pandemics such as phone visits, video visits if possible, exam rooms with phone or video capabilities, etc. • Assure that food and water supplies are available for health facilities and patients. • Identify and plan for pharmacies with 24 h services, or places for medical supplies, sanitation or cleaning materials, and warehouses for emergency supplies. • Identify all potential private healthcare providers and facilities in your camp/community to reach out to if needed and explore their resources.
School-level	• Identify potential areas that could be used to isolate infectious students or staff. • Assure basic infection control plans and have protective gears at hand in the school during an epidemic or other health emergencies.

Community-level	• Promote prevention and protection measures in regards to infectious and noninfectious agents during epidemics or other health emergencies such as chemical exposure, flooding, or earthquake is an important step.
	• Such measures should be empowering for the community and aim to be well accepted.
	• Emotional and psychological support during epidemic or disasters are important for the community.
	  – There will be guilt, horror, fears, anger, demoralization, paranoia, sleeplessness, substance abuse, acute stress disorder, etc.
	  – People may experience helplessness and hopelessness, and an increase in careless behaviors that put oneself or others at risks.
	• There may be an increase in child neglect and abuse including domestic abuse. Have some form of plans to address them.

Appendix 9: Case Management for SARS-Cov-2/Covid-19 at the Household and Facility Levels [15, 20, 21]

Household-level care	<ul><li>Nonspecific measures include basic antipyretic, antitussive, and anti-pain medications.</li><li>Encourage drinking more fluid to help thin and loosen mucus so it is easier to cough up phlegm.</li><li>Liquids such as water, fruit juice, and broth will help keep the patient hydrated.</li><li>Soothe a sore throat by helping the patient gargle with warm salt water that could be made by dissolving ¼ teaspoon salt in 1 cup of warm water (8 ounces).</li><li>You can also recommend to older children and adults to use throat lozenges, ice chips, or other sore throat remedies available.</li><li>Humidifying air increases moisture and makes it easier for patients to breathe and help decrease coughing. Any type of warming water to evaporate should help with this.</li><li>Do not allow smoking cigarettes and cigars to avoid worsening symptoms.</li><li>Nasal drops could help relieve congestion if available. Vaseline/Petroleum-based jelly around the outside of nostrils could help decrease irritation from blowing the nose.</li></ul>
Health Facility	<ul><li>You may need to provide care for patient with respiratory failure.</li><li>This would need oxygen and or other supportive respiratory devices. If available, start with nasal cannula oxygen therapy and avoid ambo-bag.</li><li>Non-rebreather masks are better than ambo-bag to prepare for intubation.</li><li>If patient's Oxygen saturation drops below 92% on 6 litters of NC oxygen or high non-rebreather mask, they may need intubation depending on resourecs and possibilities.</li><li>If available, then prepare for intubation and have sedation available.</li></ul>
Separation/Isolation	<ul><li>Covid-19 patients should be placed in a single room if possible. If not, then they should ideally be placed in communal room but separated from others by 6 ft/182 cm and by physical barriers such as privacy curtain or partitions.</li><li>These barriers and all equipment and devices that are used to care for an infected patient should be cleaned and disinfected regularly as described above.</li><li>For most patients the decision to discontinue isolation practices should follow the recommendations in Appendices 4 and 6.</li><li>In general, you can discontinue isolation after the following are met: no symptoms such as cough, sore throat, runny nose, or fatigue, and more than at least 7 days after patient's first symptom, and no fever within the past 72 h without taking any medicine.</li><li>Isolation: separation of ill persons from others until the ill person is no longer considered infectious.</li><li>Quarantine, separation of exposed persons from others to reduce the risk of transmission of the virus from known exposed persons to other susceptible individuals in the community.</li></ul>

Categories of patients	Some basic helpful definition or terminologies to use could include different categories of:
	• Patient Under Investigation (PUI), meaning a person who has above Covid-like symptoms and is awaiting testing results or no test is available.
	• Exposed Person, meaning a person who had close contact, <182 cm for >10 min, with Covid-19 positive or individuals with Covid-19 like illness
	• Infectious Person, a person who has onset of Covid-like illness or who is laboratory diagnosed with Covid-19 and who has not gone 7 days since onset or whose fever is not resolved and respiratory symptoms not improving for 3 days, whichever is longer.

References

1. Medecins Sans Frontieres. Refugee health: an approach to emergency situations. Oxford: Macmillan Education; 1997. ISBN: 0333 72210 8.
2. Martin AA, Moore J, Collins C, Beillik R, Kattel U, Tool MJ, Moore PS. Infectious disease surveillance during emergency relief to Bhutanese refugees in Nepal. JAMA. 1994;272(5): 377–81.
3. Moren AM, Bitar D, Navarre I, Gactellu Etchegorry M, Brodel A, Lungu G, Hakewill P. Epidemiological surveillance among Mozambican refugees in Malawi, 1987-1989. Disasters. 1991;15(4):363–72.
4. Moore PS, Toole MJ, Nieburg P, Waldman RJ, Broome CV. Surveillance and control of meningococcal meningitis epidemics in refugee populations. Bull World Health Organ. 1990;68(5):587–96.
5. Wharton M, Chobra TL, Vogt RL, Morse DL, Buehler JW. Case definitions for public health surveillance. MMWR Recomm Rep. 1990;39(RR-13):1–43.
6. Toole MJ, Waldman RJ. An analysis of mortality trends among refugee populations in Somalia, Sudan, and Thailand. WHO Bull. 1988;66:237–47.
7. World Health Organization (WHO). Water, sanitation, hygiene, and waste management for the Covid-19 virus. Technical Brief, 3 Mar 2020. Available at: https://www.who.int/publications/i/item/water-sanitation-hygiene-and-waste-management-for-covid-19.
8. World Health Organization (WHO). Rational use of PPE for COVID-19. Available at: https://apps.who.int/iris/bitstream/handle/10665/331215/WHO-2019-nCov-IPCPPE_use-2020.1-eng.pdf.
9. Nurses on the frontline: preparing for and responding to health emergencies and disasters. Educational Module at George Washington University School of Nursing. Revised by Asgary R (Senior Advisor) in 2020. Available at: https://nnepi.gwnursing.org.
10. Resolve to save lives: prevent epidemics. https://preventepidemics.org/coronavirus/insights/.
11. Liu Y, Funk S, Flache S. The contribution of pre-symptomatic infection to the transmission dynamics of COVID-19. Wellcome Open Res. 2020;5:58. Available at: https://www.ncbi.nlm.nih.gov/pmc/articles/PMC7324944/.
12. Kucharski AJ, Russell TW, Diamond C, Liu Y, Edmunds J, Funk S, et al. Early dynamics of transmission and control of COVID-19: a mathematical modelling study. Lancet Infect Dis. 2020;20(5):553–8.

13. Linton NM, Kobayashi T, Yang Y, Hayashi K, Akhmetzhanov AR, Jung S, Yoan B, Kinoshita R, Nishiura H. Incubation period and other epidemiological characteristics of 2019 novel coronavirus infections with right truncation: a statistical analysis of publicly available case data. J Clin Med. 2020;9(2):538.
14. Wu Z, McGoogan JM. Characteristics of and important lessons from the coronavirus disease 2019 (COVID-19) outbreak in china: summary of a report of 72 314 cases from the Chinese Center for Disease Control and Prevention. JAMA. 2020; https://doi.org/10.1001/jama.2020.2648. Available at: http://www.ncbi.nlm.nih.gov/pubmed/32091533.
15. Dahab M, van Zandvoort K, Flasche S, Warsame A, Ratnayake R, Spiegel PB, Waldman RJ, Checchi F. COVID-19 control in low-income settings and displaced populations: what can realistically be done? Confl Heal. 2020;14:54. https://doi.org/10.1186/s13031-020-00296-8.
16. Russell TW, Hellewell J, Jarvis CI, Van-Zandvoort K, Abbott S, Ratnayake R, CMMID Covid-Working Group, Flasche S, Eggo RM, Edmunds WJ, Kucharski A. Estimating the infection and case fatality ratio for COVID-19 using age-adjusted data from the outbreak on the Diamond Princess cruise ship. Euro Surveill. 2020;25(12):2000256.
17. Nishiura H, Linton NM, Akhmetzhanov AR. Serial interval of novel coronavirus (COVID-19) infections. Int J Infect Dis. 2020;93:284–6.
18. Moore D. "We fear, but have to work": isolation not an option for the poor of Nairobi | Global development | The Guardian. 2020. Available at: https://www.theguardian.com/global-development/2020/mar/27/we-fear-but-have-to-work-isolation-not-an-option-for-the-poor-of-nairobi-coronavirus.
19. Gilman RT, Mahroof-Shaffi S, Harkensee C, Chamberlain AT. Modelling intervention to control Covid-19 outbreaks in a refugee camp. BMJ Glob Health. 2020;5:e003727.
20. Centers for Disease Control (CDC). Prevent the spread of Covid-19 if you are sick. Available at: https://www.cdc.gov/coronavirus/2019-ncov/downloads/sick-with-2019-ncov-fact-sheet.pdf.
21. Centers for Disease Control (CDC). Caring for someone sick at home. Available at: https://www.cdc.gov/coronavirus/2019-ncov/if-you-are-sick/care-for-someone.html.

Ramin Asgary, MD, MPH, FASTMH started working in refugee and conflict settings with Doctors Without Borders (MSF) and other agencies in the 90s as field physician, project director, medical coordinator, and health advisor in assignments in Eurasia, South East Asia, Sub-Saharan/East/South Africa, and South/Central America. He served on multiple MSF committees and as senior medical referent or advisor for MSF operational centers, and on the Board of Directors, MSF-USA. He is Associate Professor of Global Health and International Affairs and Director of Humanitarian Health Program at George Washington University. As Associate Professor of Medicine at Weill Cornell Medical College, he teaches clinical medicine, performs health disparities research, and provides healthcare to the homeless populations. He is Vice-Chair of IRB for the International Rescue Committee, Governing Councilor of APHA, and Past-President of Global Health of ASTMH. His expertise includes Refugee Health, Humanitarian Assistance, Global Health Curriculum, Cancer Screening, Ethics and Accountability, and Healthcare of the Underserved Populations.

Data Management Systems for Migrant and Refugee Children

Siyana Mahroof-Shaffi and Bruce Murray

Introduction

Key questions to be addressed:

1. Why keep patient records at all?
2. What are the broad considerations in refugee health care settings?
3. How can pitfalls be considered, prepared for, and avoided?
4. Do we need to bear in mind any legal or ethical issues?
5. What are the currently available systems or standards (e.g., by UNHCR/WHO)?
6. What needs to be considered when developing EHR systems in a refugee health-care setting?
7. What would data collection look like in an ideal situation?

The Challenge of Record-Keeping: To Write or Not to Write

In the earliest stages of response to a humanitarian disaster, when urgent triage and treatment of the sickest children are of immediate concern, accurate and consistent registration, data collection, and record-keeping may not feel like the highest priority.

A traditionally trained healthcare worker placed in the field of disaster relief or a temporary camp setting will find themselves having to adapt to the situation in several ways. This may occur despite how well prepared they or their organizations

S. Mahroof-Shaffi
Kitrinos Healthcare, London, UK
e-mail: director@kitrinoshealthcare.com

B. Murray (✉)
Josephine County Public Health Department, Grants Pass, OR, USA

Medical Teams International, Portland, OR, USA

© Springer Nature Switzerland AG 2021
C. Harkensee et al. (eds.), *Child Refugee and Migrant Health*,
https://doi.org/10.1007/978-3-030-74906-4_18

think they might be. Clinicians may be working surrounded by the dangers of natural disasters or even in war zones amidst a sea of ailing, traumatized, or wounded patients (Fig. 18.1). Challenges include trying to maintain adequate medical documentation, assuming of course that there is some lighting or a working pen while trying to complete a crude paper chart. A simple paper record to be kept with the patient as they are processed and treated with the most basic but crucial information recorded is likely to be as much as can be expected in the critical emergency phase of a disaster. With hundreds of patients needing care and the medical response team being significantly understaffed, there may seem to be no time at all to make a credible medical record. It may even appear that the best that can be done is to "see and treat" and move along to the next person.

A core medical assessment which consists of taking a basic history may need to be obtained in another language or through trying to decipher barely legible or soiled reports which have been carried through long arduous journeys. Physical examinations may be impossible to do in the dark, wet, cold, or undignified surroundings—especially in the case of shy children and sensitive adolescents. One such example was the case of a teenage girl who was found to be writhing around with what appeared to be severe abdominal pains while patiently queueing in a line

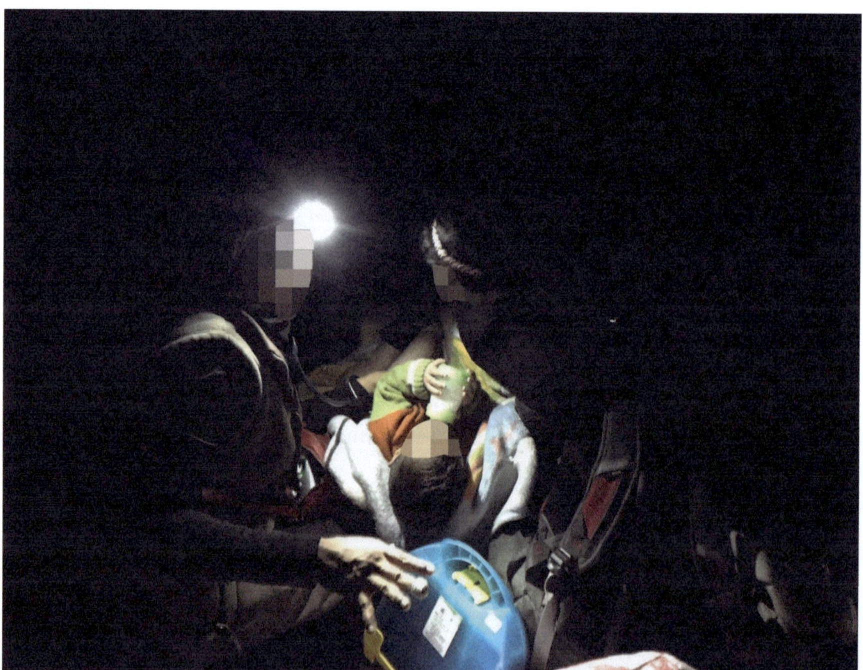

Fig. 18.1 During an evening "ward-rounds" on the hills of Camp Moria in Greece in October 2015, a volunteer physician does assessments for families stranded in queues for up to 10 days at its peak carrying only a backpack of medication and basic equipment. This demonstrates the limitations in the field for clinicians who have to be prepared to adapt and may need to compromise on other standards such as clinical documentation

to register as a new arrival to the camp. A quick assessment on-site revealed what the problem was. She had been afraid to lose her position in the queue and so decided not to pass urine for most of the day. In a make-shift camp, there are no toilets and so a carefully screened corner behind the police barracks was all that was needed to provide the shy child with much-needed and fortunately instant relief. In the early days, in some camps, a record may be made of the type and quantity of medication dispensed (probably more for ensuring that the stock is accurate for the needs and adequately replenished). In the case of pediatric suspensions—once made up there may not be the possibility of refrigeration—rendering it of doubtful efficacy. There may be a need to consider giving shorter courses of therapy with higher doses; if only to improve parental compliance.

No one would doubt the importance of even a minimum amount of documentation not only to provide the best patient care but also for research purposes to better understand the needs of populations in these difficult settings. Initiating or maintaining such systems of record-keeping does not come without its challenges.

Difficulties that may be encountered in the field in data management apply to both the initial phase as well as to the next phases in disaster response, where the immediate urgency of a situation has started to subside and migrant families are settled into abodes (however humble) with access to a static clinic facility. In the developed world, this would be an equivalent of a primary community-based health center with a multidisciplinary workforce. In the remote setting, this would likely be the back of a vehicle or in a tent where running water, electricity or even Internet access would be considered a luxury. The authors believe that recording and collating data should be prioritized no matter what the setting. We hope the reasons for this will be presented forthwith.

Surprisingly, there is still no universally recognized international data standard or even coordinated system for collecting vital patient-encounter information on refugee children. Assuring continuity and quality of data collection on pediatric populations across health care non-governmental organizations, UNHCR agencies, and health ministry representation remains an elusive goal.

In addition, there is a need for the purposes of organizational service planning and delivery, to keep some statistical data on the number and type of patient visits, basic demography, and diagnosis or treatment prescribed. Even such simple data could provide a means of surveillance for infectious disease outbreaks, particularly relevant during preparatory stages that need to be made in the refugee setting when planning for an impending outbreak. Such a situation occurred when the world was grappling with the novel coronavirus pandemic (COVID-19). It became even more imperative that some form of record-keeping was maintained. In the spring of 2020, as worldwide cases of the disease increased exponentially, an urgency prevailed to try and identify the earliest stages of an impending outbreak in the refugee setting. While well-equipped hospitals in more affluent parts of the world were brought to their knees with the high numbers of patients requiring intensive hospital treatment and rising mortality rates. The outcome for average refugee camps with limited access to hospitals (many without ventilators or even the capacity for more than a handful of patients) looked bleak.

At the time of the initial outbreaks, there was a notable absence of formal testing due to lack of availability of suitable kits as well as isolation facilities. Consequently, the medical teams on-site used a simple tally system to monitor the presenting symptoms of those attending the primary healthcare facilities. In particular, careful attention was paid to the presentation of suspicious symptoms such as fevers or coughs. The authors observed that in a typical refugee camp, respiratory infections are endemic in winter months anyway. In observing a sharp rise in the number of patients with respiratory illness, there was the hope of identifying the presence of a potential outbreak. In an overcrowded, refugee camp where relatively poorly nourished residents lived, a grave sense of an impending humanitarian catastrophe was at hand. The Health Information Service (HIS) described later in this chapter was developed by the UNHCR in an attempt to address this need. This process may require additional administrative or technical support staff as this data collection service is not driven by immediate clinical priorities. Instead, the recording of the vital data is for sharing with other healthcare providers as part of the continuity of patient care or facilitating longer term patient outcomes. Collecting this information is also helpful for anticipating the needs of the clinical service for equipment and stocks of medication and even for recruiting the correct number and type of staff. All in all, data collected can become a crucial part of service planning and delivery.

Medical Passports

Children and their guardians often leave a clinic with follow-up instructions and medication use instructions that are handwritten in what is to them a foreign language. This admittedly poor system usually evolves in the first days to weeks to the printing of individual patient records in a booklet form (a "medical passport") for a specific foreign medical team (Fig. 18.2). However, this is usually done without standardization and vital data is often not consistently recorded. At times, long sentences may result in pages running out. Additionally, the use of medical jargon (which varies from country to country even if it is in English) can become a

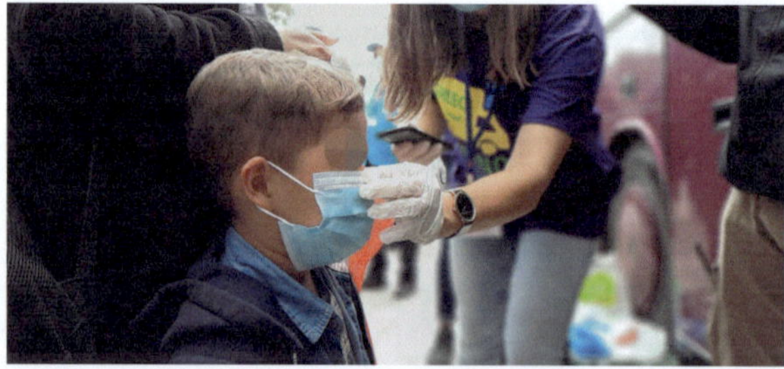

Fig. 18.2 One of the luckiest children and his family who were able to be prioritised for evacuation during the coronavirus pandemic from Camp Moria, Lesvos where just under twenty thousand residents lived at the time. The value of electronic medical records to identify the most vulnerable families was key to this process

confounding factor. The best outcomes would be possible if this process of producing booklets can be done in coordination with other healthcare providers in the region in the hope for some standardization. These booklets are usually retained by the caregivers of refugee children. The desired outcome would be that they bring the booklet, as patient-held records, for any clinical consultation. In dealing with a population not accustomed to systematic, longitudinal medical care there is a frequent lack of understanding or even desire for continuity of care. Without a coordinated response, multiple medical opinions may be sought in order for desperate families to eventually obtain a crucially heart-wrenching diagnosis can be given. This, in theory, would facilitate medical advocacy, leading to the child and the immediate family receiving a more favorable outcome during their asylum procedures. Ultimately, this could lead to prioritization to be evacuated out of the camp setting and ideally legally relocated to another country (Fig. 18.3).

As well-equipped hospitals in more affluent parts of the world were struggling with high numbers of patients requiring intensive hospital treatment and rising mortality rates, the outcome for average refugee camps with limited access to hospital (many without ventilators) looked bleak.

This vacuum of an overall plan for quality medical records, consistency of data collected, protection of patient confidentiality, and interagency coordination is recognized as a crucial deficiency in existing systems based on broad reviews of the literature on record-keeping in sudden onset natural disasters as well as for migrant and refugee settings [1, 2]. Unfortunately, this applies not only in the acute phase of a disaster but even as the refugee or migrant setting matures and evolves. Moreover, children will likely be evaluated at different acute care settings within the same location, and they may even be relocated to other distant camp environments with each healthcare facility doing child record documentation in a different and probably equally incomplete manner.

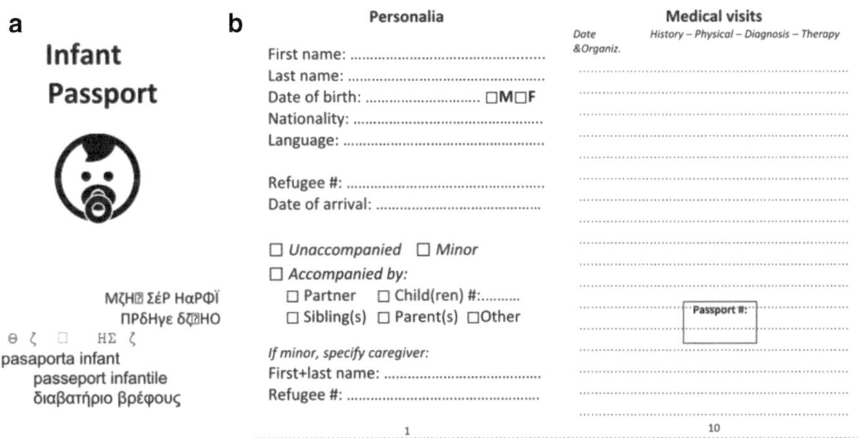

Fig. 18.3 (**a–c**) Samples of a typical UNHCR templates for the 'medical passport', including pediatric growth charts, which could be printed and distributed to all new patients as patient-held records

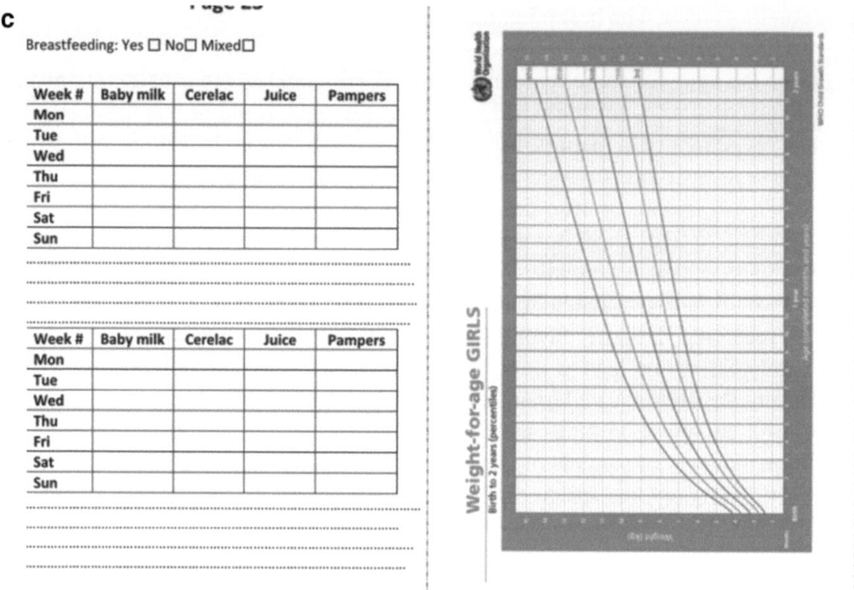

Fig. 18.3 (continued)

World Health Organization Standards

In 2016, WHO published minimum standards of medical record-keeping as a part of their application process for NGOs desiring Emergency Medical Team (EMT) recognition [3]. This is a crucial designation to be included in UNHCR's sudden onset disaster plan. It is a general roadmap of required key elements that NGOs should incorporate without endorsing any specific model or template. For recognition as a Type 1 mobile team (seeing >50 patients/day in remote areas) and a fixed team primary care team (seeing >100 patients a day in a fixed out-patient setting), essential components include:

- System identified to maintain confidentiality such as individual patient records with unique identifiers.
- Clinical care documentation records in accordance with accepted international standards.
- Discharge and referral documentation (in appropriate language) with the ability to provide duplicate copies to the patient and Ministry of Health if so required.
- Documentation of informed consent (in an appropriate language if required).

Presently, it is left to each NGO applying for EMT status to write clinical guidelines and Standard Operating Procedures for each of these four categories. Whether this will ultimately lead to the development of a coordinated system of data collection, entry, analysis, and sharing with other key players while maintaining confidentiality is not known yet.

As a result of these problems, a wide range of electronic health record (EHR) platforms available for commercial and institutional use has proliferated which have been designed to address the recording of legible key demographic data as well as the pertinent acute and chronic health care problems of children. Being able to capture acute care encounters, prior diagnoses, family medical histories, vaccination status, laboratory and imaging results, medication use, drug utilization, growth charts, and inventory management are all attractive components of a useful electronic system to aid pediatric care. However, each EMR option may come with its own proprietary software requirements or with unique hardware platforms individually adapted by the vendor to a low resource environment. The sharing of patient data presents significant confidentiality and legal issues that have not been satisfactorily resolved [2].

Again, there is no one evidence backed system or EMR product that has been validated, endorsed, or even structured to communicate much less integrate data regarding the care of a child across aid organizations and longitudinally over time and changing locations. As a result, supervising entities such as UNHCR, UNICEF, and host Ministries of Health are trying to make crucial planning and logistic decisions based on often incomplete or duplicated information. Two current systems used in UNHCR sponsored refugee settings for collection of broad demographic data as well as clinical information to shape early reporting and response are the Health Information System (HIS) and WHO's Early Warning and Rapid Response Network (EWARN). Each represents a hybrid of paper documents initially that are later entered into electronic formats as the data leaves the basic field clinic environment.

UNHCR Health Information System (HIS)

In 2005 UNHCR started a uniform system of collecting and reporting selected patient-encounter information within a refugee setting, known as a Health Information System (HIS) [4]. This documentation program allows for uniform daily collection and entry of data from each health care setting serving refugees, including information on numbers of patients seen, gender, age, type of encounter (new or follow-up), the general category of illness, the administration of vaccinations, vitamins, as well as other disease and syndrome specific data. Usually, a standardized HIS form is tailored to the specific camp setting and population characteristics. It is meant to interface with the Early Warning Alert and Response Network (EWARN) [5] system to record the priority epidemic diseases encountered including the alert thresholds for those conditions or syndromes. The same case definitions for these key conditions are used by both EWARN and HIS for uniform reporting purposes. Although the system is evolving towards greater use of electronic medical record-keeping in most refugee settings, the data is still primarily gathered by hand at the primary health post setting on a standardized form that is then entered daily and weekly into a proprietary data system for the camp at large. This allows for rapid analysis of information that permits monitoring trends such as disease incidence, current vaccination status and anticipated needs, and evaluation of health impact interventions which may then facilitate appropriate allocation of resources, and development of common guidelines tailored to the needs of each refugee setting.

One major challenge of HIS is how best to interface and collaborate with the host country's Ministry of Health data collection process since national patients are often seen along with the refugee population at clinics within the camp. Cooperation, sharing of data, agreeing on minimum standards of care, and agreeing on when a "suspected" case of measles or cholera becomes a confirmed case are all issues to be resolved specific to each humanitarian emergency. With planning, agreed upon standardization of necessary data collection and cooperation at all levels, electronic record systems to capture this data can be well-suited to innovation going forward.

Early Warning Alert and Response Network (EWARN) Approach in a Refugee Setting

In addition to HIS, another essential data collection system utilized in the earliest phase of a disaster is the Early Warning Alert and Response Network (EWARN), set up by the WHO in coordination with the host country and the health sector [5]. Designed to be set up and fully functional within the first 3 weeks of a disaster, EWARN provides the guidance and blueprint for early epidemic outbreak detection and coordinated response. This system provides for early and broad surveillance of previously identified sentinel diseases or syndromes at the field clinic level. Using daily and weekly standardized reporting, as well as training key refugee community leaders and CHWs to notify health personnel of any public health concerns or rumors of concern, serves to signal an early epidemic or clusters of similar health problems.

In the early stage of a humanitarian crisis, data collection at the field can be done as paper records and submitted quickly to head off the spread of epidemics especially dangerous to children. These would include diarrheal syndromes, measles, malaria, and meningitis among other highly contagious diseases.

Standardized case definitions of each category of reportable disease are created that are necessarily sensitive enough to include almost all of those affected by the priority diseases yet specific enough to be distinguishable from non-priority, self-limited diseases. For example, a case of suspected measles would be a patient with fever, a non-vesicular maculopapular rash, and one or more of the following findings: conjunctivitis, cough, and/or coryza. Reporting channels have to be set up to allow for the swift transmission of information up the chain of command in order to launch an appropriate investigation and laboratory confirmation. Although the data collected on-site at the field clinic will likely be recorded on paper templates initially, the transmission and coordination with other reporting facilities are ideally suited for electronic data methods, as was widely utilized in the early weeks of the Rohingya refugee crisis in Bangladesh in 2017, as just one example.

In addition to immediate (same day) notification of key health events, aggregate data should be collected weekly to indicate trends in presenting complaints of broader concern. There are minimum alert thresholds that are established for each disease or syndrome that will identify early potential outbreaks. For example, in the case of measles, acute flaccid paralysis, or suspected hemorrhagic fever syndrome only a single afflicted child is cause for concern and immediate reporting is necessary. A review of the key diseases or syndromes and their case definitions targeted in the EWARN system are included in the WHO Guidelines [5].

Considerations for Developing Electronic Health Records

The first rule of technology used in a business is that automation applied to an efficient process will magnify the efficiency. The second is that automation applied to an inefficient operation will magnify the inefficiency. Bill Gates, Founder, Microsoft

In striving for efficiency and productivity, the authors dared to dream that no problem and no amount of chaos should exclude the systematic application of practical solutions when it comes to implementing electronic health record (EHR) systems in the refugee healthcare setting. Why should something that works reasonably well in modern medical practice not work so well in a low resource setting and with variable manpower? In fact, the compulsion should be that best practice should be brought to children and families in the most vulnerable setting as a priority and not a last resort. Mistakes in this scenario on the background of malnutrition and other vulnerability criteria (i.e., physical and psychological disabilities), with minimal diagnostic testing and monitoring facilities could lead to more serious consequences. EHR can help avoid mistakes by providing a narrative for each patient, in chronological order that is easier to follow than barely legible or potentially damaged paper records, which are more than likely to be in several different foreign languages.

A paperless system reduces the risk of data being lost, produces less paper waste, and reduces the need for secure storage of confidential medical records. After a destructive fire in Camp Moria in September 2020, there was much regret by the local asylum services that much of the information acquired had not been stored electronically. Many asylum cases were set back years as a result of this loss. As medical providers who kept scant records at least for the most vulnerable, such as those children on long-term epilepsy medication, there is a window of opportunity for the influence of medical advocacy.

In the author's experiences, several systems were tried and tested from grassroots experiences in nearly 20 different locations in various camps which began during the 2015 European Migration Crisis. Families from different countries speaking a multitude of different languages and dialects meant an additional layer of complexity in this scenario which necessitated simple, reliable, flexible systems that were easy to produce with minimal technology, inexpensive and transferable.

Consultations needed to be painstakingly translated into and documented in English. A clinician would have spent precious time and much effort in extracting this information. Additionally, by offering predefined choices in the form of electronic drop-down menus, medical jargon can be avoided and the data becomes more standardized and measurable.

In our experience, one of the earliest drivers for recording systems was brought about by the need to identify gaps in childhood immunizations in refugee children. For many children from war-torn countries like Syria or Afghanistan, access to vaccines was limited and records were even more scarce. Without such a simple healthcare intervention and accurate documentation, many children were denied access to local educational facilities often shared with children from the host population. In this example, the power of a formal vaccination record card stamped and signed was self-evident. Indeed, the vaccination record became a passport for many children to start the next phase of their lives denied by years of war and conflict in their countries of origin by being able to join local schools (Fig. 18.4).

The benefits of such diligent and organized record-keeping are even greater in children with more complicated needs. Electronic recording systems can support caregivers' decisions, communication between specialists, and improve patient

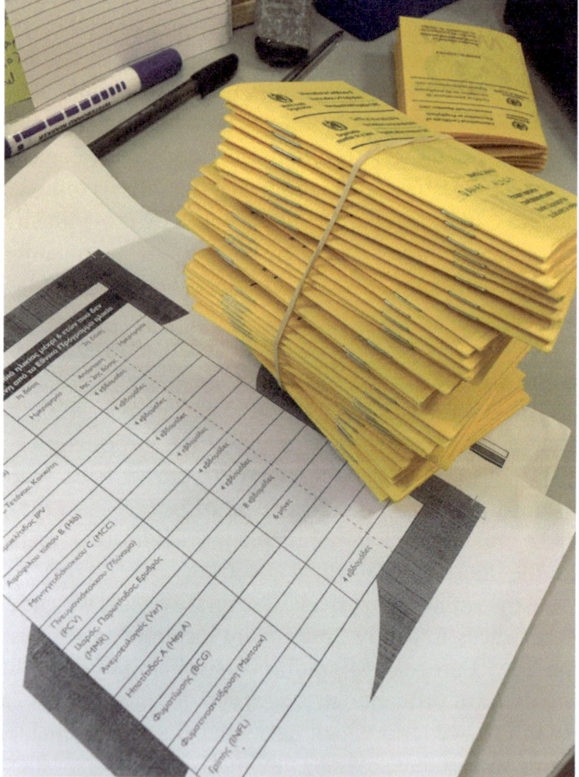

Fig. 18.4 Sample WHO Immunization Record booklets which effectively served to certify that the refugee children were fully vaccinated and therefore fit to join host country schools

outcomes [6]. Children and infants (especially those with special health care needs) are at higher risk than adults for medical errors and their consequences [7].

This is demonstrated in the management of a pair of 14-year-old twins with complex needs learning to live with a range of new onset and progressive disabilities. Their parents had already lost one son to a deadly, as yet undiagnosed disease process causing severe neuromuscular degeneration. They anguished about making the perilous journey by land towards Europe as they watched their children who were phenotypically normal at birth gradually started to develop serious symptoms including loss of vision and speech. The family's treacherous journey, escaping war, and across rough terrains were undertaken to find a possible cure and to potentially try and save their children's lives as well as hoping to prevent the disease in their youngest as yet unaffected child (Fig. 18.5).

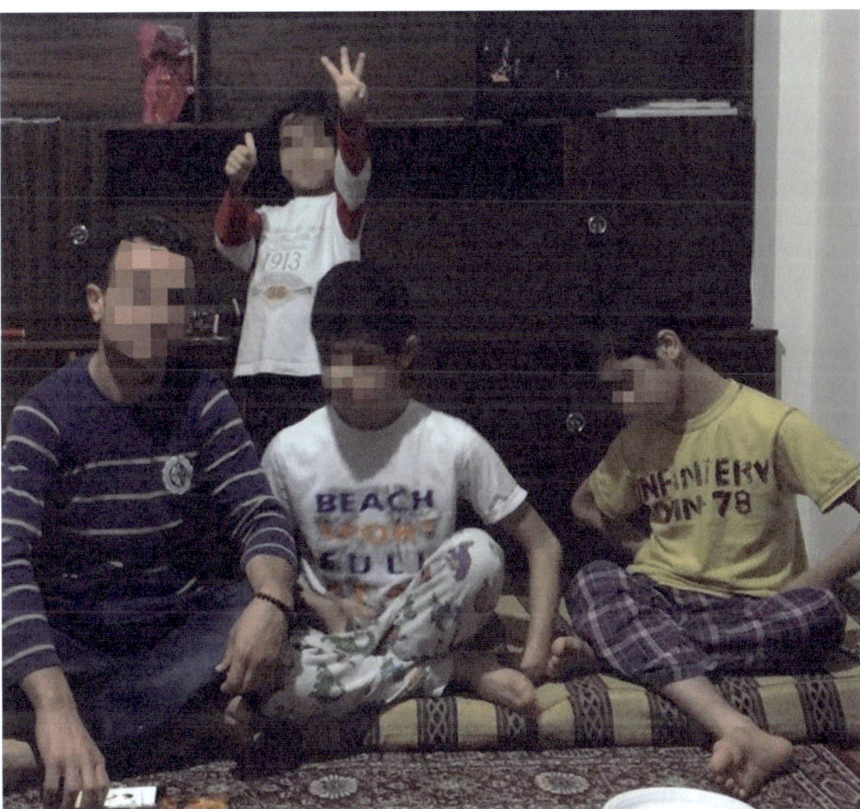

Fig. 18.5 The case of twin boys, disabled by blindness, progressive muscular weakness, and frequent seizures are an example of how chronologically organized electronic data played an important role in helping their medical providers identify the cause of their mysterious and possibly fatal illness. The hope was to prevent the development of similar symptoms in their youngest and so far healthy little brother

Initially, they started to become visually impaired; then developed weakness with loss of bladder and bowel control, spasticity in their limbs, and seizures necessitating upward titration of their anti-epileptic medication. The growing pile of paper records was becoming harder to piece together and each volunteer clinician seemed to extract a gem of medical data to add to their story. Their health data (including digital images from scans) was collected and organized in chronological order, over a period of 2 years while direct care was being provided in a host country with its own healthcare limitations. In an electronic format, this data could have been shared with specialists across the world ultimately leading to a healthcare conference being facilitated between multiple specialists across the world collaborating to elucidate a diagnosis.

The simplest form of an "e-record" could be in the form of a typed, spelling-checked document—which was little more than an electronic version of the "medical passport" booklet mentioned earlier. This simple start meant instant legibility (avoiding notorious physician "poor-handwriting" and language issues). If needed it could also be printed as hard copies or downloaded to encrypted memory sticks as a soft copy for parents or guardians to carry with them when consulting other providers. Additionally, if these were destroyed a secure cloud-based server could be accessed by the provider to make duplicates or to transfer information electronically to other healthcare providers wherever in the world the child and their family find themselves on their onward journey. This simple method had an important function of being able to be updated in an "offline" capacity and later be able to be synchronized once Internet connectivity was available.

Challenges in Using EHR in Field Medicine

The earliest considerations in terms of ambulatory care of patients will be likely to involve paper-based recording systems. Any system will struggle to be maintained when camp sizes increase, particularly when several thousand people are present. The irony of course is that if the initial hurdle of setting up a suitable system is overcome, the outcome in terms of the many advantages mentioned earlier will become automated and streamlined and allow the collection of measurable data.

The successful use of any electronic systems also depends on the availability of suitable hardware, software, and some Internet connectivity. In many countries, the use of EHR is still viewed with some skepticism where bureaucratic efficiency is gauged by how much paper workers have collected on their desks. In these situations, electronic systems would need to be used discreetly. The use of electronic tablets and smartphones might be akin to "spying" and could potentially lead to criminal charges. It is not unknown for volunteers to be charged with all sorts of offenses; the most serious could include violation of human rights and human trafficking. One way to potentially overcome this if the data that is collected remains the property of the patient themselves or their guardians. They can then choose to share this with healthcare providers or legal representatives of their choice, as and when needed.

In practice, giving patients access to EHR is not always easy due to language and technological barriers. Many would not have a suitable device and would identify with a more traditional hard copy of a medical report. Some host country asylum service systems for that matter are heavily bureaucratic and rely heavily on original paper copies ideally stamped with a multitude of colors that would be difficult to forge. These medical reports are much-needed for adding weight to their asylum procedures and the ultimate ticket to their freedom of passage.

Another consideration is the balance to be struck between being too prescriptive in record-keeping (structured data) compared to allowing a more free-flowing account on the records. There could potentially be a risk in lack of clarity with the former and the inability to measure outcomes and possible inability to analyze data at all with the latter! In practice, a large proportion of clinical data tends to be unstructured [8]. All data can be analyzed but the less organized it is, the more time-consuming and more costly this process can become. This could cause a significant administrative and financial burden on a small organization running on a tight budget and result in no improvement at all to the care of individual children.

Data Protection and Risk Management

Hand-held hard copies of patient records are easily damaged through liquid spills, burnt or lost. Lost or misplaced paper-based records can lead to a potential breach of patient confidentiality if these end up in the wrong hands. Arguably, these would more easily fail information governance criteria and be at risk of data breaches. Although encrypted devices and the world wide web with cloud-based storage have become increasingly more secure, advice given has been that nothing is 100% safe and beyond a persevering hacker. Ultimately it is the balance between improved patient care and the risk data following into the wrong hands; a risk that any healthcare provider will have to exercise careful consideration and due diligence over in terms of their preferences.

Legal and Ethical Considerations

Medical record-keeping has become an essential standard in good medical practice recommendations by the General Medical Council (UK) [6]. Kim and Lehmann state that adoption of health information technology is a path to improved quality of patient care (effectiveness, safety, timeliness, patient-centeredness, efficiency, and equity) and has been promoted by the medical community [7]. In the developed world where technology has infiltrated all aspects of our lives from shopping to banking, medical licensing bodies have provided financial and legal incentives to promote wider use of EHR (and penalties in some cases when it is not used). The clinician's accurate and contemporaneous note-keeping is almost as vital as their medical expertise, and one strongly encouraged by all medical indemnity lawyers.

As projects become serious and some level of grant funding needs to be applied for, "proof of service delivery" can only be identified through rigorous record-keeping in some capacity. Ultimately, EHRs will improve caregivers' decisions and patients' outcomes and have become a core duty of modern medical practice.

However, application of these standards in other countries faces multiple challenges. For example, skepticism and concerns about data protection can exist among patients themselves who can have false beliefs that everything electronic will end up on "face" (i.e., Facebook and other social media platforms) and therefore in the hands of their pursuers. For some fleeing war and persecution, their lives may conceivably be endangered if personal information such as their location ends up in the wrong hands.

A clear and pragmatic process of informed consent in practice helps us to overcome most of these issues. One possible argument and one used by the author is the importance of EHR for patient safety. In particular, the importance of citing previously tried interventions and their therapeutic outcomes—especially in the case of adverse outcomes. Additionally, extremely vulnerable patients may not volunteer sensitive information at every single visit (such as disclosure of childhood sexual abuse or other psychological trauma). Children may have aggressive or violent families, raising safeguarding concerns necessitating meticulous documentation. Practitioners may judiciously choose where to see their patients based on this knowledge, for their own well-being and safety.

The Ultimate Value of Electronic Records

As mentioned earlier, during the 2020 Covid-19 pandemic, an example of such information gathering and strategic action occurred in an overstretched camp on the Greek island of Lesvos where mathematical modeling had been done on the potential impact of the new coronavirus infection. The aggregate population at the time was about 18,000 refugees [8]. This illness, with its anticipated disruption in normal supply chains, could have had devastating consequences particularly on those with noncommunicable diseases receiving regular medication. This is a particularly vulnerable subgroup that would have been identified in the rest of the world as warranting "shielding."

In one of the camps, a system of electronic recording of the patients being provided "refill" or "repeat" medications had already been implemented for pharmaceutical dispensing and monitoring. From this electronic data in the form of a spreadsheet, those receiving regular medication such as for epilepsy and asthma were identified as some of the most vulnerable people in the camp. With this information many children and their families were identified and prioritized for immediate evacuation; a maneuver that could be considered lifesaving.

Despite the many daunting challenges to constructing a comprehensive and accessible electronic health records program for refugee care application, there is no question about the need and urgency for this to be prioritized. Currently, there is no uniform opinion on the goals or scope of such a system, much less agreement on the specific platform to be used. Progress going forward will require building on the success of individual tested projects, learning from the lessons and limitations of prior experience, and developing a comprehensive and collaborative effort across governmental and non-governmental agencies. The critical requirement for better management of data and patient records, especially of children, will only accelerate as refugee numbers and needs vastly increase in the years ahead as has been forecasted. There is probably no greater need nor greater opportunity before us than the successful management of information to serve and to protect one of the most vulnerable populations in our world: migrant and displaced children.

Learning notes:

- Do explain and obtain informed consent from the patient to make electronic records as they may be sensitive about who the information is shared.
- Do consider an electronic system to avoid having storage issues for paper records which are most at risk of being misplaced, ending up in wrong hands, or destroyed.
- Do choose software that has the ability to be used in an "offline" mode and be able to be synchronized at a later time when connectivity is available.
- Do keep templates short with quick drop-down menu options to make it easier for consistency and provide for structured data collection without the use of medical jargon.
- Do give clinicians protected time to complete medical data records.
- Do consider portable hardware such as tablets or laptops that can be used at the bedside, as this has been shown to be time-saving for clinicians [9].

References

1. Jafar A, Norton I, Lecky F. A literature review of medical record keeping by foreign medical teams in sudden onset disasters, Cambridge core. Prehosp Disaster Med. 2015;30(2):216–22. https://doi.org/10.1017/S1049023X15000102.
2. Chiesa V, Chiarenza A, Mosca D, Rechel B. Health records for migrants and refugees: a systematic review. Health Policy. 2019;123(9):888–900. https://doi.org/10.1016/j.healthpol.2019.07.018.
3. World Health Organization. Global emergency medical team classification, self-assessment minimum standards checklist type 1—Mobile V1.5. 14 Mar 2016.
4. Haskew C, Spiegel P, Tomzyk P, Cornier N. A standardized health information system (HIS) for refugee settings: rationale, challenges and the way forward. Bull World Health Organ. 2010;88(10):792–4. https://doi.org/10.2471/blt.09.074096.
5. WHO Guidelines for Early Warning and Response Network. Outbreak surveillance and response in humanitarian emergencies. Geneva: WHO Document Production Services; 2012. p. 45. https://apps.who.int/iris/bitstream/handle/10665/70812/WHO_HSE_GAR_DCE_2012_1_eng.pdf?sequence=1.
6. GMC. https://www.gmc-uk.org/ethical-guidance/ethical-guidance-for-doctors/protecting-children-and-young-people/keeping-records. Accessed 25 Aug 2020.

7. Kim GR, Lehmann CU, Council on Clinical Information Technology. Pediatric aspects of inpatient health information technology systems. Pediatrics. 2008;122:e1287–96. https://doi.org/10.1542/peds.2008-2963.
8. Gilman RT, Mahroof-Shaffi S, Harkensee C, Chamberlain AT. Modelling interventions to control COVID-19 outbreaks in a refugee camp. BMJ Glob Health. 5(12):e003727. https://doi.org/10.1101/2020.07.07.20140996.
9. Poissant L, Pereira J, Tamblyn R, Kawasumi Y. The impact of electronic health records on time efficiency of physicians and nurses: a systematic review. J Am Med Inform Assoc. 2005;12:505–16.

Siyana Mahroof-Shaffi, MBBS, MRCGP, DRCOG is a practicing general medical practitioner (family physician) in the UK for over 20 years and a mother of five. She changed her career to become a full-time humanitarian doctor in 2015 after a stint of volunteering as a lead physician for a medical mission during the European Refugee Crisis. Following the mission to the infamous Moria Camp on the Greek island of Lesvos for many months, she founded and continues to lead as the medical director of Kitrinos Healthcare Charity. Through this NGO, she has facilitated thousands of fellow clinicians to provide primary medical care services in over 20 different locations in Greece; ranging from a mobile clinic from the back of a used ambulance to clinic facilities in tents inside the camp. She became passionate about developing systems for the accurate and efficient collation of patient data to serve the vulnerable population she cared for.

Bruce Murray, MD, DTM&H was trained as a general internist at the University of California, San Francisco. He has practiced in academic settings, on a Native American reservation, and in private practice in rural communities California and Oregon. Since 2006 he has done volunteer work in multiple low resource settings including refugee camps in Uganda, Greece, and Bangladesh. He has written clinical protocols for both acute and noncommunicable chronic diseases for different international NGOs. He assisted in the Rohingya humanitarian disaster in Bangladesh in 2017, helping to develop early field clinics and opening a 24-bed field hospital for acute diarrheal illness. He was involved in the capacity building of Bangladeshi physicians teaching refugee medicine, tropical disease, and epidemic management on two subsequent trips in 2018. He now works for Josephine County, Oregon, as COVID-19 medical liaison and contact tracing coordinator.

Pharmacy Setup and Management in the Humanitarian Context

19

Maria Filipa Pereira

Introduction

Pharmaceutical services are an essential part of any medical operation, be it in emergency settings or regular health care services, or specifically for displaced populations or communities, all around the world. From strategic setup, to logistics management and sound clinical use of drugs, any multidisciplinary team can benefit from knowing how these services operate.

In a field humanitarian project, pharmaceutical services are even more important and slightly more difficult to manage. In any high-income country, it is expected that one can procure any drug the same day the need arises (with few exceptions). On the contrary, when in middle- and low-income countries, where most displaced populations are found, there can be months without any drug supply and/or the medical cargo is stuck at borders. This will require managers to calculate all long-term drug and disposables needs as accurately as possible.

With displaced populations, there are frequently different needs according to which stage of migration they are in. It depends on where, geographically, they are passing by and where they are settling. The setting is considered to be an emergency whenever populations are still moving and a regular project setting when a displaced population is settling—either to wait for asylum seeker status or to go back to their home country. Regardless of the type of disaster causing the population displacement, in regards to medical and pharmacy needs, the strategy and setup will often be the same.

M. F. Pereira (✉)
Faculty of Pharmacy, University of Coimbra, Coimbra, Portugal

University of Aberdeen, Aberdeen, UK

Porto Business School, Porto, Portugal

Emergency vs Regular Settings and Different Specialty Programs

In an emergency setup the level of care should be directed to decreasing the mortality and morbidity of the populations. All pharmacy setups will be basic at this stage [1]. A particularly useful tool for any set up at this stage, and afterward, is the Interagency Emergency Health Kit (IEHK) [2]. For any emergency worldwide, organizations big or small should use standardized kits.

When the emergency state is over (and mortality and morbidity have decreased considerably), there is a transitional stage where the level of care goes from basic emergency care to more specialized activities. Usually, these activities tend to cover more vulnerable populations—such as women and children—and are intended to last for a longer period. These activities are often seen in refugee or Internally Displaced People (IDP) civilian camps. These might include services such as reproductive healthcare (in recent years, sexual violence treatment kits and Post Exposure Prophylaxis (PEP) kits have become increasingly important and are included in projects that have very basic primary health care). There are also malnutrition treatment centers, mental health clinics, laboratories, and HIV treatment centers. Likewise, to set up these services, drugs, and consumables can be chosen from standardized kits already available to purchase.

Framework: Setting Up and Managing Pharmaceutical Services in the Field

In order to understand how a program's pharmaceutical service works, including all its different activities, the following framework can help healthcare workers comfortably navigate this specific department in the field. Setting up a pharmacy and managing it properly is essential for any healthcare activity in the humanitarian context, mainly because it will reduce costs and will maintain a permanent stock of essential drugs and consumables thus optimizing the work of healthcare staff [3].

The logic behind a pharmacy setup and management is always the same, irrespective of its capacity, scope, or level of care in which it is running. The same tasks and strategies apply to any situation: someone should procure drugs, arrange for the necessary logistics, manage its stock and storage conditions, and promote rational use of those drugs.

The framework below can be used as a guide and checklist for monitoring and supervising any field pharmacy activities (Table 19.1).

Procurement

Essential Medicines List

The national essential medicines list, if available, should be used to guide procurement for any medical activity. If the country does not have such a list, the WHO

Table 19.1 Framework—pharmacy setup and management in the humanitarian field

Procurement	Logistics	Pharmacy Management	Drug Clinical Management

essential medicines list will have all the references needed to set up any medical treatment center [4, 5]. It is useful to consider WHO's list recommendations because most drugs included in these lists have generic formulations available which reduce costs. The drugs included in this list are selected based on standardized medical protocols. This in turn will simplify the process of procuring drugs and allow increased rational use of medicines with more limited treatment options.

Emergency Health Kit

The IEHK is an incredibly good option for setting up a pharmacy at an emergency treatment facility. Even when procuring drugs independently, it will serve as a starting point to strategize and decide what is going to be needed at any medical project. The kit (and its contents) is designed to allow treatment for up to 10,000 people for the most common diseases for 3 months. These readymade kits can be upscaled and tailored according to the needs of the population treated, and they are regularly updated. For example, this interagency basic kit was recently updated to include drugs for non-communicable diseases (NCDs).

The IEHK guide also features a resource section in which procurement agencies and organizations are mentioned. These options can be quite convenient, even when working in high-income country operations, as these institutions have international supply channels in place. However, to manage these activities for a longer period of time, drug consumption and disease trends need to be properly monitored, and premade kits may no longer be appropriate.

Drug Procurement

Regardless of the project phase, drug orders should be as restrictive as possible. Simplifying and reducing the number of medical protocols available should be the main goal. For instance, when purchasing drugs and medical consumables, the minimum essential doses, formulations, and sizes should suffice. For example, there is no point in having nasogastric tubes of all sizes when only one size can be used for neonates, one size for pediatric patients, and one size for adult patients. Rational consumption should always be a priority even at the purchase level. Furthermore, when purchasing the same drug with different strengths, only one pediatric and one adult strength should be considered (if possible). A simple example is ibuprofen: 400 and 200 mg will allow for both a child and a young adult to be treated. If there is the need to increase the dose to 600 mg it can easily be done with these two different strengths without having to purchase it. Otherwise, unnecessary drugs will be rarely used, will expire, and will waste money.

Drug Donations

Another common situation in the field is to have donated drugs in stock. Although sometimes extremely useful, they can be quite difficult to manage [6]. The intention of having standardized clinical procedures will be disrupted if the donated drugs are not the ones doctors are used to prescribing. Either the drugs will not be used and expire, or they can be wrongly used due to lack of knowledge or because the language of the packaging is not understood. For example, in organizations where doctors rotate often there are several different prescribing trends. Doctors from one country will be accustomed to using a certain drug and doctors from another country will have another preference. This will make it exceedingly difficult to forecast all drug needs and will contribute to inconsistent use and unstable stocks. This was a very frequent issue in the current Greek camps. Due to proximity, European doctors would come to the camps often but for short periods of time. This made the task of normalizing any drug order difficult and, ultimately, led to many unnecessary and different drugs for the same pathology in those pharmacies. Moreover, these drugs may be shipped under unstable conditions, which affects their quality. It is extremely difficult to test if a certain drug is still in good condition in the field, and adverse reactions or ineffective treatment are possible outcomes. One should always assess the risks of accepting donated medications.

Counterfeit and Substandard Drugs

Another particularly sensitive topic regarding medication procurement is the existence of substandard and falsified medical products and drugs in the market. Local procurement should be avoided as much as possible when the operation is set in the middle- and low-income countries. The outcomes can be drastic with casualties reported in many countries [7]. It is plausible that patients will seek the cheapest treatment option, or that healthcare staff in charge of drug procurement will seek a readily available solution to supply any needed drug. However, surveillance and monitoring systems for these falsified products are not yet fully reliable, and one can come across this situation anywhere.

Logistics

Infrastructure

The infrastructure of a field pharmacy should have some specific characteristics, although it is exceedingly rare that it will have all the necessary requirements in place unless it is built from scratch. Additionally, the type of pharmacy needed will depend on the nature of ongoing activities. The most common setups found in the field are Project Pharmacies (commonly called central project pharmacies), Hospital/Clinic Pharmacies, Ward Pharmacies, Drug Dispensaries, and, in cases where there are mobile operations, emergency bags and transportation boxes.

There is not any rigid and mandatory design for these pharmacies. However, there is usually the need to have a main pharmacy as the primary storage site. This main pharmacy will then supply all the end-user pharmacies and should have designated areas for its essential functions. The final design and organization should encompass the following areas: Stock Arrival and Departure (In/Out Movements), work station with office desk, cold chain fridge and freezer if the project needs it, safe places for controlled drugs, and drug storage shelves and pallets for bulky stock [3].

As an example, the schemes below represent two central project pharmacies. Scheme 19.1 is of a Central Pharmacy of a big project run by MSF for IDPs in South Sudan (Schemes 19.1) and Scheme 19.2 is of a small project in the Congo (DRC) to support refugees from Rwanda (Scheme 19.2). The South Sudanese project had been established for a long time and had many regular activities such as a HIV/TB program, laboratories, mental health services, and nutrition clinics. The Congolese project was much less specialized. Storage spaces are dependent on the size of the project and population treated and affect the complexity of pharmacy layouts. However, it is interesting to notice that all of them will have the same essential areas: work desks, cold chain system, In/Out movement pallets, controlled drugs' locked cabinet and lots of shelves (grey rectangles) and pallets for bulky stock (blue squares).

Storage Conditions and Organization

Irrespective of the size and setup, storage conditions, pharmacy layout, and organization will depend mainly on three factors: temperature, humidity, and security/safety.

In an ideal situation, all pharmacies should maintain a temperature between 15 and 25 °C, and humidity levels of around 50–60% [3]. However, this is extremely difficult to achieve in certain countries. The consequences of inadequate humidity and temperature control can include decreased drug effectiveness and drug deterioration with the appearance of undetectable toxic metabolites. More fragile formulations such as liquid oral formulations, solvents, and injectables in these imperfect conditions should be used with caution. As for tablets and external use drugs, though

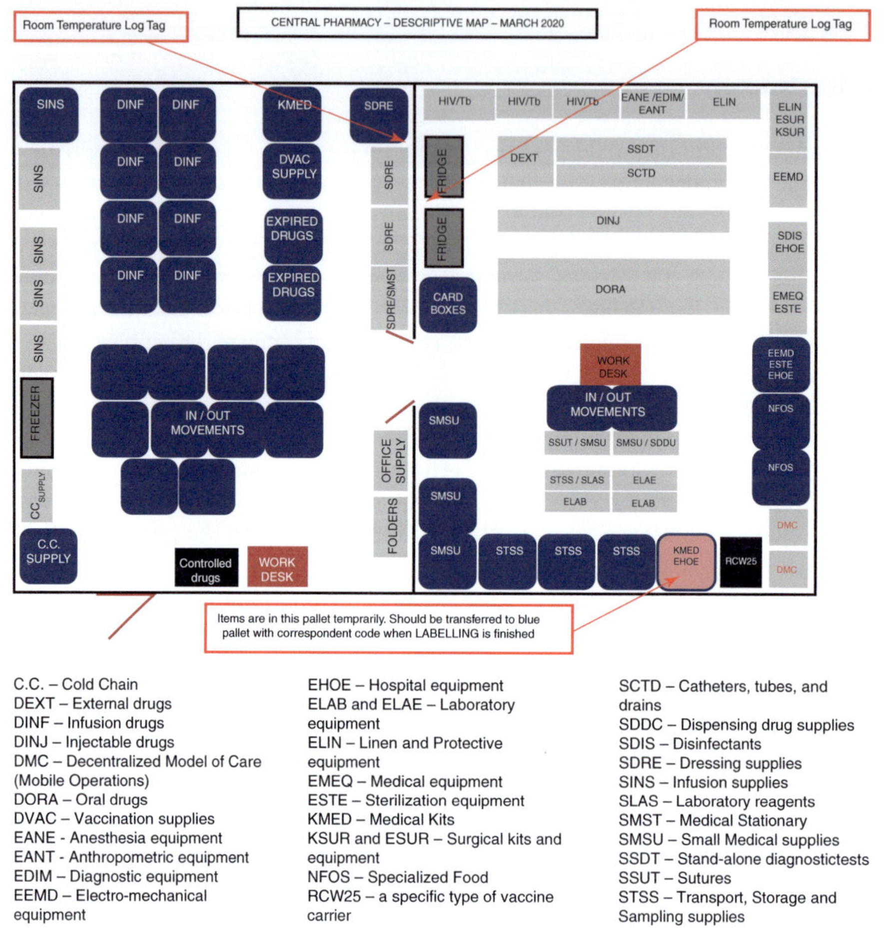

C.C. – Cold Chain
DEXT – External drugs
DINF – Infusion drugs
DINJ – Injectable drugs
DMC – Decentralized Model of Care (Mobile Operations)
DORA – Oral drugs
DVAC – Vaccination supplies
EANE - Anesthesia equipment
EANT - Anthropometric equipment
EDIM – Diagnostic equipment
EEMD – Electro-mechanical equipment

EHOE – Hospital equipment
ELAB and ELAE – Laboratory equipment
ELIN – Linen and Protective equipment
EMEQ – Medical equipment
ESTE – Sterilization equipment
KMED – Medical Kits
KSUR and ESUR – Surgical kits and equipment
NFOS – Specialized Food
RCW25 – a specific type of vaccine carrier

SCTD – Catheters, tubes, and drains
SDDC – Dispensing drug supplies
SDIS – Disinfectants
SDRE – Dressing supplies
SINS – Infusion supplies
SLAS – Laboratory reagents
SMST – Medical Stationary
SMSU – Small Medical supplies
SSDT – Stand-alone diagnostictests
SSUT – Sutures
STSS – Transport, Storage and Sampling supplies

Scheme 19.1 Pharmacy display—IDP camp in South Sudan

slightly more resistant to inappropriate temperatures and humidity levels, they usually change color and consistency when they deteriorate.

Regarding security and safety, one should always look for ways to restrict access to pharmacies and to drugs, for several reasons, including theft, misuse, and inaccurate stock control.

In the two pharmacy illustrations above, one can see that the organization of shelves and pallets considers temperature and humidity conditions. For example, in the South Sudanese pharmacy, all drugs are on the right side of the pharmacy where the lack of doors or windows allows for a more constant room temperature. Additionally, the left side of the pharmacy stored consumables and intravenous infusions which can be exposed to higher temperatures without deteriorating as easily. On the contrary, the Congolese pharmacy was not set up with those characteristics mainly because the temperature was not a problem in that region, but the

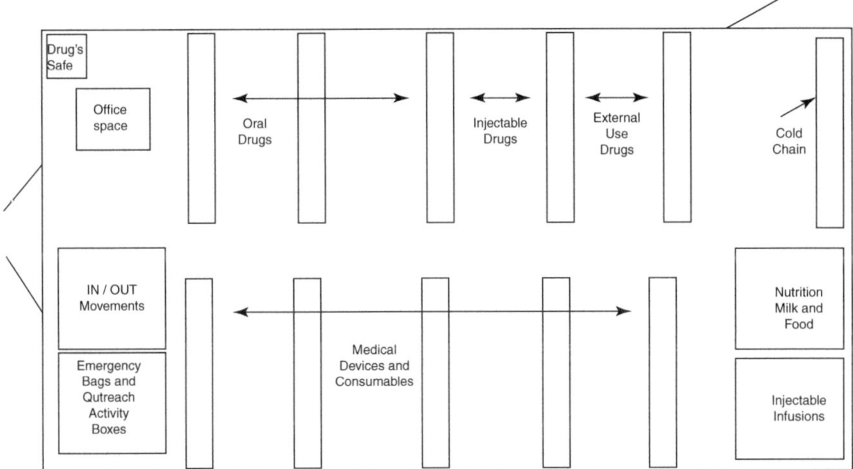

Scheme 19.2 Pharmacy display—project in DRC

humidity was a problem. Another consideration worth pointing out is that controlled drugs are close to the working desk/office space in both pharmacies.

As for shelves and/or pallet organization inside a pharmacy or cabinet, the most used methods are: by active ingredient, alphabetically ordered, organized by formulation class, and arranged by security level. For example, diazepam is generally available in tablets and injectable form however because it is a benzodiazepine, it will be considered a controlled drug. For that matter, all diazepam will need to be locked in a cabinet or box, away from all other oral and injectable drugs, but still divided by its formulation class and alphabetically ordered. Another common way of organizing drugs is by pharmacological family. Although a possible organizational method, experience suggests that it works better in ward and clinic pharmacies that supply to end-users, as that is where prescribers will be working, and they usually understand the difference between categories.

Cold Chain Products

Cold chain (CC) product management is a particularly important task in any project, and it entails a great level of responsibility from logisticians and pharmacy managers. CC product is the term used to refer to any medication or consumable (usually vaccines, rapid test reagents, insulins, antivenoms, etc.) that needs to be stored in colder temperatures, usually between 2 and 8 °C. (If there is a blood bank at project level, human blood needs to be stored at temperatures between 2 and 6 °C). A fridge, freezer, and temperature monitoring tools will be needed to set up a CC system. However, depending on where the project is located, or if there are mobile medical operations going on, a fridge will not be an option because there may not be any electricity available. In these cases, a passive cold chain should be arranged, which is a vaccine carrier that has been conditioned with icepacks to maintain the required temperature for a few hours, and monitoring tools inside to track temperature [8].

Water, Sanitation, and Hygiene (WASH) and Sterilization Procedures

WASH control measures and sterilization procedures are essential to any medical project. WASH allows for effective infection control, access to safe drinking water, proper sanitation, and overall hygiene and comfort of patients and staff [9]. At the pharmacy level, potable water is a concern when reconstituting an oral solution.

Regarding sterilization and disinfection procedures, even though they may not be carried out at the pharmacy level, it is the pharmacy manager who often must procure cleaning supplies. There are many options available according to the level of care provided and facility-specific infrastructures. There are varying protocols used by different organizations. However, methodologies tend to be the same. Autoclaves (including their hardware) and chemical detergents are the most common products procured by pharmacy managers in the field for WASH and sterilization activities [10].

Waste Management: Drug/Device Disposal and Destruction

Health facilities produce potentially infectious and hazardous waste that needs to be managed properly. Pharmaceutical waste management should be handled as much as possible by local authorities. In the absence of such programs, there are protocols that could be implemented locally to destroy this waste. Even though there is no universal methodology guideline for medical waste disposal, the two most common types of procedures are incineration and encapsulation [11]. These will allow for the complete destruction of hazardous pharmaceutical waste and posterior disposal in proper landfills (encapsulation procedure). Logistically, the pharmacy's responsibility will be to properly separate and store expired and deteriorated drugs and consumables (pharmacies are crucial for this specific task). Also, sometimes it falls under the pharmacy's responsibility to supply and collect safety boxes for sharps from wards and mobile clinics. The disposal of medical sharps and any potential infectious waste coming from the health facilities will follow similar protocols to pharmaceutical waste disposal, where incineration is the most used methodology [12].

Pharmacy Management

Forecasting of Needs

For medical operations to run smoothly it is essential to have proper needs forecasting and proper follow-up of consumption. Accurate data gathering and data analysis are crucial, though often difficult to produce. Nevertheless, there are a few tools that could be put in place to track the entire path of a given drug within a project. Examples of this can be found in the IEHK annexes and MSF guidelines [2, 3]. Different tools include stock cards (and any software or excel spreadsheet an organization is using); consumption sheets; inventory sheets; and order sheets. Usually, in smaller operations, medical staff tend to dismiss these tools, but they are extremely useful and will help prevent any out-of-stock situation and spot any unusual trends in consumption that may indicate public health issues and other useful trends.

Consumption and order sheets will help to evaluate how the project's clinical guidelines are being followed. When this information is cross-checked with medical records from the clinics and hospitals, a clearer picture of the population profile and their medical needs can be produced. Gathering and analyzing this data will allow for a pharmacy manager to forecast and prepare a coherent and cost-effective drug and consumables order.

Reception of Medical Cargo

Receiving medical cargo is an exceedingly difficult task in some parts of the globe, and often one must charter proper transportation. Logistically, it can be difficult to receive the cargo and often there are legal constraints and clearance delays imposed by local health authorities. Frequently, medical cargo is quarantined at the country border causing considerable delays in cargo reception, which can disrupt all medical operations. Therefore, anticipating the project needs and accounting for setbacks and security stocks is crucial (Figs. 19.1 and 19.2).

Stock Management and Inventory

Finally, managing the stock of any project pharmacy will probably be the most time-consuming task but the most essential one. Of all the mentioned tools, stock cards and inventories are by far the most important. The stock card usually has the drug or product and its strength and formulation type, all the movements in and out of the pharmacy, and the quantity counted when the inventory was performed. This will allow for a comparison between theoretical stocks and actual stocks. It will also help to identify any discrepancies, to where the products are going, how much is needed for security stock, how much is being consumed, and for what purpose the drugs are being used. Stock cards and inventories can help track expired items and spot deterioration in drugs.

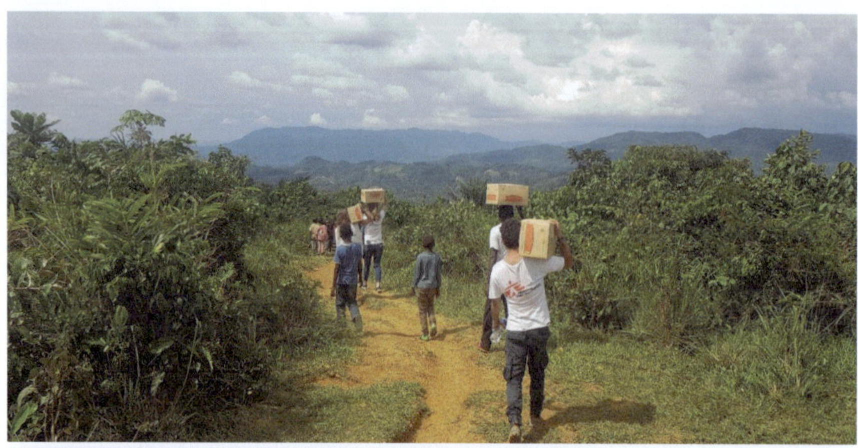

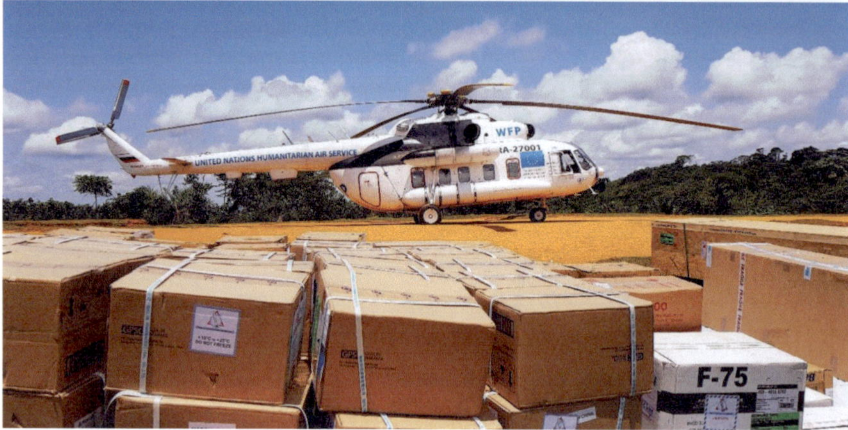

Figs. 19.1 and 19.2 Receiving medical cargo—Democratic Republic of Congo 2018

Given all these managerial activities and tools, something that should be set up straight away is a chronogram of all pharmacy activities. This helps with overall organization of the operation and helps the medical teams organize their monthly tasks.

Drug Clinical Management

Treatment Compliance

There are several reasons to promote rational use of drugs: judicious, careful choice of medications can help reduce pharmacy costs and improve efforts towards Antimicrobial Resistance (AMR) control.

There are a few common guidelines that can be applied in the field, that will allow medical teams to promote safe and rational use of medications and consumables. For example, the use of injectable drugs should be limited. Some patients regard injectable treatments as the only ones strong enough to be effective, but the medical staff knows this is false. Different perceptions among certain populations can make this task difficult. Sometimes it is difficult to convince patients of a particular treatment procedure because it is against their cultural beliefs. Clinicians should make efforts to understand the cultural and social aspects of the treated populations to better understand how to increase treatment adherence.

Clinical Protocols and Preventing Drug Misuse

In order to increase the rational use of medications and reduce antimicrobial resistance (AMR), it is important that clinicians respect approved treatment protocols. Failure to do so is harmful to patients, likely to impact pharmaceutical operations and planning, and leads to AMR. Medical and pharmacy directors should consider holding regular meetings to discuss antibiotic use with clinicians.

For example, the prescription in the figure below (Fig. 19.3) is considered by many an example of excessive empirical prescription. The patient was stable and afebrile. The prescriber decided to treat immediately for possible bacterial gastroenteritis and an intestinal parasitosis. In addition to potential adverse side effects for the patient, this decision might reduce the availability of these medications for patients who truly need them.

MSF clinical guidelines are available to help implement clinical protocols in a medical setting [13]. These can help to understand where weaknesses exist in rational use of drugs.

Antimicrobial Resistance

It is extremely important to tackle antimicrobial resistance (AMR) in all medical settings. Antimicrobial Stewardship (AMS) has been broadly implemented and frameworks have been proposed to decrease the rate at which bacteria are becoming resistant to existing antibiotics [14]. There are a few strategies aimed at reducing the burden of AMR that should be present in any field operation. These include

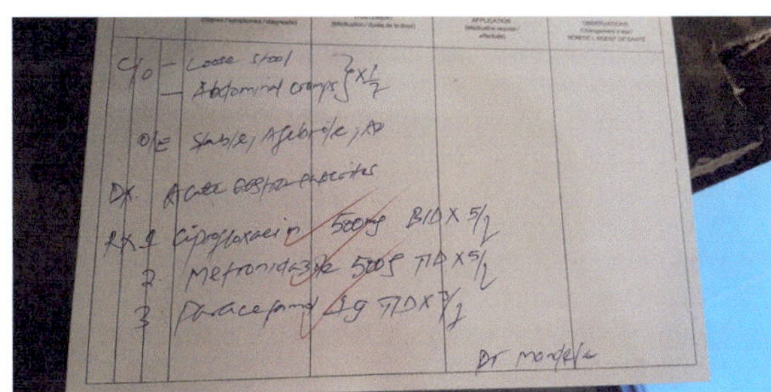

Fig. 19.3 Prescription paper—South Sudan 2019

diagnostics that identify causative bacteria, and indicate if said bacteria is resistant to certain antibiotics, as well as infection control and prevention measures (WASH activities are essential to achieving this), immunization coverage, and better education on AMS among healthcare workers and patients [15].

Traditional Healers and Common Drug Interactions

Traditional healers are often found in displaced communities. Although they are a very important pillar of any community, they may prescribe treatments that interact negatively with drugs prescribed in other clinics. Patients may fail to mention the traditional treatments. There are many known interactions between drugs and herbs. However, traditions differ geographically, and thus a comprehensive study of traditional healing practices in the project's region is recommended.

Conclusions and Useful Resources

Pharmacy operations can be daunting and complex in any part of the world. In the humanitarian field, there are increased difficulties and challenges. Standardization of protocols and procedures make pharmacy programs much easier to run and navigate.

Many useful resources can be stored on a phone, tablet, or laptop, and there is no longer the need to go to the field with heavy pharmacy books and notebooks. A few of the most useful resources and guidelines are mentioned throughout this chapter and can be found in the bibliography. WHO, MSF, Physician Colleges and Associations, and Pharmaceutical Councils all have available apps with useful, user-friendly resources, all of which result in increased efficiency and effectiveness in the field.

References

1. The Johns Hopkins and The International Federation of Red Cross and Red Crescent Societies. Public health guide in emergencies. 2008.
2. World Health Organization. The interagency emergency health kit 2011. Geneva: World Health Organization; 2011.
3. Médecins Sans Frontières. Essential drugs: practical guide intended for physicians, pharmacists, nurses and medical auxiliaries. 2020.
4. World Health Organization. 21st WHO model list of essential medicines. Geneva: World Health Organization; 2019.
5. World Health Organization. 7th WHO model list of essential medicines for children. Geneva: World Health Organization; 2019.
6. World Health Organization. Guidelines for medicine donations revised 2010. Geneva: World Health Organization; 2011.
7. World Health Organization. WHO global surveillance and monitoring system. Geneva: World Health Organization; 2017.

8. Townsend M, Grandclément G. Cold chain management guideline. Geneva: Médecins Sans Frontières; 2013.
9. General Secretariat Malteser International. WASH guidelines for field practitioners. Cologne: Malteser International; 2014. p. 1–130.
10. Choquenet P, Dimeglio S. Sterilization in Médecins Sans Frontières healthcare facilities. Geneva: Médecins Sans Frontières; 2017.
11. van den Noortgate J. Hazardous waste management of health structures within low-income countries. Geneva: Médecins Sans Frontières; 2013.
12. ICRC. Medical waste management, vol. 59. Geneva: International Committee of the Red Cross; 2009. p. 451.
13. MSF. Clinical guidelines—diagnosis and treatment manual. 2016.
14. World Health Organization. Antimicrobial stewardship programmes in health-care facilities in low- and middle-income countries: a WHO practical toolkit. Geneva: World Health Organization; 2019.
15. O'Neill J et al. Tackling drug-resistant infections globally: final report and recommendations. 2016.

Maria Filipa Pereira, PharmD, MBA, CEFA is a Community and Humanitarian Pharmacist. She has a Pharmacy degree from the University of Coimbra, Portugal, an MBA in International Healthcare Management from the University of Aberdeen, Scotland, and a Postgraduate degree in Financial Analysis from Porto Business School, Portugal. She has worked as both pharmacist and researcher at Erasmus MC Hospital in the Netherlands; with the pharmaceutical industry in pharmaceutical marketing and market research at Bial, in Spain; and in community pharmacy as a Senior Pharmacist and General Manager in Portugal. For the past few years, she has extended her experience into the humanitarian field, having worked with many international organizations: first in Greece, setting up clinic pharmacies in different refugee camps and, since 2018, with Médecins Sans Frontières/Doctors without Borders, in South Sudan and the Democratic Republic of Congo, where she has been in charge of overseeing both projects' entire pharmaceutical operations.

Working with Interpreters in a Humanitarian Setting

20

Christian Harkensee

Introduction and Background

The oral translation of spoken language (interpretation) is a critical link in the humanitarian response. The response should be driven by the needs and preferences of the beneficiaries, and it can only do so if actors fully understand these needs and preferences in their cultural context on all levels. The humanitarian workers should do all they can to learn the language of the people they are working with as part of their preparation for deployment or "on the job" to reduce their reliance on the need for interpreters. Here we are focusing on how to best work with interpreters in the field in a humanitarian healthcare setting.

Definitions

Interpreter: someone whose job is to change what someone else is saying into another language.

Translator: a person whose job is changing words, especially written words, into a different language.

Cultural Mediator: a person who can speak and interpret a language (perhaps not to the skill level of an interpreter), has deep insight into the cultural context of this language, and is able to communicate this to someone from another cultural background.

In this chapter, the focus is on interpretation in a humanitarian context, which may contain elements of translation and cultural mediation.

C. Harkensee (✉)
Queen Elizabeth Hospital, Gateshead, UK

© Springer Nature Switzerland AG 2021
C. Harkensee et al. (eds.), *Child Refugee and Migrant Health*,
https://doi.org/10.1007/978-3-030-74906-4_20

Types of Interpreters

In humanitarian settings there are mainly three types of interpreters. These include expatriates, which can be volunteers or professionals from overseas, often with good mastery of the language and sometimes a professional interpreter who may or may not have the same cultural background or insight into the culture. Secondly, these could be locally recruited interpreters from the host community; these might be host country citizens who learned the language or members of the diaspora living in the host country. Finally, interpreters could be volunteers (or professionals) from the refugee population itself; this is probably the most common situation in many settings.

The work of an interpreter or translator goes well beyond a technical translation of words into another language—they "interpret" the spoken or written word or text within a cultural context. This is why there is no single version of a particular interpretation, and why interpretation is a skill and an art that takes training and experience to master. In the humanitarian setting, we seldom have the luxury of independent, professional interpreters and translators—most commonly they are recruited from the refugee population itself or from the host country. This brings particular challenges.

The Relationships Between Interpreters, Patients, and HealthCare Workers

In order to understand the potential ethical pitfalls, it is helpful to look at the barriers and the power imbalances in the triangular relationships between interpreters, patients, and healthcare workers.

Patients come to the healthcare worker with a health need. The patient depends on the services that the healthcare worker provides. If the healthcare worker is from a different culture and does not speak their language, this puts up an immediate barrier—they cannot express their health concerns or needs, and they cannot be sure the healthcare worker understands their experience of health and illness.

The healthcare worker comes with the intention to help and understand the needs of the patient. Not understanding the culture and language puts a barrier between fully understanding and addressing the needs. Despite the lack of understanding, the healthcare worker is in a position of power. Healthcare workers usually rely on interpreters as a scarce resource and may not be in a position to judge their skill, training, and quality of interpretation.

The interpreter could find herself or himself in a conflicted position: Their language skills put them in a privileged situation; they may control what information is interpreted, and how. This hierarchy may be conscious or sub/unconscious. Interpreters may also be subjected to harassment, bullying, and abuse for the position they are in, by both patients and healthcare workers. There may be conflicts of loyalty, especially if they have personal relationships with patients. These could be enhanced by the status of interpreters—in particular, if they are formally paid rather than work as volunteers. Nonprofessional interpreters may have limited skill and experience and may not understand fully their potential conflicts of interest, which could put them under stress and pressure.

Ethical Principles of Interpreting in a Humanitarian Setting

Interpreters form part of a humanitarian team, and the same ethical principles that apply to all humanitarian actors should apply to them. Below are ethical principles specifically for humanitarian interpreters, adapted from the humanitarian principles of the International Committee of the Red Cross (ICRC) [1]:

- *Humanity*: The commitment and desire to assist without discrimination, prevent and alleviate suffering, protect life and health, promote mutual understanding, cooperation, and lasting peace among all people.
- *Impartiality*: An obligation to serve both parties in the encounter, not to seek any advantage from their position or knowledge they gain from their work, and not to exercise power/influence over their listeners. Interpreters should be in a position to reject/end assignments if they feel their impartiality is breached.
- *Neutrality*: Interpret what is "factually" said, separating this from the interpreter's own opinion about what is said.
- *Accuracy*: Interpreting as accurately as possible the words, but also the intention/context of what is being said.
- *Transparency:* There should be full transparency in any encounter between the patient, healthcare professional, and interpreter. There should be no untranslated "side conversations" between patient/interpreter or healthcare worker/interpreter.
- *Confidentiality*: All conversations are kept confidential and their content must not be shared without the explicit, informed, voluntary consent of all parties involved.
- *Respect*: Respect for culture and customs, nondiscrimination, tolerance, and compassion for both the patient and healthcare worker. Likewise, the interpreter has a right to expect the same towards him from the healthcare worker and the patient.

Practical Tips for Working with Interpreters

How healthcare workers can make the most out of working with interpreters:

- Explain to the interpreter that the way they translate the communication, and how they listen to the patient's concerns are crucial for building trust and creating an atmosphere of well-being. In this sense, the interpreter is very much an essential part of the team rather than simply providing a service.
- Before the interaction begins, make sure to introduce the interpreter as a professional (perhaps stating the organization they work for), who has agreed to respect the patient's privacy and confidentiality.

- Try to provide as much confidentiality as possible—recognize the limitations to do so in a busy crowded clinic.
- Cultural awareness: Ask the patient at the beginning of consultation if he/she is comfortable with the interpreter—consider gender roles (e.g., a woman with a male doctor and a male interpreter—consider getting a female chaperone). It is sometimes necessary that the interpreter needs to leave the room (or draw a curtain) when examining women. However, make sure the patient knows they can ask questions and give feedback during the exam. Communicate this clearly.
- Face the patient, and talk to the patient directly, not the interpreter. Position the interpreter to your side, which makes it easier to maintain eye contact with the patient while making sure the interpreter can hear you clearly.
- Break it down—talk for no more than 2–3 sentences or 10–15 s, to allow the interpreter to interpret timely, and not to omit important information. Allow the interpreter to finish interpreting before speaking.
- Do not allow for "side conversations"—i.e., untranslated communication between both yourself and the interpreter in a language the patient does not understand, or likewise between the interpreter and the patient that you do not understand.
- Do not allow the interpreter to answer questions on the patient's behalf; inquire if an interpretation is longer or shorter than expected. Likewise, do not let the interpreter ask questions on your behalf to the patient.
- Be aware of social and family dynamics in the encounter. Parents tend to interpret how their child feels and some expect their child to be silent. On the other hand, children often learn a new language quicker than their parents and become their interpreters, but may not fully understand what they are asked to interpret. If the child is a teenager, the interpreter should be encouraged to speak with the teenager directly. However, this may be difficult for both the parent and the teenager, and the notion of speaking with the teenager in the absence of the parent will not be tolerated by some parents. When discussing consent for major treatments (e.g., surgery) be aware that it may not necessarily be the parents but another person (e.g., community leader) who would have to be consulted.
- Most volunteer interpreters do not have a medical background. Ensure that your language is simple and understandable. Explain terminology and concepts to the interpreter if requested. Keep in mind that some medical questions may be embarrassing for both the patient and the interpreter to ask or answer. Make sure you are getting the full information you need.
- Ask the interpreter for clarification of cultural concepts and differences if necessary.

Lost in Translation!
One editor's fondest memories of language misinterpretation comes from her experience working in a children's hospital in the US with refugees from Laos. She had been stopping in to chat with a Lao boy each day although he was not her patient. He was usually alone. His father was working and his

mother had several other children to care for. Late one day a nurse came to the doctor's office to say that he had been crying for an hour. The doctor went to his room and he told her that he had not eaten, *"Bo kin khao, bo kin khao"* (I have not eaten). She asked the nurse if he had received his dinner. She said he had eaten everything on the tray. She asked if there was rice in the meal. She said no. Traditionally, most Lao do not regard a meal as a true meal unless it contains rice. Rice is so important that "kin khao" (eat rice) is also the phrase for a meal. This child was crying because he had not received rice. The doctor called the hospital kitchen. They had closed. So she called her husband who made a batch of rice and brought it to the boy. He was all smiles!

Training, Education, and Ongoing Support for Interpreters

It is important for interpreters not only to have language skills but also to follow a set of basic ethical principles of interpreting in a humanitarian setting, as outlined above. This can be achieved through a structured education program that should encompass the following elements:

- Orientation or induction training, including understanding and applying the ethical principles of interpreting in a humanitarian setting, and training on the goals and principles of the organization they are working with
- Regular language and interpreting training, including medical terminology
- Sessions about cultural awareness
- Regular feedback and appraisal; ongoing education and support

Furthermore, organizations working with interpreters have a moral duty to support the well-being of interpreters. This should include adequate working conditions—adequate working hours, breaks, and off-days, and supporting interpreters in upholding ethical principles. The workplace should nurture a culture of respect and support, making a clear stance against any form of discrimination, bullying, harassment, and racism. Interpreters should be provided with adequate supervision, of both day-to-day supervision and exploration of professional development opportunities as well. As interpreters are exposed to many traumatizing conversations, they should have regular debriefings and mental health support, as discussed below.

How to care for the well-being of interpreters:

- Be aware of the standing of your interpreter in the community—they may be in a vulnerable position.
- Briefing with your interpreter before consultation: Emphasize the ethical ground rules (e.g., no side conversations) and encourage the interpreter to voice if you speak too fast, too long, not clear enough, or if they feel uncomfortable or exhausted. Encourage the interpreter to voice any concerns that may arise for them during the consultation.

- Some interpreters may find it uncomfortable to witness a medical examination or procedures—allow them to leave the room or turn their back if they prefer.
- Check with your interpreter beforehand to gauge how comfortable they feel about translating questions that can be sensitive for the patient and to the interpreter. Respect if they do not want to interpret those (and ask for another interpreter who may).
- Debriefing after the consultation—check in with them if they are ok, and ask for feedback if there is anything you can do to make their work easier. Asking them for their views and perceptions about the consultation is a great learning opportunity in cultural understanding.
- Ensure interpreters get regular breaks. If you feel physically or emotionally exhausted, so do they. Check on their well-being regularly, show kindness and compassion, and allow for breaks, food, and drink.
- Inform interpreters where they can find psychological support if needed.
- Maintain a professional distance: Interpreters are often the closest link that healthcare workers will have with the community they work for. They will become friends, confidants, and often companions for healthcare workers. However, there remains an imbalance of power (especially if the interpreter is a volunteer from the community), which makes the interpreter vulnerable as long as the working relationship persists. It would be best to keep a professional distance to protect both the integrity of the interpreter and the healthcare worker.

Tips for Interpreters to Enhance Their Skills
Skills practice:

Use short articles from magazines or newspapers to translate directly into spoken word. Practice in front of a mirror or to another person. Practice reading a paragraph and then translate a summary or paraphrasing of the content directly into spoken language.

Memory training: Ask someone to read to you a text (initially for 1 min, increase to 3 min) and then write down the entire text from memory. Compare to the original and spot your gaps. Identify your patterns of attentive/inattentive listening and memory gaps. Practice this at regular intervals. Start with same language, then do this with the translated language, back and forth.

Practice speed, tone voice, and confidence: Record a short text, e.g., a radio program. Verbally translate and record your translation. Listen to this and identify any deficiencies (e.g., intonation, diction, clarity, sounds of hesitation or nervousness). Learn to like your own voice—this will give you confidence and enjoyment.

Taking notes:

Taking notes during consecutive interpretation will help you to retain information more accurately and complete, especially if feeling tired.

Provides a way of paraphrasing and checking accuracy of the information with both the patient and the healthcare worker.

Note names, dates, figures, facts, descriptions, or other detailed information.

Purpose of the notes is to serve as an "aide memoir" for reading, not as written documentation.

Reference

1. Luchner CD, Kherbiche L. Ethics training for humanitarian interpreters working in conflict and post-conflict settings. J War Cult Stud. 2019;12(3):251–67.

Further Reading

Interpreting in a Refugee Context (RLD3). UNHCR. 1993.
Larson DN. Guidelines for barefoot language learning: an approach through involvement and independence. 1984.
Translators without Borders: field guide to humanitarian interpreting & cultural mediation. 2016.

Christian Harkensee, MD, PhD, MSc, DLSHTM, DiMM, MAcadMEd, MFPHC (RCSEd), FHEA, FRCPCH Made his first humanitarian experience in Central America in 1987. Since, he became a medical doctor (Humboldt University Berlin, Germany, 1997), pediatrician and pediatric infectious diseases and immunology specialist (UK, 2012), researcher (PhD in immunogenetics, UK, 2012), medical educator (2003), and mountain and expedition doctor (2017). He has participated in humanitarian disaster relief, development, and capacity building work in many countries ever since; and currently he is leading a health service for refugee children and families in the North East of England.

Food and Nutrition Survey

Christine Fernandes and Minh Tram Le

Introduction

Nutrition assessment provides timely and evidence-based information for setting targets, planning, monitoring, and evaluating programs aimed at reducing the burden of malnutrition in a population and providing access to treatment for children and women in need. It is also a way to determine whether people's nutritional needs are effectively being met once the program has started. In emergencies and in refugee or migrant settings, food and nutrition securities are often first to be impacted and severely threatened. Urgent actions are often required to save lives and ensure that all members of the community have access to adequate food, taking into consideration the additional needs of vulnerable people. Children and women are more at risk of malnutrition and its complications, and thus need urgent screening and nutritional rehabilitation. The nutrition situation will often determine the mechanisms for food assistance (in-kind, cash-based interventions, etc.) and the feasibility of selective feeding and therapeutic programs.

Rapid Nutrition Assessments and Coordination

As early as possible after the onset of the emergency, a primary assessment will take place to collect general information on the affected population (demographic data, vulnerabilities, number of children under five, pregnant and lactating women, etc.), as well as the immediate and urgent basic needs (access to food and water, clothing and shoes, shelter, etc.), and will help to make quick decisions in terms of

C. Fernandes (✉)
Save the Children, Amman, Jordan
e-mail: christine.fernandes@savethechildren.org

M. T. Le
UNICEF Regional Office for South Asia (ROSA), Kathmandu, Nepal

© Springer Nature Switzerland AG 2021
C. Harkensee et al. (eds.), *Child Refugee and Migrant Health*,
https://doi.org/10.1007/978-3-030-74906-4_21

programming. At this stage, it is important to include selected key nutrition questions in rapid multi-sectoral assessments, which will help collect useful information that will depict the nutritional situation. This first analysis coupled with an analysis of the situation before the emergency (if possible) will help rate the severity level of the population's nutritional status and shape the emergency response in terms of existing risks and vulnerabilities. This initial assessment and analysis will also help decide whether a more in-depth nutrition assessment is required, should the risk be high.

In refugee camps, the planning, organization, and implementation of rapid multi-sectoral assessments are led by the sector coordinator or manager, to ensure that duplication does not happen, and resources are adequately shared and used between agencies. Each organization will contribute to the assessment by bringing expertise, human resources (e.g., community workers, nutrition specialists), and equipment (e.g., vehicles, measuring boards) for the assessments. Final findings and reports will be owned and signed off by the coordination group or sector cluster. In most of the cases, a UN agency and/or ministry is designated as lead. Globally, UNICEF is the cluster lead agency (CLA) for nutrition and works in collaboration with other stakeholders present on the ground. The lead agency ensures emergency response coordination with other agencies, to minimize overlap in humanitarian assistance and optimize the use of resources, often scarce during emergencies. In refugee settings, UNHCR is often the lead agency and coordinates with all stakeholders to ensure the same. In situations where no specific lead is appointed or present, a local or international organization can take the lead to ensure coordination and collaboration are in place during the emergency response. If UNICEF or UNHCR is not present in an emergency the cluster lead can be any inter-agency standing committee (IASC) member, provided it has the resources, expertise, and is accountable to fulfill the duties required of a CLA, described in the Global Nutrition Cluster Handbook 2013 and the Nutrition Cluster Coordination Toolkit [1].

The type of emergency and context will determine the indicators to be collected during the rapid assessment and the type of survey that will be used. For example, in the Greek island of Lesvos in 2015 during the European refugee and migrant crisis, it was quickly decided that a rapid assessment should take place to collect indicators relating to Infant and Young Child Feeding practices which were identified as an immediate emergency and threat for the youngest children. An assessment of the nutritional status of the population to determine the prevalence of stunting and wasting was not deemed a priority in the first phase, but rather in response to information collected on the ground in the early days of the response and secondary information from people arriving in these camps from many different backgrounds.

Key considerations during these nutrition assessments are to ensure that a standardized and agreed-upon method will be used, to ensure high-quality data and results. These types of assessments are usually expensive to carry out and happen only once in a year in refugee settings. Proper expertise and training are needed, for example, for enumerators to properly understand the questionnaires and goals of each question, to make sure the findings can respond to initial questions and indicators (e.g., IYCF assessments), and to get accurate and precise measurements in child anthropometric assessments (temperature, weight, height, MUAC, etc.). A lack of accuracy can lead to an incorrect interpretation of the nutritional situation and invalid findings of the nutrition survey. The inter-agency standing committee (IASC) has developed tools and gathered information on Multi-sector Initial Rapid Assessment (MIRA) that can be useful and quickly adaptable to the context of emergencies. For a rapid nutrition survey, the SMART methodology has also been adapted to a more simplified version using MUAC measurements only, provided a number of criteria are gathered and a more comprehensive (and accurate) survey cannot be conducted [2]. If resources do not exist for this level of technical nutrition surveys, a simple transect walk, key informant interviews, or focus group discussions can be implemented. However, all nutrition enumerators must be efficiently trained prior to any type of nutrition assessment.

Other key considerations during the roll-out of a nutrition survey are to set up a referral system if not in place (i.e., when a child is detected with severe acute malnutrition and will need a higher level of care). Also, remember that the population must give their informed consent before being questioned. Finally, the meaningful, ethical use of data collected must be agreed-upon, and the methodology must respect recognized standards in order to be statistically representative of the population.

Nutrition Programs to Prevent and Treat Child Malnutrition

Children detected with acute malnutrition need urgent life-saving treatment. In refugee settings, the most common approach is to use the *Community-based management of acute malnutrition* (CMAM) protocol where community health workers are trained in early detection to recognize cases and refer them to the nearest health centers. Consider recruiting people from the affected population who meet the requirements and can receive quick training. This will help empower the community in need and minimize the gaps due to cultural and language differences. It is likely that some are already trained health workers, and willing to support their communities while earning an income during this situation. This is the case in the Rohingyas' settlement in Cox's Bazar, where many community workers are from the Rohingya communities, and often the only ones able to speak the same language as mothers and caregivers.

While RUTF is often the preferred choice for the treatment of acute malnutrition, it is important that adequate supplementary foods (ideally local foods) are provided in the camps for the rest of the population and children at risk of undernutrition. The food distributed should be selected based on the nutritional needs and the cultural choice of the population. An acceptable food basket is critical to maintaining the nutritional status of the affected people and ensuring that the service provided fulfills its primary objective. In some crises, the food provided was deemed inappropriate or inedible by the population and was given to livestock instead. To avoid this, key considerations for the design of an appropriate food basket are:

- Cultural preferences of the population vs availability in local markets. This can be assessed during the initial survey, or while the distribution is taking place as a readjustment measure.

- The demographic profile of the population: pregnant and lactating women, people with disabilities, elderly, and children between 6 and 24 months have special dietary needs that must be considered when developing the program.
- The context: climatic conditions, level of activity of the population (e.g., how far do they have to walk each day on average).
- If people are fully dependent on food assistance, 2100 calories per person per day should be provided (including 10–12% protein, 17% fat, and micronutrients). If people also have access to other sources of food, the basket will aim at providing a top-up ration and should be designed accordingly.
- An example of a food basket could be: a staple such as wheat flour or rice; lentils, chickpeas, or other pulses; vegetable oil (fortified with vitamin A and D); sugar; and iodized salt.

Indiscriminate distribution of infant formula, milk powder, and commercial baby foods is discouraged in food baskets and any time during emergencies as stipulated under the international code of marketing of breastmilk substitutes, because of the likelihood to displace breastfeeding practices and increase potential physical harms to infants when clean water, fuel, and other resources are limited for hygienic preparation [3]. Nutrition support for non-breastfed infants must be in accordance with global guidelines and administered by staff trained in Infant Feeding in Emergencies and Breast Milk Substitute (BMS) Programming [3, 4].

Often, a *supplementary ration* of food will be given to the most vulnerable groups such as small children and pregnant and lactating women, aimed at providing the additional nutritional needs required during these periods of life. Based on initial assessments and in order to prevent a worsening of the nutritional status of the population, a list of the most vulnerable individuals within a population should be developed to ensure that additional support will be provided.

Mother and baby areas can be set up in refugee and migrant camps to protect, promote, and support infant and young child feeding practices. These safe spaces are designed in a way where mothers and their babies can come on a daily basis and receive targeted or group nutrition counseling, take the time to play and feed their babies (especially important in a context where privacy is an issue), meet with other caregivers of young children, and rest when needed. Nutrition workers are present in the space to provide necessary support to caregivers and their babies, and refer them to other services if relevant. These spaces provide specialized support on breastfeeding and optimal complementary feeding for infants and young children, and contribute to the prevention of malnutrition. These spaces were seen in refugee camps across Europe, Turkey, and Iraq in 2015 during the European refugee and migrant crisis and are also included in some hospitals as part of the Baby-friendly Hospital Initiative [5].

Overall, it is critical to have a thorough understanding of the causes and complexities of malnutrition to provide appropriate solutions for affected persons, primarily PLWs and children under 5 years. Comprehensive services require a multi-sectoral lens to address the material, physical, and behavioral components of acute, chronic malnutrition, and micronutrient deficiencies. This is especially important in the first 1000 days of life when the cycle of malnutrition can be broken. Therefore, accurate nutrition assessments and high-quality coordination of food and nutrition interventions are important to ensure a timely and appropriate nutrition response, critically in humanitarian contexts, such as refugees and migrants, due to the increased vulnerabilities of the population [6]. Providing treatment and other evidence-based interventions and best practices for the malnourished must also offer sustainable solutions to both the immediate and long-term consequences of malnutrition, to appropriately reduce morbidity and mortality rates around the world.

References

1. Global nutrition cluster. https://www.nutritioncluster.net/Coordination_Toolkit.
2. SMART. https://smartmethodology.org/survey-planning-tools/smart-methodology/rapid-smart-methodology/.
3. WHO. Available from: https://www.who.int/nutrition/publications/code_english.pdf.
4. IFE Core Group. Infant feeding in emergencies: operational guidance for emergency relief staff and programme managers, vol. 3. Oxford: Emergency Nutrition Network; 2017.
5. Gribble K, Fernandes C. Considerations regarding the use of infant formula products in infant and young child feeding in emergencies (IYCF -E) programs. World Nutr. 2018;9(3):261–83.
6. WHO. https://www.who.int/nutrition/topics/bfhi/en/.

Christine Fernandes, MSc is a Maternal, Infant and Young Child Nutrition specialist with significant experience in humanitarian contexts ranging from fieldwork such as nutrition counseling with mothers and infants during emergencies, to global policy and guidance development. She is a member of the Infant Feeding in Emergencies (IFE) Core Group, based in Oxford, UK, and was on the editorial board to produce the Operational Guidance on Infant Feeding in Emergencies (Version 3.0, 2017), in which the revisions she spearheaded were heavily influenced by nutrition contexts in the Middle East. Areas of focus include training curricula on IYCF-E, breast milk substitute program management, complementary feeding program design for the first 1000 days, and technical support to nutrition clusters (UNICEF and UNOCHA) in the Middle East region. She is currently working as Director of Program Development and Quality at Save the Children, Jordan.

Minh Tram Le is a public health nutritionist with more than 10 years of experience in development and humanitarian settings. She has worked with several non-governmental organizations (Action Contre la Faim, Save the Children) as a nutrition adviser in different contexts including emergency responses (Pakistan floods, Afghanistan conflict, European refugee and migrant crisis, Horn of Africa drought, Rohingyas' crisis, etc.). She is currently working as a nutrition specialist with UNICEF with a focus on child wasting and nutrition in emergencies in the South Asian region.

Nutrient Deficiencies

22

Christine Fernandes and Minh Tram Le

Introduction

Often referred to as vitamins and minerals, *micronutrients* are vital to healthy development, disease prevention, and overall well-being. Only a very small amount is required daily, but micronutrients must be derived from the diet as the body does not produce them. Deficiencies in micronutrients such as iron, iodine, vitamin A, folate, and zinc can have devastating consequences. In 2019, at least half of children younger than 5 years of age worldwide suffered from vitamin and mineral deficiencies.

During an emergency, micronutrient deficiencies can easily develop or deteriorate due to loss of livelihoods and food crops, interruption of food supplies, increase in food prices, increases in diarrheal diseases or infectious diseases resulting in malabsorption and nutrient losses. For these reasons, it is essential to ensure that the micronutrient needs of people affected by a disaster are adequately met. To do so, it is critical that general food aid rations are adequate and well-balanced to meet daily nutrition needs, and that their distribution is regular and in sufficient quantities to cover the population's needs [1]. Commonly seen is the provision of foods fortified with micronutrients such as corn-soya blend, biscuits, vegetable oil enriched with vitamin A, and iodized salt. Those are usually provided as part of food rations during emergencies to prevent micronutrient deficiencies, but fortified foods can also be found in local markets.

Parts of the population may be more vulnerable to micronutrient deficiencies and will need additional supplementation, such as pregnant and lactating women and children under the age of 5. Iron and folic acid should be supplied to pregnant and

C. Fernandes (✉)
Save the Children, Amman, Jordan
e-mail: christine.fernandes@savethechildren.org

M. T. Le
UNICEF Regional Office for South Asia (ROSA), Kathmandu, Nepal

C. Harkensee et al. (eds.), *Child Refugee and Migrant Health*,
https://doi.org/10.1007/978-3-030-74906-4_22

lactating women. Micronutrient supplements are often distributed to pregnant women and should be given until the emergency is over and access to nutrient-rich foods restored. Vitamin A supplements should be given to young children and post-partum mothers, according to existing recommendations.

As the diagnosis of one or more micronutrient deficiencies requires the integration of clinical, nutritional, and biochemical data, it is important to be able to recognize the clinical signs of deficiencies especially when working in a refugee camp. The diseases to look for are described in Table 22.1, and some common deficiencies are further detailed thereafter:

Iron Deficiency Anemia

Iron is an essential mineral, needed for motor and cognitive development. Iron deficiency is the most common and widespread nutritional disorder in the world and affects many children, adolescents, and women in developing countries [2]. Anemia during pregnancy increases the risk of maternal and perinatal mortality and low birth weight; therefore, women should be systematically screened during their prenatal consultation. Anemia can be due to inadequate diet, trauma involving blood loss, childbirth, chronic diseases, or parasite infection such as hookworm, schistosomiasis, or tuberculosis.

Clinical signs of anemia can be fatigue, faintness, headache, and susceptibility to infections. The child can look very pale, especially in the conjunctiva, tongue, palms of the hands, and fingernails.

WHO has developed a comprehensive package of public health measures addressing all aspects of iron deficiency anemia. This package can be implemented in camps when the population is known to have a high prevalence of iron deficiency and includes the following elements:

- Dietary diversification including iron-rich foods, food fortification, and iron supplementation.
- Control infection through immunizations and programs addressing malaria, hookworm, and schistosomiasis.
- Improve the nutritional status of the population with focus on the most vulnerable, including the prevention of other nutritional deficiencies such as vitamin B12, folate, and vitamin A.

Foods that are rich in iron include: meat (especially red meat), fortified cereals, iron-fortified blended foods, dark leafy greens, eggs, cashew nuts, and lentils, and should be prioritized if available and culturally acceptable.

Table 22.1 Micronutrient deficiency diseases

Common disorders/ diseases	Deficient nutrient	Treatment/ prophylaxis/ requirements	Food recommendations (should be local, affordable, and culturally acceptable)
Anemia, low birth weight, increased maternal and infant mortality	Iron	Iron deficiency anemia: 3–6 mg/ kg/day of elemental iron for 2–4 months	Meat (lean beef, chicken, liver) beans, lentils, spinach, fortified cereals and breads, seeds and nuts, dried fruits
Xerophthalmia, night blindness, immunosuppression	Vitamin A	Prophylaxis: 6–11 months: 100,000 IU single dose 12–59 months: 200,000 IU every 4–6 months	Dark green leafy vegetables (spinach, kale, lettuce); orange and yellow fruits and vegetables (sweet potatoes, butternut squash, apricots, pumpkin), broccoli, liver
Iodine deficiency disorders, goiter, high risk of stillbirth, infant mortality, birth defects	Iodine	Daily requirements: 0–6 months: 90 µg/ day 7–12 months: 110 µg/day 1–8 years: 90 µg/ day 9–13 years: 120 µg/day 14–18+ years: 150 µg/day Pregnant women: 220 µg/day Breastfeeding women: 270 µg/ day	Fish (especially cod), shrimp, canned tuna, seaweed, milk, yogurt, iodized salt
Beriberi	Thiamine	Daily requirements: <1 year: 0.3 mg/ day 1–3 years: 0.5 mg/ day 4–6 years: 0.7 mg/ day 7–9 years: 0.9 mg/ day Male 10–19 years: 1–1.2 mg/day Female 10–19 years: 0.9–1.0 mg/day	Meat, fish, beans, peas, asparagus, seeds
Pellagra	Niacin	100–300 mg/day	Beef, chicken, pork, fish, peanuts, brown rice

(continued)

Table 22.1 (continued)

Common disorders/ diseases	Deficient nutrient	Treatment/ prophylaxis/ requirements	Food recommendations (should be local, affordable, and culturally acceptable)
Scurvy	Vitamin C	Daily requirements: 0–6 months: 40 mg/day 7–12 months: 50 mg/day 1–3 years: 15 mg/day 4–8 years: 25 mg 9–13 years: 45 mg Male 14–18 years: 75 mg Female 14–18 years: 65 mg	Guava, sweet peppers, broccoli, kale, kiwis, oranges, tomatoes, papaya, strawberries
Ariboflavinosis	Riboflavin	Daily requirements: 0–6 months: 0.3 mg/day 7–12 months: 0.4 mg 1–3 years: 0.5 mg/day 4–8 years: 0.6 mg/day 9–13 years: 0.9 mg/day Male 14–18 years: 1.3 mg/day Female 14–18 years: 1.0 mg/day	Meat (beef, turkey), soybeans, spinach, almonds, eggs, yogurt, mushrooms, asparagus
Rickets, osteoporosis	Vitamin D	Prophylaxis: 0–48 months: 400 IU/day Consider prophylaxis for breastfeeding mothers	Oily fish, fortified milk, yogurt, red meat, egg yolks, fortified cereals, liver, mushrooms

(continued)

Table 22.1 (continued)

Common disorders/ diseases	Deficient nutrient	Treatment/ prophylaxis/ requirements	Food recommendations (should be local, affordable, and culturally acceptable)
Pregnancy complications, impaired growth (stunting), genetic disorders	Zinc	Daily requirements: 0–6 months: 2 mg/day 7–12 months: 3 mg 1–3 years: 3 mg/day 4–8 years: 5 mg/day 9–13 years: 8 mg/day Male 14–18 years: 11 mg/day Female 14–18 years: 9 mg/day	Beef, chicken, shellfish (oysters, crab, shrimp, lobster), beans, nuts, seeds, egg yolk, oats, brown rice

Iodine Deficiency

Iodine is taken from the diet and is used by the body to produce thyroid hormones. Iodine is one of the most important minerals required by a fetus for brain and cognitive development. The lack of iodine can result in goiter, physical deformities, and reduced mental and physical development. Iodine deficiency disorders during pregnancy can lead to increased risk of perinatal and neonatal mortality.

Clinical signs of iodine deficiency disorders can be assessed by looking or palpating for the presence of a goiter, or testing urine or blood.

To prevent iodine deficiency, it is recommended to use iodized salt. Iodized salt fortification is one of the most successful and cheapest nutrition interventions. Today, it is estimated that 71% of households globally have access to iodized salt. In refugee camps, it is recommended to ensure the use and distribution of fortified salt.

Vitamin A

Vitamin A deficiency is a public health problem in more than half of all countries, mostly in Africa and South-East Asia. It affects the youngest children and pregnant women in low-income countries. Vitamin A is necessary for vision (especially at night), growth and development, and strong immune systems. Deficiencies in vitamin A can lead to blindness and death from infections, such as death from measles in malnourished children (hence, it is useful to combine the measles vaccination with a single dose of vitamin A). In pregnant women, vitamin A deficiencies mostly occur during the last trimester and can also cause night blindness, as well as increased risk of maternal mortality.

Clinical signs of deficiency in vitamin A can be seen in the eyes, as xerophthalmia. To confirm the deficiency, a blood sample is necessary.

Because it can reduce child mortality by 23%, WHO recommends the supplementation in vitamin A of children aged from 6 to 59 months twice in a year, using health system contacts or other public health programs when possible (e.g., polio or measles national immunization days) [3]. The administration of vitamin A should be recorded on the child's health card and the caregiver should be informed. For children enrolled in nutrition programs (e.g., CMAM), vitamin A is often administered at inpatient or outpatient settings. Recommended dosage is 100,000 IU once for children aged 6–11 months, and 200,000 IU every 4–6 months for children aged 12–59 months. Proper infant feeding practices have shown highly effective interventions in combating vitamin A deficiencies and reducing child mortality. Combined nutrition interventions include breastfeeding and vitamin A supplementation, coupled with vitamin A-rich diets and food fortification. Breast milk is also a natural source of vitamin A for infants and young children. Good sources of vitamin A include liver and some fish, palm oil, carrots, and yellow maize. Vitamin A is also found in fortified blended foods and is often given to children in capsules.

Vitamin D

Vitamin D builds healthy bones and helps the immune system resist bacteria and viruses. Deficiencies in this vitamin can therefore cause bone diseases, including rickets in children and osteomalacia in adults. Newborn infants are at an elevated risk of vitamin D deficiency and thus must have a vitamin D supplement if exclusively breastfeeding. Recommendations for vitamin D intakes in infancy are typically 5–10 µg daily.

Very few foods naturally have vitamin D, but it can be found in fortified foods such as fish, cheese, eggs, mushrooms, and milk. The body also makes vitamin D when the skin is directly exposed to the sun, and most people meet at least some of their vitamin D needs this way.

Zinc

Zinc is a mineral that promotes immunity, resistance to infection, and proper growth and development of the nervous system. 17.3% of the global population is at risk for zinc deficiency due to dietary inadequacy, though up to 30% of people are at risk in some regions of the world [4].

Supplementation with zinc reduces the incidence of premature birth, decreases childhood diarrhea and respiratory infections, lowers all causes of mortality, and increases growth and weight gain among infants and young children.

Folate

Folate is a vitamin that is essential in the earliest days of fetal growth for healthy development of the brain, spinal cord, and skull. Ensuring sufficient levels of folate in women prior to conception can reduce neural tube defects (a serious birth defect) by up to 50%.

Supplementations of women 15–49 years old with folic acid and fortification of foods such as wheat flour with folic acid are effective interventions for the reduction of birth defects, as well as decreasing morbidity and mortality in newborns. Flour can be fortified with folic acid at low cost, helping prevent birth defects and some forms of anemia.

Summary

In conclusion, several interventions can be implemented in refugee settings to treat and prevent micronutrient deficiencies:

- Ensure nutrient-rich foods in the general food ration with adequate portions
- Provision of fresh food items with vegetables and fruits
- When possible, promotion of gardening in the camp (refer to Case Study 2—Community Gardening Project, in Chap. 12)
- Provision of fortified foods and distribution of nutrient supplements
- Home fortification with micronutrient powders added to family foods
- Improve access to markets with adequate availability of foods
- Promotion of optimal infant and young child feeding practices, emphasizing exclusive breastfeeding, and appropriate dietary diversity after the age of 6 months.

Nutrition education of the affected population about food choices and cooking methods are also essential to ensure the best use of available foods. If people understand the importance of different nutrients, in which food they can find them, and how to prepare them, it will help them take ownership of their diet and their health, and thus prevent nutritional disorders such as those mentioned above.

Similarly, public health interventions such as promoting good general health, ensuring vaccinations are up to date, proper hygiene and sanitation, and access to quality healthcare are key actions to support good nutrition and prevention of micronutrient deficiencies in difficult contexts.

References

1. WHO, WFP, UNICEF. Preventing and controlling micronutrient deficiencies in population affected by an emergency, Multiple vitamin and mineral supplements for pregnant and lactating women, and for children aged 6 to 59 months. 2007.
2. CDC. Micronutrient facts. https://www.cdc.gov/nutrition/micronutrient-malnutrition/micronutrients/index.html.
3. UNICEF. Vitamin A supplementation A decade of progress. 2007.
4. Wessells KR, Brown KH. Estimating the global prevalence of zinc deficiency: results based on zinc availability in national food supplies and the prevalence of stunting. PLoS One. 2012. https://journals.plos.org/plosone/article?id=10.1371/journal.pone.0050568.

Christine Fernandes, MSc is a Maternal, Infant and Young Child Nutrition specialist with significant experience in humanitarian contexts ranging from fieldwork such as nutrition counseling with mothers and infants during emergencies, to global policy and guidance development. She is a member of the Infant Feeding in Emergencies (IFE) Core Group, based in Oxford, UK, and was on the editorial board to produce the Operational Guidance on Infant Feeding in Emergencies (Version 3.0, 2017), in which the revisions she spearheaded were heavily influenced by nutrition contexts in the Middle East. Areas of focus include training curricula on IYCF-E, breast milk substitute program management, complementary feeding program design for the first 1000 days, and technical support to nutrition clusters (UNICEF and UNOCHA) in the Middle East region. She is currently working as Director of Program Development and Quality, at Save the Children, Jordan.

Minh Tram Le is a public health nutritionist with more than 10 years of experience in development and humanitarian settings. She has worked with several non-governmental organizations (Action Contre la Faim, Save the Children) as a nutrition adviser in different contexts including emergency responses (Pakistan floods, Afghanistan conflict, European refugee and migrant crisis, Horn of Africa drought, Rohingyas' crisis, etc.). She is currently working as a nutrition specialist with UNICEF with a focus on child wasting and nutrition in emergencies in the South Asian region.

Respiratory Illnesses

23

Ante Wind and Daniel Martinez Garcia

Introduction

Respiratory illnesses are among the most common pathologies seen in children in refugee and resource-limited settings. In 2017 pneumonia was the cause of 15% of all deaths in children under 5 years old worldwide, second only to newborn deaths [1]. Infectious etiologies are the most common respiratory pathologies, but asthma, respiratory symptoms secondary to systemic disease, exposures (smoke), oncologic processes, and congenital conditions should also be considered.

While much of this chapter is focused on treatment strategies, prevention of respiratory illnesses is equally important. Immunization programs, hygiene promotion, simple interventions such as soap distribution, education on breastfeeding and nutrition, and addressing environmental factors are important elements of the global approach to minimizing the morbidity and mortality related to respiratory illnesses.

Being informed of some key context-related information will help better guide your diagnosis and management of common respiratory ailments.

Disease Burden

Familiarize yourself with the national and regional disease burden. Use sources such as the WHO Country Profiles, the National Ministry of Health website, and mandatory monthly epidemiological data or reports from the local health center or hospital (i.e., data reported from health centers to the local health authorities) [2, 3].

A. Wind (✉)
Unity Health Care, Washington, DC, USA

D. M. Garcia
Médecins Sans Frontières (MSF), Geneva, Switzerland

EveryWhereSchools (EWS), Geneva, Switzerland

© Springer Nature Switzerland AG 2021
C. Harkensee et al. (eds.), *Child Refugee and Migrant Health*,
https://doi.org/10.1007/978-3-030-74906-4_23

Of note, obtaining a variety of data sources will minimize the bias sometimes seen in humanitarian settings. The best source to provide you with a better understanding of the local disease burden is the target population including local staff and community health workers. If you get to know the local staff and community members by slowing down and spending some time talking and establishing a level of mutual respect and understanding, you will gain a much better insight into the health context than from formal sources alone. The importance of local knowledge cannot be overstated.

Vaccination Information

It will also be helpful to have a basic understanding of the national vaccination program and vaccination schedule. On arrival, the local ministry of health, other NGOs, and local staff can give you an idea of the vaccination rate, vaccine availability, the reliability of the vaccine supply chain, and community acceptance of vaccinations. Again, do not rely on only one source, some data may be biased. Depending on the context and country, some patients or parents may have vaccination cards or know the anatomical location of the vaccines that the patient received. This can provide further information about the actual vaccination coverage. This will help narrow down the most likely respiratory pathogens that you will come across in clinical practice (for example, Streptococcus pneumoniae, Haemophilus influenza B (HiB), pertussis, measles, and diphtheria are vaccine-preventable diseases). Knowing whether your patients have received the BCG vaccine will also guide your evaluation and management for tuberculosis (TB). Please refer to the UNICEF website for more information [4].

Resources

A very important practical matter impacting care is the resources available to the medical team. Your ability to provide care will be dramatically different in a remote clinic without electricity or running water versus an established hospital. For example, will you have supplemental oxygen and a reliable supply of electricity? Are there pediatric size nasal prongs, face masks, ventilation bags, and masks? Do they have electric or a manual/penguin suction (a small portable suction device that can be easily cleaned)? Are there ultrasound capabilities? Are there sufficient staff and have they been trained in pediatric care? What are the referral options? Is there an isolation ward or tent for suspected measles, pertussis, tuberculosis, or other contagious diseases? Are there clear hygiene and infection protocols in place? Is there a contingency plan in case of a surge of respiratory cases?

History Taking

When taking a patient's history, it is important to remember some questions that you may not be accustomed to asking. Always ask about potential tuberculosis (TB) exposure and be explicit when you ask these questions. Do not ask simply about family members, but also anyone who shares the same tent/house/shelter/compound. Always ask, in a culturally sensitive way, about HIV status and vaccination status. Ask whether any home remedies or traditional medicines have been given, as some could cause harmful side effects or delay in seeking urgent medical care. Note that some caregivers will be reluctant to admit having given their child traditional medications prior to presentation.

Systematic Approach

Lastly, as with all pediatric pathologies, remember to take a systematic approach: Start with the initial assessment using standardized tools such as the "pediatric assessment triangle" to ensure that the most critical issues are addressed first. The "pediatric assessment triangle" is a 30 second method to evaluate the appearance, breathing, and circulatory status of a patient to determine how urgently the patient needs to be seen. It is incredibly useful in emergency contexts where at times you may have tens to hundreds of patients waiting to be seen. Once the emergent cases have been determined, the ABCDE (airway, breathing, circulation, disability, exposure) approach can be used to identify and manage the most emergent symptoms first. Once patients are stabilized, make sure to screen for malnutrition as this will change your management.

The country where you will be working may have adopted the WHO IMCI (Integrated Management of Childhood Illnesses) strategy. IMCI is a simple and standardized algorithm-based approach to the most common childhood illnesses using resources available in most outpatient settings. Some familiarity with it will help with your integration into the medical team.

Overview of the Most Common Respiratory Pathologies

Since antibiotic recommendations change over time, for the best antibiotic choice and dose for age, please refer to the technical sources mentioned at the end of this chapter. In general, it is prudent to follow national guidelines. At times, due to medication availability, exceptional clinical presentation, or proven resistance patterns, it may be appropriate to deviate from these protocols, but always with a strong rationale.

The following sections will provide a brief overview of the most common respiratory problems in children, including pneumonia, upper respiratory tract infections, TB, asthma, bronchiolitis, croup, and pertussis.

In your differential diagnosis, remember that common non-respiratory patholo-gies can often present with respiratory distress: malaria, anemia, acute chest syn-drome from sickle cell disease, cardiac insufficiency, sepsis, metabolic derangements (diabetic ketoacidosis), and micronutrient deficiencies (beriberi and vitamin D deficiency).

Cough

Cough is a very common presenting complaint as it is a symptom of many pediatric illnesses. The differential for cough is broad. Start by taking a good history. The duration of cough, the nature of the cough, and the associated symptoms can help you distinguish between various causes of cough, many of which are described in further detail below. Remember that most cough syrups are not indicated for chil-dren and can be harmful. You may want to ask the local staff what is locally avail-able for symptomatic management of cough. This can include homemade remedies such as warm water with honey (for children >1 year old), ginger, and/or pepper-mint. Reassure caretakers that the cough may last several days to weeks and, that as long as there are no signs of respiratory distress, fatigue, persistent fever, or worsen-ing clinical condition, there is no cause for alarm.

Upper Respiratory Tract Infections

An upper respiratory tract infection, or a "cold," may present with a runny nose, sore throat, cough, general malaise, and/or low-grade fevers. The child will usually not be tachypneic. The most important part of the evaluation and management is to rule out more serious diseases such as measles or pneumonia. Once you have done that, offer education about supportive care including plenty of fluids, sleep, and acetaminophen or ibuprofen as needed for comfort and fever management. Treating nasal congestion with nasal saline drops can help ease difficulty breathing, espe-cially for infants. Because upper respiratory infections are most often caused by viruses, antibiotics are not helpful and should not be given. It is also important to discuss danger signs, which will indicate to the caregiver that he or she should bring the child back to the health center. These danger signs should include the appear-ance of a rash as this could indicate that the upper respiratory tract infection may have been a measles prodrome.

Pneumonia

Pneumonia most often presents with cough, fever, tachypnea, and occasionally with associated abdominal pain, vomiting, or diarrhea. Crackles are a specific but not sensitive finding. In more severe cases, signs of accessory muscle use, grunting,

Table 23.1 Normal respiratory rate per age in breaths per minute (Adapted from the Harriet Lane Handbook) [5]

Age	Rate
0–3 months	30–60 bpm
3–6 months	30–45 bpm
6–12 months	25–40 bpm
1–3 years	20–30 bpm
3–6 years	20–25 bpm
6 –12 years	14–22 bpm
>12 years	12–18 bpm

central cyanosis, and altered consciousness may be seen. In settings with limited diagnostic modalities, tachypnea will be the most useful indicator to help you differentiate between an upper and lower respiratory illness. Please see Table 23.1 for normal respiratory rate values per age group.

The most common causes of pneumonia are viral pneumonia, including influenza and respiratory syncytial virus, and bacterial pneumonia, such as Streptococcus pneumoniae and HiB. COVID-19 should also be considered. There is often no reliable way to differentiate between viral and bacterial pneumonia in these settings. Note that children may have coinfections with multiple viruses or a mix of viral and bacterial pathogens. Take into account local immunization rates and the prevalence of severe acute malnutrition as you are deciding how to manage these cases.

If the child is tachypneic, without signs of significant accessory muscle use or grunting (remove the shirt to be able to fully appreciate respiratory status in a child), and is tolerating oral intake, the child probably has simple pneumonia and could be managed with oral antibiotics in an outpatient setting. Providing information to the caretaker with explicit instructions to guide when to bring the child back to the clinic or health post is vital. These instructions should include looking for danger signs such as inability to tolerate oral fluids or medications, worsening tachypnea, cyanosis, or lethargy.

If the child is not able to tolerate fluids by mouth, has signs of accessory muscle use or respiratory distress, central cyanosis (of tongue or oral mucosa), decreased oxygen saturation, altered consciousness, sepsis, or moderate to severe malnutrition, the child should be treated with IV antibiotics, in an inpatient facility if possible. For general antibiotic dosage guidance please see Table 23.2. When possible, please refer to the most updated guidelines for the management of community-required pneumonia as these recommendations will regularly change based on local resistance patterns, immunization coverage, comorbidities, and the child's nutrition status. If the oxygen saturation is less than 90–92%, provide supplemental oxygen. If there is no pulse oximeter, then start oxygen if there are any signs of respiratory distress such as grunting, head bobbing, or accessory muscle use. Ensure adequate fluid intake orally (PO), via nasogastric tube (NG), or via intravenous catheter (IV). If IV fluids are given, please make sure that they are isotonic. Address aggravating factors such as fevers, dehydration, anemia, hypo- or hyperglycemia, and comorbid conditions such as malaria, malnutrition, influenza, sickle cell disease, TB, HIV, and diabetes. Throughout inpatient management, the child should be monitored closely to ensure resolution of symptoms. If their condition worsens or does not improve,

Table 23.2 Suggested antibiotic dosing for simple and severe pneumonia antibiotic dosing for simple and severe pneumonia [6]

Simple	Amoxicillin PO 90 mg/kg/day (max 1.5 g) divided in 2 daily doses
Severe, fully immunized child	Ampicillin IV 150–200 mg/kg/day divided every 6 h
Severe, inadequately immunized child	Ceftriaxone IV 50–100 mg/kg (max 1 g) daily
School-aged child at higher risk for atypical pneumonia	Consider adding azithromycin PO or IV 10 mg/kg daily × 1 day then 5 mg/kg daily
Complicated (effusion, empyema, sickle cell disease, other concurrent infections)	Consider adding staphylococcal coverage with clindamycin IV 40 mg/kg/day divided every 6–8 h or vancomycin IV 40–60 mg/kg/day divided every 6–8 h

consider pleural effusions, empyema, TB, HIV, or other regional pulmonary conditions.

Note: If possible, always ask about HIV status during the initial history taking. If the child has any risk factors or if you are in a country or area with high HIV prevalence (>1% of the population), test for HIV. There may, ideally, be a counseling program to which you can refer patients. If not, make sure to obtain consent from the caregiver prior to testing the patient. This can get complicated if, for example, couples are discordant, so ask your organization and local staff for help in how they usually approach HIV testing

Children with HIV are at higher risk for typical pneumonia-causing pathogens including Streptococcus pneumoniae, HiB, and staphylococcus, but are also at risk for pneumocystis jiroveci, fungal infections, pulmonary Kaposi's sarcoma, and TB. Remember to inquire whether the child is receiving HIV medications and whether he/she is receiving cotrimoxazole prophylaxis. Always refer to the national guidelines for HIV management and inquire about existing longitudinal HIV programs in the area. Refer the child for hospitalization if possible. Please refer to the infectious disease chapter for further detail about risk factors, screening, treatment, and comorbidities.

Tuberculosis

Pediatric TB continues to be a substantial public health challenge. One million children are diagnosed with TB annually, of whom 233,000 die. Of those eligible for preventative treatment, only 23% receive it [7].

Some children may be vaccinated with the BCG vaccine. This vaccine offers protection against, but not immunity to, TB infection. It also reduces the risk that infection will lead to disease, especially the more severe types of disease including meningitis and disseminated TB. Lastly, it reduces the absolute mortality risk from TB and seems to reduce absolute mortality risk in children below 5 years of age [8, 9]. Of note, the BCG may cause false positive TB skin tests [10].

Diagnosing a child with TB is very difficult. Symptoms can be nonspecific, diagnostic modalities for pediatric TB are very limited, and children present with extra-pulmonary TB more often than adults making diagnosis even more difficult. Of note, TB scoring systems have not been proven reliable in children.

Consider TB in any child who presents with 2 weeks of cough that is unresponsive to antibiotics, has unexplained weight loss, and/or persistent fevers. Also, consider TB in any child with severe acute malnutrition who is not responding to treatment. Sputum or NG aspirates are difficult to obtain in a child and laboratory facilities for advanced diagnostics may be lacking. Thus, diagnosis in these settings is often made based upon clinical presentation and history.

In general, if the child has a known exposure to a member of the household with active TB plus respiratory symptoms, the child should be started on anti-TB medications. Remember that in children you may not always be able to trace the contact. Not having a known contact with TB does not rule out TB infection. Children less than 5 years old with a known exposure but without respiratory symptoms, weight loss, fevers, or night sweats should be started on anti-TB prophylaxis.

Children on effective anti-TB treatment do not need to be isolated.

Always refer to the national guidelines for TB management, always inquire about existing national TB programs, and refer the child if possible. Enquire about the TB drug supply system to be sure the patient will not face gaps in treatment and will have access to age appropriate formulations [11].

Asthma

The prevalence of asthma is highly variable from region to region. Conditions during migration and/or in camps or resettlement areas, such as stress and exposure to traumatic events, wood or coal fires, crowded and unhygienic conditions, cigarette smoke, fuel or chemical fumes, physical exertion, and dust, can all exacerbate symptoms and frequency of asthma exacerbations and its complications. Additionally, an unstable political context and unpredictable migrations limit access to medications and proper follow-up for all chronic conditions including asthma.

In resource-limited settings, asthma often presents with an acute exacerbation. In absence of a good clinical exam, these exacerbations might be confused with pneumonia and unnecessary antibiotics might be prescribed. Obtaining a good history plus a thorough clinical exam will usually help to make an accurate diagnosis. The child may present with nighttime cough, shortness of breath exacerbated by activity, sensitivity to smoke and other irritants, wheezing, chest tightness, difficulty speaking in full sentences, and prolonged expiration. There may be crepitations during auscultation but, unlike pneumonia, these will shift and change location over time. Remember to rule out other causes of shortness of breath, stridor, and wheezing, such as foreign body, bronchiolitis (especially in wheezing children less than 2 years old), croup, pertussis, reflux, strongyloidiasis, and congenital disorders [2].

Depending on the context, medical staff familiarity and competency with asthma management will vary. Staff education and close surveillance are vital to providing adequate care. Severe asthma exacerbations are managed with salbutamol every 15–20 min × 3 treatments, then are weaned to every 2–4 h as tolerated, along with steroids and oxygen therapy as needed. Please see Table 23.3 for steroid dosing guidance. If you have access to ipratropium bromide, this should be administered concurrently with the first three doses of salbutamol. Ensure adequate hydration. If these measures cannot control the asthma exacerbation, the child may need magnesium sulfate, or in rare cases, epinephrine [2]. Consider adding acid suppression if you are using IV steroids.

Mild or moderate exacerbations can be managed in the clinic or as an outpatient. Provide salbutamol every 4 hours until follow-up or until symptoms abate, and also prescribe oral steroids. If symptoms are recurrent, the child may additionally need to be on an inhaled corticosteroid daily. Oral salbutamol is still available in some countries but is never indicated and will cause unwanted side effects. Additionally, asthma is not infectious and antibiotics are not indicated unless there is a comorbid infection.

Please see the asthma management algorithm, Fig. 23.1, for more detailed guidance.

Table 23.3 Steroid dosing for acute asthma exacerbation [5, 12]

Prednisone	PO: 1–2 mg/kg × 3–5 days (max 60 mg)
Prednisolone	PO: 1–2 mg/kg × 3–5 days (max 60 mg)
Dexamethasone	IV: 0.6 mg/kg every 24 h × 1–2 doses (max 16 mg)
	PO: 0.6 mg/kg once with repeat dose in 24 h (max 16 mg, may give IV formulation orally)
Methylprednisolone	IV: 1–2 mg/kg/day divided into q6 or q12 h dosing (max 60 mg, switch to PO as soon as patient can tolerate it)
Hydrocortisone	IV: 8 mg/kg/day divided into q6 h dosing (max dose 250 mg, switch to PO as soon as patient can tolerate it)

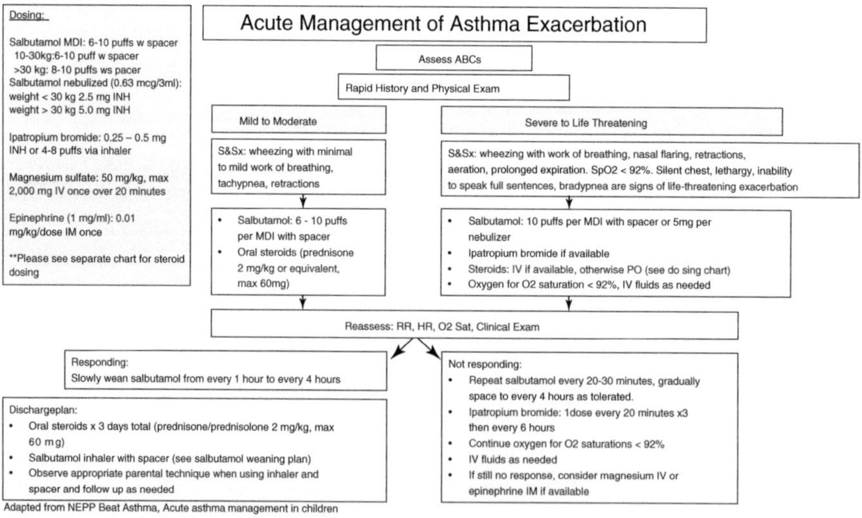

Fig. 23.1 Management of an acute asthma exacerbation [12, 14]

Fig. 23.2 Example of a homemade spacer using a plastic bottle. (Credit Heather Zar, South Africa) [13]

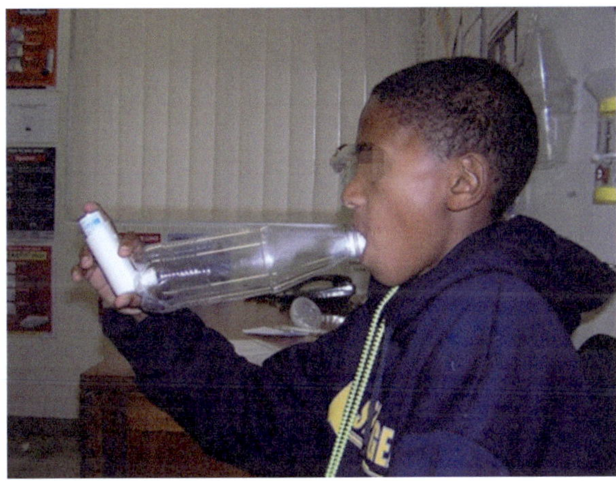

Table 23.4 How to make a low cost spacer

1. Find a clean water bottle or soda bottle and cut a hole in the bottom. You can also melt a hole using a hot wire bent into the shape of a circle. Depending on the inhaler and bottle type, you may be able to fit the inhaler mouthpiece into the top opening of the bottle without cutting to size.
2. Cut the opposite end open and cover the rough edges with medical tape or duct tape.
3. Wash the bottle with water and one drop of liquid soap, do not rinse, and let dry. This minimizes static charge and prevents the medication from adhering to the sides.
4. Fit the inhaler mouthpiece into the small circular opening of the bottle (or the bottle top).
5. Place tape around the inhaler mouthpiece and bottle to ensure a leak-free seal.
6. Prior to use ensure that the area in contact with the mouth has been washed of soap residue and prime with two puffs of salbutamol.

Because children have difficulty coordinating their breath to allow for optimal inhalation of aerosolized albuterol into the lungs, administration devices should be used. Salbutamol can be administered by nebulizer (ensuring hygiene measures are maintained), commercially available spacers (one per patient—do not share between patients), or homemade spacers (see Fig. 23.2 and Table 23.4).

As in high resource settings, asthma education and follow-up with medication titration are key to preventing and alleviating symptoms. Please see the salbutamol weaning algorithm and home asthma management plan in Figs. 23.3 and 23.4 for further detail. Ensure that all children with asthma are given an inhaler and spacer. Attempt to link them with a local clinic or long-term follow-up option.

Patients with asthma and their caregivers need support, education, and follow-up after the initial presentation. Make sure to address aggravating factors such as second-hand smoke, animal dander, indoor cooking, and environmental pollution. For patients and families who are actively migrating, consider upcoming movements and ensure that the child has sufficient medication to make it to their next destination. If possible, provide the patient's caregiver with information on medical services available along their route, as well as what to do in emergency situations where health workers might not be accessible. Given the link between asthma and stress, consider counseling or screening for mental health conditions.

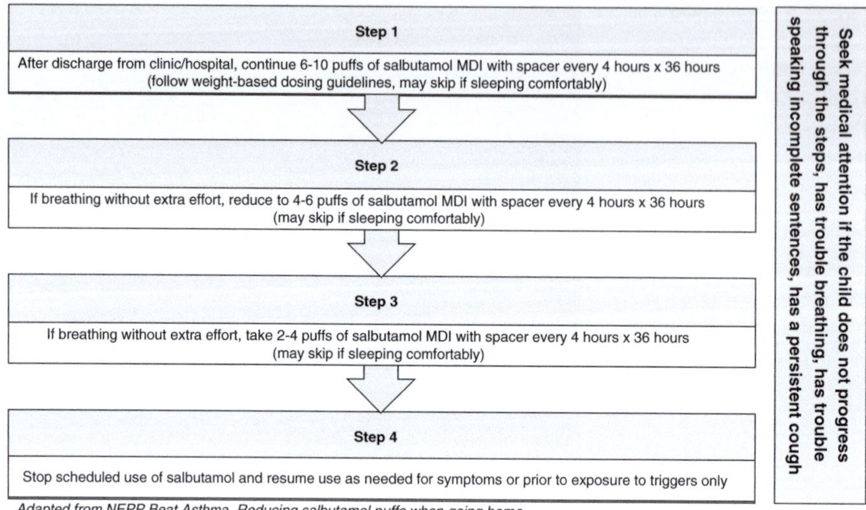

Fig. 23.3 Guidance for weaning salbutamol [14]

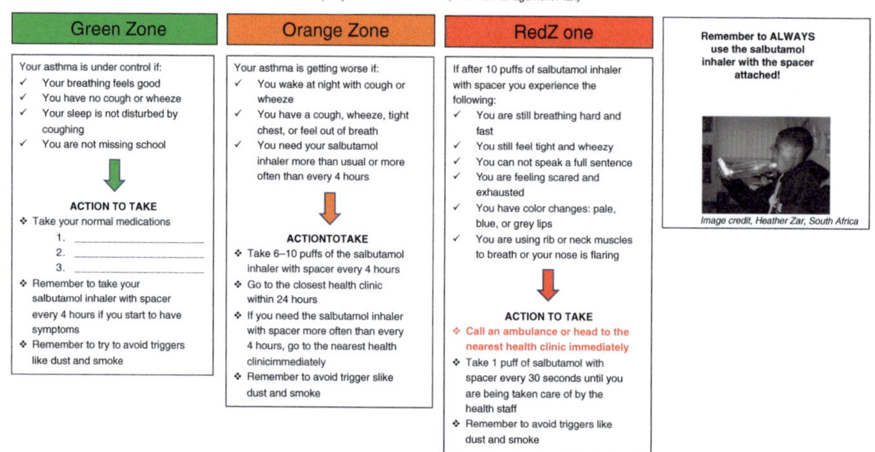

Fig. 23.4 Home asthma management plan [14]

Bronchiolitis

Bronchiolitis is very common and is frequently misdiagnosed as pneumonia. Bronchiolitis presents in children less than 2 years old. In children <12 months old the most prominent features are tachypnea, cough, and widespread crepitations plus or minus wheezing. Children aged 1–2 may have more prominent wheezing and crepitations that move from place to place with each exam. The child is often very "wet," meaning that the child has copious nasal and oral secretions, nasal congestion, and a persistent hacking cough. Simple suction using the penguin or bulb suction goes a long way to ameliorate symptoms in these children. Maintain adequate hydration by encouraging breastfeeding or liquids by mouth. If the respiratory rate is above normal for age, consider placing an NG tube to administer fluids or IV access to run maintenance fluids. Provide supplemental oxygen if the O_2 saturation is low, or, in the absence of a pulse oximeter, if there are signs of severe respiratory distress. If the clinical condition worsens and you do not have the diagnostic means to rule out pneumonia, treat for comorbid pneumonia with antibiotics. In these settings, when a child in respiratory distress is worsening clinically and advanced treatment modalities are limited, it is acceptable to add antibiotics tailored to cover the most frequent pathogens. Children aged 1–2 years old with atopy (eczema, food allergies) may respond to salbutamol and steroids, but for classic bronchiolitis these medications are not indicated.

Pertussis

Due to inconsistent vaccination coverage, crowded migrant and refugee conditions are prime conditions for pertussis outbreaks (and other respiratory viruses). Pertussis presents with a 1–2-week catarrhal phase with cold-like symptoms, followed by a 2–8-week paroxysmal phase of coughing fits, and finally a convalescent phase lasting weeks to months, with cough occurring at lesser and lesser frequencies. During the paroxysmal phase, bouts of coughing may cause the child to become cyanotic and appear to be struggling to breathe. These bouts are often (but not always) followed by a classic whooping sound, which is the sound of forced inspiration. Post-tussive emesis is moderately sensitive and specific for pertussis. Pertussis can be particularly severe in infants younger than 6 months. They are at higher risk of apnea, bradycardia, pneumonia, and sudden infant death. Closer observation in an inpatient setting is recommended.

Children with pertussis should be well hydrated and be placed on oxygen as needed. Make sure to isolate the child (with droplet precautions) for 21 days if not treated, or for 5 days after initiation of antibiotics (see Table 23.5). Treatment with a macrolide antibiotic may not shorten the length of the illness but will decrease transmission. If a macrolide is not available or contraindicated, cotrimoxazole is a reasonable alternative. Post-exposure prophylaxis should be provided to all close contacts, and any unimmunized or under-immunized contacts should be vaccinated. Do not forget to report all pertussis cases to the local health authorities and consider local vaccination coverage [15].

Table 23.5 Suggested antibiotic dosing for pertussis [15]

Infants 1–5 months	Azithromycin 10 mg/kg × 5 days
Child 6 months and older	Azithromycin 10 mg/kg (max 500 mg) × 1 day followed by 5 mg/kg (max 250 mg) × 4 days

Table 23.6 Suggested dexamethasone dosing for croup [5]

Dexamethasone	0.6 mg/kg/dose PO/IV/IM × 1 dose (max 16 mg/dose, IV formulation may be given PO)

Croup (Viral Laryngotracheobronchitis)

Croup will present with a very acute onset of fever, cough, hoarseness, head bobbing, and worsening stridor. The child appears ill but not toxic. Try not to aggravate the child and allow him/her to remain comfortable in the caregiver's arms. Optimize fluid intake, ideally by mouth. Administer a dose of dexamethasone (see Table 23.6) and, if you have a nebulizer, administer nebulized epinephrine. In the case of croup, after appropriate management symptoms usually resolve within 24–48 h. If they do not, consider other diagnoses.

If the child assumes a tripod position (sitting up and leaning forward on both arms) with excessive drooling, consider epiglottitis, especially in contexts of low vaccination rates. If you suspect epiglottitis, do not try to examine the posterior oropharynx or aggravate the child but treat presumptively and aggressively.

Other Respiratory Pathologies

You may be faced with less common respiratory pathologies or syndromes with respiratory manifestations such as diphtheria, measles, COVID-19, rickets, cardiac disease, or others. If your organization does not have preestablished disease-specific protocols, refer to the most recent edition of the following resources: national protocols, the *Harriet Lane Handbook*, the American Academy of Pediatrics *Red Book*, *WHO's Pocket Book of Hospital Care for Children*, Nelson's *Pediatric Antimicrobial Therapy*, MSF Clinical Guidelines, or the WHO's disease-specific guidelines [5, 15–17].

References

1. World Health Organization. Pneumonia. 2019. Available from: https://www.who.int/news-room/fact-sheets/detail/pneumonia.
2. Nadimpalli A, Boulle P. Respiratory illness. In: Kravitz AS, van Tulleken A, editors. Oxford handbook of humanitarian medicine. 1st ed. Oxford: Oxford University Press; 2019. p. 631–46. (Oxford handbooks).
3. World Health Organization. Countries. Available from: http://www.who.int/countries/en/.
4. UNICEF. Where we work. Available from: http://www.unicef.org/infobycountry.
5. Harriet Lane Service (Johns Hopkins Hospital), Flerlage J, Engorn B, Johns Hopkins Hospital, Children's Medical and Surgical Center. The Harriet Lane handbook: a manual for pediatric house officers. 2015 [cited 2019 Nov 4]. Available from: https://www.clinicalkey.com/dura/browse/bookChapter/3-s2.0-C20110078213.
6. Bradley JS, Byington CL, Shah SS, Alverson B, Carter ER, Harrison C, et al. The management of community-acquired pneumonia in infants and children older than 3 months of age: clinical

practice guidelines by the Pediatric Infectious Diseases Society and the Infectious Diseases Society of America. Clin Infect Dis. 2011;53(7):e25–76.
7. World Health Organization. Tuberculosis (TB). Available from: https://www.who.int/tb/areas-of-work/children/en/.
8. Roy P, Vekemans J, Clark A, Sanderson C, Harris RC, White RG. Potential effect of age of BCG vaccination on global paediatric tuberculosis mortality: a modelling study. Lancet Glob Health. 2019;7(12):e1655–63.
9. Garly M-L, Martins CL, Balé C, Baldé MA, Hedegaard KL, Gustafson P, et al. BCG scar and positive tuberculin reaction associated with reduced child mortality in West Africa. Vaccine. 2003;21(21–22):2782–90.
10. Roy A, Eisenhut M, Harris RJ, Rodrigues LC, Sridhar S, Habermann S, et al. Effect of BCG vaccination against Mycobacterium tuberculosis infection in children: systematic review and meta-analysis. BMJ. 2014;349(5):g4643.
11. WHO Global TB Programme. Guidance for national tuberculosis programmes on the management of tuberculosis in children. 2nd ed.
12. Patel SJ, Teach SJ. Asthma. Pediatr Rev. 2019;40(11):549–67.
13. Global Asthma Network. Global asthma report 2018. Aukland: Global Asthma Network; 2018.
14. Beat asthma. Beat asthma resources. Available from: https://www.beatasthma.co.uk/resources/.
15. Long SS, Brady MT, Jackson MA, Kimberlin DW. Red Book 2018: report of the committee on infectious diseases. Elk Grove Village: American Academy of Pediatrics; 2018. [cited 2019 Nov 4]. Available from: http://public.eblib.com/choice/publicfullrecord.aspx?p=5391883.
16. World Health Organization, editor. Pocket book of hospital care for children: guidelines for the management of common childhood illnesses. Second edition, 2013 edition. Geneva, Switzerland: World Health Organization; 2013. p. 412.
17. Bradley JS, Nelson JD, editors. Nelson's Pediatric Antimicrobial Therapy. S.l.: American Academy of Pediatrics; 2021.

Ante Wind, MD is a general pediatrician with an interest in global and immigrant health. She completed medical school at the University of Virginia and pediatric specialty training at Virginia Commonwealth University. Dr. Wind spent 6 years working for Médecins Sans Frontières in various roles including clinical pediatrician, deputy medical coordinator, and pediatric educator. She was based in Haiti, Honduras, Niger, South Sudan, the DRC, Tanzania, and Switzerland. She now lives in Washington, DC and works at the Upper Cardozo Clinic of Unity Health Care and at the National Institutes of Health.

Daniel Martinez Garcia, MD, MPH is a pediatrician and Pediatric Advisor in the Medical Department of Médecins Sans Frontières (MSF), GVA, Switzerland. He is clinical coordinator of MSF's Telemedicine platform and part of MSF's Paediatric Days organizing committee. He is an affiliate of the Johns Hopkins School of Public Health Centre for Humanitarian Medicine, as well as Chair of the Strategic Advisory Group for Children in Disasters for the International Paediatric Association (IPA). He has participated in the AAP Pediatrics in Disasters Course. He received his medical degree from UNAM, Mexico City, completed pediatric residency training at INP, Mexico City, and an MPH from Johns Hopkins Bloomberg School of Public Health, Baltimore, MD. His research focus is pediatric care in resource-limited, humanitarian and disaster settings, telemedicine in pediatrics, nutrition in critically ill children, and pediatric early warning systems. He has 15 years of experience in humanitarian and resource-limited settings. In 2016, he founded EveryWhereSchools, an NGO dedicated to Education in Emergencies and Humanitarian crisis.

Gastrointestinal Diseases in Humanitarian Settings

24

Philip Bruce Murray

Diarrhea: An Overview

After lower respiratory tract infections, diarrhea is one of the leading causes of death worldwide of children ages 1 month to 5 years old. Although impressive strides have been made in reducing overall child mortality since 1990, diarrhea still claims about 500,000 deaths per year, more than from malaria, HIV/AIDS, and measles combined [1]. Children from overcrowded disadvantaged settings, often faced with inadequate clean water and sanitation facilities and lacking understanding of the impact of basic hygiene on their health, are at particular risk. Malnutrition is also directly linked to diarrheal diseases as both are a cause of and the result of acute and persistent diarrhea [2]. Although diarrhea can kill directly due to systemic infection and sepsis seen with GI diseases such as bacterial dysentery and typhoid fever [3], the most common cause of death in a child with severe diarrhea is dehydration resulting in hypovolemic shock and multi-organ system failure.

The challenge of reducing the morbidity and mortality due to childhood diarrheal diseases rests primarily with broad public health initiatives to prevent the diseases and to respond with measured urgency to treat the catastrophes of various outbreaks. Vaccinations, especially against rotavirus and cholera, have emerged as a crucial tool in reducing the burden of disease. Unfortunately, the challenge of antibiotic resistance to bacterial causes of childhood diarrhea is also emerging, which will be discussed in Chap. 19 (Field Pharmacy).

P. B. Murray (✉)
Josephine County Public Health Department, Grants Pass, OR, USA

Medical Teams International, Portland, OR, USA

© Springer Nature Switzerland AG 2021
C. Harkensee et al. (eds.), *Child Refugee and Migrant Health*,
https://doi.org/10.1007/978-3-030-74906-4_24

Diarrhea Prevention and Control Strategies Once an Outbreak is Detected

Since the fecal-oral route is the most common mode of transmission for infectious diarrhea, prevention strategies must focus on broad public health measures. Culturally appropriate messaging on the transmission of diarrhea causing agents should focus on soap and water hand washing after defecation or after touching someone with diarrhea and prior to food preparation and eating. The "F-diagram" (see Fig. 24.1) is an easily conveyed public hygiene message emphasizing some of the ways that infection may be transmitted. The diagram also shows where points of the transmission cycle may be interrupted by using toilet, safe water, and hygiene "barriers."

Identifying the source of an infectious diarrhea outbreak requires considering drinking water contamination, inadequacy of toileting facilities, and public spaces where close person-to-person contact could augment the spread of infection (i.e., food distribution sites or childcare areas). Simultaneously, hand washing stations and oral rehydration posts need to be manned by informed community health workers, who can disseminate hygiene information relevant to the transmission of diarrhea and instruct residents on the proper use of low osmolality oral rehydration salts or solution (ORS). ORS may be used with clean water for repletion of fluid losses

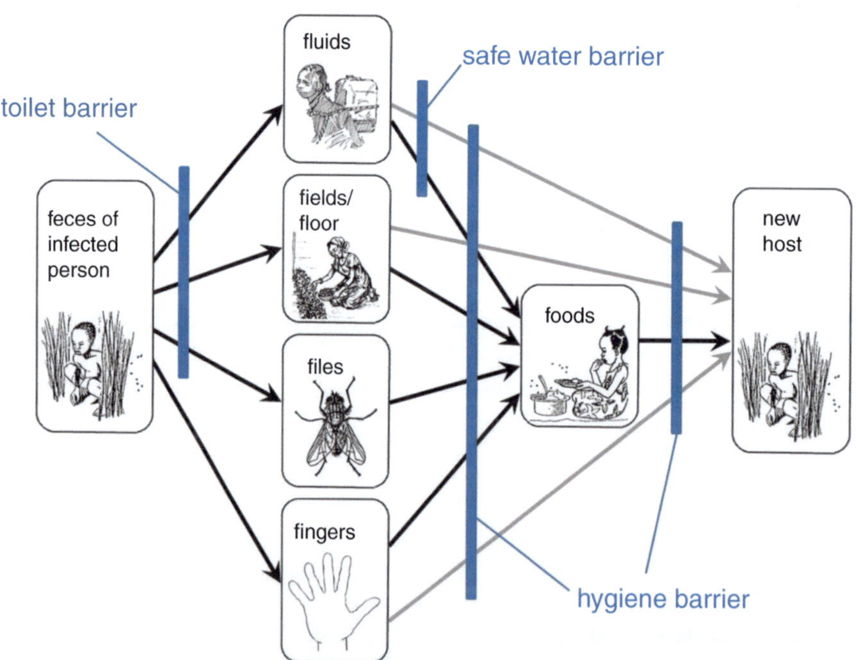

Fig. 24.1 F-diagram of Water First1st International. (Written permission granted) [4]

at any point in the course of a diarrheal illness and are especially important for use in young children.

The key role of *handwashing* and easily accessible wash stations with soap has been shown by meta-analysis of 30 published studies to be effective in diminishing outbreaks of diarrhea by 31% [5]. Notably, antibacterial soaps have been found to be no more effective than non-antibacterial soaps [6]. Teaching handwashing hygiene and technique is an inexpensive and effective public health intervention. Convenient handwashing stations using chlorinated water or bars of soap (or both) are usually placed at strategic points in refugee camp settings, such as outside latrines, homes, clinics, camp cafes, or other congregate settings (see Figs. 24.2 and 24.3).

Hand disinfection strength chlorine solution, recommended at 0.05% dilution, can be made with standard household 5% chlorine bleach (sodium hypochlorite) by mixing 14 tablespoons of bleach to 20 liters of clear water. The solution should be stirred and allowed to rest for 30 min before use and needs to be clearly labeled for hand cleaning not for drinking. HTH powder and Aquatabs chlorine tablets are dry, commercially available products that are available for hand washing purposes and are much simpler and easier to measure than liquid chlorine solution. Instructions for use in making safe drinking water as well as disinfecting solution are included in the package inserts. If chlorination is used, a fresh container of solution needs to be made daily as it quickly degrades with air and light exposure and particulate contamination.

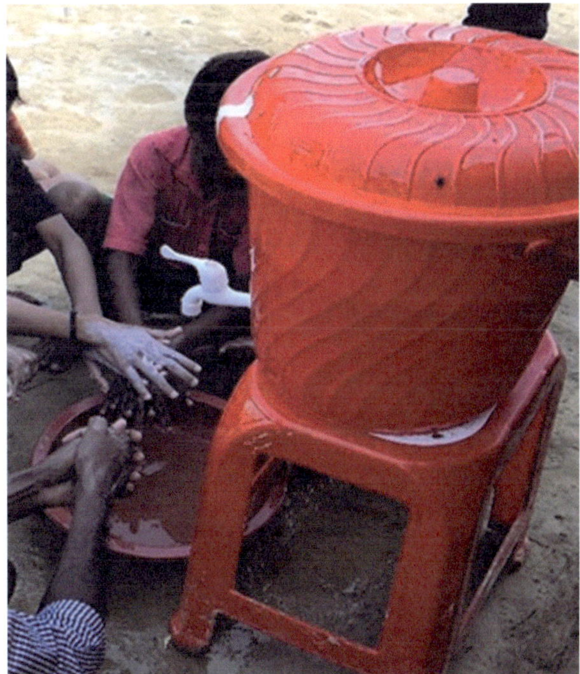

Fig. 24.2 Chlorinated handwashing stations outside of medical clinic in Rohingya Kutupalong Camp, Cox's Bazar, Bangladesh 2017. Problem is that the white valve could recontaminate the hands of the user. (Photo courtesy of Rebecca Duskin, RN, Medical Teams International)

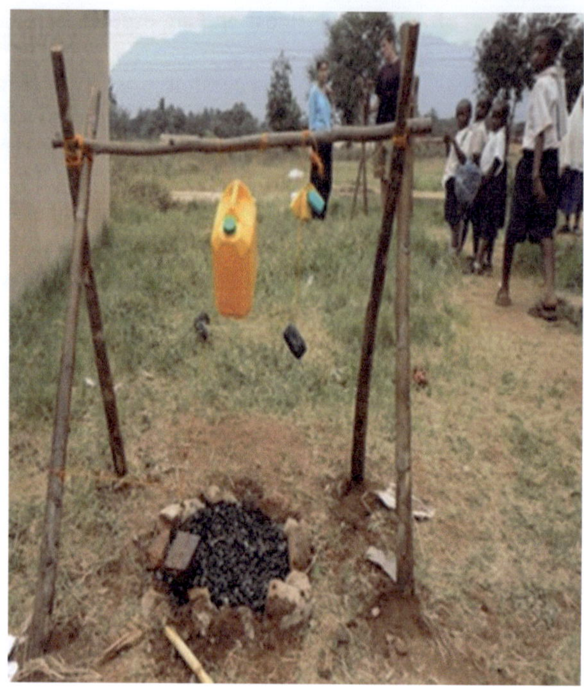

Fig. 24.3 A "tippy tap"—the foot pedal (lower left) would tilt the can so water comes out without having the user touch the can. Used water runs through a charcoal patch on the ground which absorbs/eliminates pathogens and toxins while the water is draining into the ground. If the can would be a transparent one, UV light would provide additional sterilization. Instead of a cap you could use a clean hose similar to one for petrol cans that makes the water run out more smoothly. The next step of invention would be a unidirectional valve that would prevent anything from entering the can—that would obviate the necessity for having to remove and put back the lid with the (contaminated) hand! (Photo and description courtesy of Chris Harkensee)

Syndromic Approach to Diarrhea and Dehydration in Low Resource Settings

Often the causative agent responsible for an outbreak of infectious diarrhea in low resource settings is not known due to lack of access to immunologic or culture identification of the offending organism. Fortunately, grouping the clinical presentation of diarrheal illnesses by their time course, symptoms, appearance, and severity allows an approach that does not require microbiological certainty but often leads to a successful clinical outcome.

Childhood diarrhea can be divided into three main categories. The most common cause of epidemic diarrhea is *acute watery diarrhea* (AWD), defined as three or more loose or watery stools per day for less than 14 days. Second, *dysentery* is diarrhea with visible blood, and the third category is *persistent or chronic diarrhea* characterized as lasting >14 days. The primary focus for this chapter will be on

AWD and dysentery which are responsible for the bulk of diarrhea-related illness and deaths in children under 5 years old. Typhoid or enteric fever will be addressed separately due to its often-nonspecific presentation and significant contribution to childhood morbidity and mortality in endemic areas. Rather than a disease presenting with primarily diarrhea, enteric fever in a child may manifest as a fever of unexplained origin.

Acute Watery Diarrhea (AWD)

The causes of AWD are commonly viral. Rotavirus is the primary cause of the morbidity and mortality of acute diarrhea in infants and young children in camp epidemics, but adenovirus and norovirus may be seen as well. Other frequent causes of AWD in children include bacterial agents such as enterotoxin-producing *E. coli* (ETEC) and campylobacter spp. [7]. The parasite cryptosporidium may be a serious and frequent pathogen as well and is often seen in children less than 1 year old. Generally, any of these agents (viral, bacterial, or parasitic) may cause a wide range of clinical illness and severity. Cholera, due to Vibrio cholerae bacteria, is usually an epidemic disease but in a few countries may be endemic as well. Cholera may be the most important feared cause of a fulminate secretory AWD in refugee settings and will be addressed further below (see *Cholera*).

The AWD syndrome, consisting of loose stools, at times nausea and vomiting, and low-grade fever is graded from mild to severe based upon the degree of the resulting dehydration [8]. The primary therapeutic approach is to correct the lost fluids, electrolytes, and glucose through the use of standard low osmolality oral rehydration solution (ORS). The majority of AWD episodes in children are self-limited infections that are best treated with hydration and ongoing adequate nutrition (especially breastfeeding). Routine use of antibiotics is to be discouraged generally. However, in the case of severely ill children with diarrhea, dehydration, and malnutrition the use of empiric antibiotics (such as azithromycin) may well be appropriate [4].

Surviving AWD is still largely dependent on replacing fluid losses orally. Giving small volumes (e.g., 3–5 ml by cup feeding or syringe) more frequently, such as every 10 min, may help young children tolerate fluids better and reduce vomiting. Oral ondansetron (from age >6 months) can be used for excessive vomiting. Dopamine receptor antagonists should be avoided or used with caution because of neuroleptic side effects. If the child cannot take fluids orally or vomits them back repeatedly then the orogastric or NG tube route of administration may be necessary, depending on the severity of the dehydration. Attempts at oral or tube administration are clearly preferable before considering IV administration of fluids in an infant or small child. If the IV route is required then Ringer's lactate with Dextrose 5% is the preferred IV solution of choice, although normal saline is an acceptable second-line therapy [8].

In addition to ORS, continued nutrition, and zinc (discussed separately in section *"Role of zinc in the management of diarrhea"*), the drug racecadotril may play a complementary role as well in the management of significant diarrhea (see

Weight	Less than 9 kg	9 kg to less than 13 kg	13 to 27 kg	More than 27 kg
Dose (3 times a day)	10 mg	20 mg	30 mg	60 mg
Sachets per dose	1x10 mg	2x10 mg	1x30 mg	2x30 mg

Fig. 24.4 Dosing regimen for racecadotril in infants (over 3 months age) and children [9]

Fig. 24.4). This is an antisecretory medication licensed for use in infants >3 months old and in children to be used to shorten the duration of diarrhea when used along with ORS, increased fluid intake, and dietary advice. Recommended doses and duration are as follows [9]:

Treatment should be continued until two normal stools are recorded and use should not exceed 7 days. Reported adverse effects include severe skin reactions such as erythema multiforme, erythema nodosum, urticaria, and angioedema.

Of key importance in the care of a dehydrated child with diarrhea is prompt institution of adequate nutrition, especially breastfeeding in the unweaned child, during the early phase of diarrhea and afterwards. If the child is vomiting, this will generally lessen after a few hours of appropriate fluid repletion. Early feeding (starting with the initial treatment of dehydration) is preferred over late refeeding [10]. Weaned children should receive frequent small amounts of high-quality locally available nutrition as soon as the initial vomiting is under control. There is a paucity of quality data that any food group, liquid or solid, is harmful in the setting of acute diarrhea. No form of milk should be withheld, unless it clearly makes diarrhea worse, as it is an important way to prevent malnutrition at a critical time [10].

Dysentery

Even in the case of dysentery, dehydration is still the chief threat to the child. However, since the blood in the stool is felt to represent intestinal mucosal disruption with bacterial invasion, antibiotics are usually recommended in addition to appropriate fluid resuscitation. The most common etiologic agent for dysentery in the low resource world is *Shigella* spp. (especially *S. dysenteriae* serotype 1) which produces Shiga-toxin and can lead to intestinal perforation, toxic megacolon, and systemic infection with sepsis and death. Other bacterial causes of bloody diarrhea may include campylobacter, and non-typhoidal *Salmonella* species. Enterohemorrhagic *E. coli* (EHEC) can produce a Shigella-like toxin and may present in a similar manner to Shigella. Ideally, antibiotic choices should be governed by access to culture and sensitivity results from a reliable regional lab, especially in this era of widespread antibiotic resistance. Unfortunately, refugee and migrant children do not commonly reside in resource-rich environments. Therefore, reasonable first-line empiric antibiotic choices include oral ciprofloxacin (15 mg/kg 2 times a day for 3 days; maximum dose 500 mg 2 times a day) or ceftriaxone (50–100 mg/kg/day IV/IM, max dose 1 g/day, for 3 days). If no clinical improvement is seen within 48 h, then switching to azithromycin (one dose of 12 mg/kg on day 1 then 6 mg/kg once daily from day 2 to day 5) is recommended [11]. If still no clinical improvement is seen after the second antibiotic and bloody diarrhea persists, transfer to a regional hospital is indicated. Just as with AWD, continuing nutrition throughout the illness and giving zinc for 14 days remain essential measures.

Treatment of Diarrhea and Dehydration

Use of ORS for Treatment of Diarrhea and Dehydration

ORS is often the key to survival in a child with diarrhea. The commercially available WHO-approved low osmolality ORS formulation contains sodium chloride (75 mmol/l), potassium chloride (20 mmol/l), glucose (75 mmol/l), and has an osmolality of 245 mOsm/l. It is often packaged in premeasured packets designed for reconstitution with 1 liter of clean water, but one should always follow the directions on the ORS package.

An alternate *simple home recipe* that has also been suggested where commercial ORS is not available, is to use six level measured teaspoons of white sugar with ½ teaspoon of table salt added to 1 liter of clean water. Because of the critical nature of getting each of these measurements correct, as well as having clean water containers, some authors no longer recommend this route of therapy [12]. Commercially made ORS is fortunately widely available now even in the most resource-limited areas.

Dehydration Triage and Management Under IMCI Guidelines

Recognition and appropriate management of dehydration is key to saving the lives of children with critical fluid losses, no matter the infectious cause. The World Health Organization's "The Treatment of diarrhea: a manual for physicians and other senior health workers (2005)" [8] is a useful resource and is incorporated in the 2014 version of the Integrated Management of Childhood Illnesses (IMCI) [13]. The IMCI is an algorithmic treatment approach to many common illnesses afflicting children in low resource areas and is particularly applicable to displaced children living in crowded conditions. In regards to diarrhea, the IMCI guidelines recognize the key physical signs of dehydration (sunken eyes, skin tenting or decreased skin turgor,[1] irritability vs lethargy, and avidity for drink) to triage children into red (high urgency), yellow (treat and observe), or green (treat at home with specific directions) categories with ensuing management recommendations.

---

[1]Assessed by pinching the skin of the abdomen and seeing if the "tenting" resolves slowly (over 2 s). See Fig. 24.5.

Once the category or grade of severity of dehydration has been evaluated then the route of fluid administration, the volume of fluids to be given, and the timing are determined. The oral route is always preferred in children compared with the parenteral especially in infants. WHO guidelines indicate that in diarrhea with absent or mild signs of dehydration that the child be treated at home, under "Plan A" management, which includes conveying key information to the mother, such as proper use of ORS, continuing breastfeeding or nutrition in the weaned child and use of zinc (see Fig. 24.6).

For children classified as having moderate dehydration (diagnosed by observing two of the following: restless/irritable, sunken eyes, drinks eagerly, skin pinch goes back slowly) then Plan B is followed using ORS in the volumes indicated, either orally or via a pediatric feeding tube, over an initial 4-hour period. This implies a period of continued observation at the clinic setting, with frequent small volume ORS administration as well as a nutrition or breastfeeding trial. If there is satisfactory improvement, the child may go home under the Plan A recommendations, including 14 days of zinc therapy. The key observation in mild to moderate dehydration is that the children affected remain interested in trying to drink. If a child appears listless or lethargic and shows little or no interest in drinking, that is a true danger sign and is indicative of severe dehydration (see Fig. 24.7).

If the child does not tolerate oral fluids, breast milk, or other nutrition during the observation period under Plan B and signs of dehydration worsen, then the child is treated under the recommendations of Plan C. Severe dehydration in a child 2–59 months old is characterized as having two of the following signs: lethargy or unconscious state, sunken eyes, not able to drink or drinking poorly, or skin pinch going back very slowly.

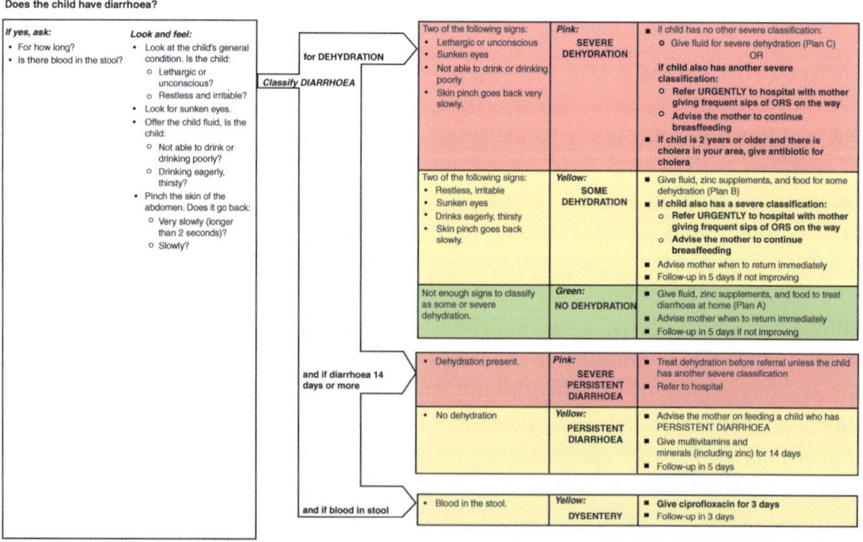

Fig. 24.5 Clinical evaluation of dehydration from Integrated Management of Childhood Illnesses [13], March 2014. (Permission granted by the World Health Organization)

Plan C eligible children generally show an apparent lack of thirst and therapy is directed at correction of fluid losses in a supervised manner using IV fluids (Ringer's Lactate with 5% glucose is preferred); if not available then normal saline is acceptable) [9]. Intravenous fluids must be given carefully, in a monitored setting by experienced personnel and only until adequate PO intake is restored. Under Plan C the child is readied for transport to a local referral inpatient facility unless 24/7 care by trained staff is available on site (see Fig. 24.8).

PLAN A: TREAT DIARRHOEA AT HOME
Counsel the mother on the 4 Rules of Home Treatment:
  1. **Give Extra Fluid**
  2. **Give Zinc Supplements (age 2 months up to 5 years)**
  3. **Continue Feeding**
  4. **When to Return.**

1. *GIVE EXTRA FLUID* **(as much as the child will take)**
   ▪ **TELL THE MOTHER:**
     • Breastfeed frequently and for longer at each feed.
     • If the child is exclusively breastfed, give ORS or clean water in addition to breast milk.
     • If the child is not exclusively breastfed, give one or more of the following:
      ORS solution, food-based fluids (Such as soup, rice water, and yoghurt drinks), or clean water.
   ▪ **It is especially important to give ORS at home when:**
     • *the child has been treated with Plan B or Plan C during this visit.*
     • *the child cannot return to a clinic if the diarrhoea gets worse.*
   ▪ **TEACH THE MOTHER HOW TO MIX AND GIVE ORS. GIVE THE MOTHER 2 PACKETS OF ORS TO USE AT HOME.**
   ▪ **SHOW THE MOTHER HOW MUCH FLUID TO GIVE IN ADDITION TO THE USUAL FLUID INTAKE:**

Up to 2 years	50 to 100 ml after each loose stool
2years or more	100 to 2000 ml after each loose stool

Tell the mother to:
   • Give frequent small sips from a cup.
   • If the child vomits, wait 10 minutes. Then continue, but more slowly.
   • <u>Continue giving extra fluid until the diarrhoea stops.</u>
2. *GIVE ZINC* **(age 2 months up to 5 years)**

  ▪ **TELL THE MOTHER HOW MUCH ZINC TO GIVE (20 mg tab):**

2 moths up to 6 monts	1/2 tablet daily for 14 days
6 monts or more	1 tablet daily for 14 days

  ▪ **SHOW THE MOTHER HOW TO GIVE ZINC SUPPLEMENTS**
     • Infants - dissolve tablet in a small amount of expressed breast milk, ORS or clean water in a cup.
     • Older children - tablets can be chewed or dissolved in a small amount of water.
3. *CONTINUE FEEDING* **(exclusive breastfeeding if age less than 6 months)**
4. *WHEN TO RETURN*

Fig. 24.6 Integrated Management of Childhood Illnesses chart booklet [13], March 2014. (Permission granted by World Health Organization)

PLAN B: TREAT SOME DEHYDRATION WITH ORS

In the clinic, give recommended amount of ORS over 4-hour period

▪ DETERMINE AMOUNT OF ORS TO GIVE DURING FIRST 4 HOURS

WEIGHT	< 6kg	6 - <10kg	10 - <12 kg	12 - <19 kg
AGE*	Up to 4 months	4 months up to 12 years	12 months up to 2 years	2 years up to 5 years
In ml	200 - 450	450 - 800	800 - 960	960 - 1600

** Use the child's age only when you do not know the weight. The approximate amount of ORS required (in ml) can also be calculated by multiplying the child's weight (in kg) times 75.*
- If the child wants more ORS than shown, give more.
- For infants under 6 months who are not breastfed, also give 100 - 200 ml clean water during this period if you use standard ORS. This is not needed if you use new low osmolarity ORS.

▪ SHOW THE MOTHER HOW TO GIVE ORS SOLUTION.
- Give frequent small sips from a cup.
- If the child vomits, wait 10 minutes. Then continue, but more slowly.
- Continue breastfeeding whenever the child wants.

▪ AFTER 4 HOURS:
- Reassess the child and classify the child for dehydration.
- Select the appropriate plan to continue treatment.
- Begin feeding the child in clinic.

▪ IF THE MOTHER MUST LEAVE BEFORE COMPLETING TREATMENT:
- Show her how to prepare ORS solution at home.
- Show her how much ORS to give to finish 4-hour treatment at home.
- Give her enough ORS packets to complete rehydration. Also give her 2 packets as recommended in **Plan A.**
- Explain the 4 Rules of Home Treatment:
    1. **GIVE EXTRA FLUID**
    2. **GIVE ZINC (age 2 months up to 5 years)**
    3. **CONTINUE FEEDING (exclusive breastfeeding if age less than 6 months)**
    4. **WHEN TO RETURN**

Fig. 24.7 Integrated Management of Childhood Illnesses chart booklet [13], March 2014. (Permission granted by World Health Organization)

Role of Zinc in Diarrhea Management

Oral zinc administration is now standard adjunctive therapy for children 2 months to 5 years old with acute diarrhea [14]. A 2016 Cochrane Database review of available studies [15] confirmed that zinc may reduce duration and severity of diarrhea; however, it appears to be most beneficial wherever malnutrition and zinc deficiency are endemic. The likelihood of recurrence of diarrhea for 3 months after zinc therapy has also been noted to be reduced as well [16]. Current WHO recommendations for zinc administration is for age 6 months up to 5 years use a 20 mg tablet daily for 14 days. For ages 2 months up to 6 months use 1/2 tablet (10 mg) daily for 14 days [13].

The mechanism of action is felt to be multifold including repairing the intestinal mucosal barrier, augmenting the antibody response against GI pathogens, and inhibiting chloride secretion into the gut. Zinc is not of proven benefit in infants less than 6 months old and vomiting is a potential side effect that may limit its usefulness at all ages.

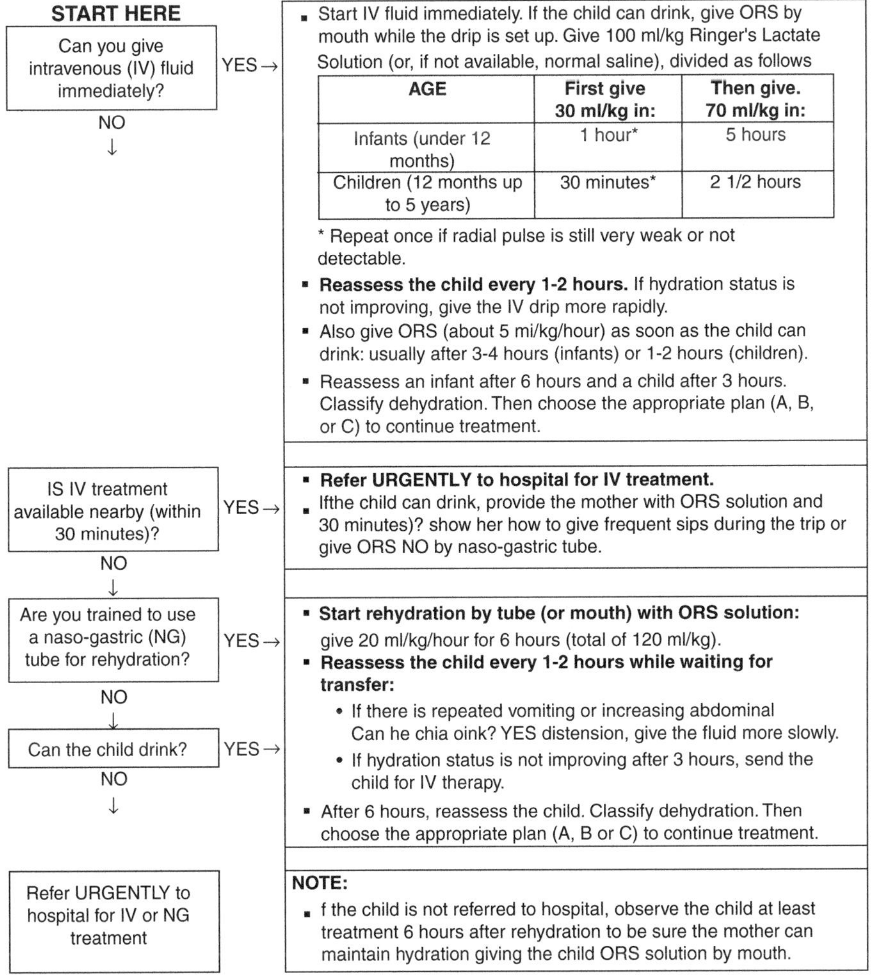

Fig. 24.8 Integrated Management of Childhood Illnesses chart booklet [13], March 2014. (Permission granted by World Health Organization)

Vitamin A Supplementation in Children with Diarrhea

Vitamin A deficiency is common in low resource areas as a part of micronutrient malnutrition. Since diarrhea and malnutrition have a direct relationship, it is recommended that infants and children with diarrhea, especially those with persistent or chronic diarrhea or suspected malnutrition, be treated with a single oral dose of vitamin A (100,000 units for infants 6–12 months and 200,000 units for children 12–59 months). A Cochrane review of the impact of vitamin A supplementation found that Vitamin A significantly reduced not only the incidence of diarrhea in children 6 months to 5 years old but mortality from diarrhea by 28% [17].

Cholera

Cholera, caused by Vibrio cholerae, is one particularly violent form of secretory AWD. In an endemic location, cholera may cause a range of symptoms from an asymptomatic carrier state to profuse watery diarrhea with rapid dehydration, hypovolemic shock, and ultimately death within several hours if not treated aggressively. In addition, vomiting, abdominal pain, and the well-described "rice water" appearance of the stool are commonly seen with symptomatic disease. Contaminated drinking water is usually the cause of the epidemic but person-to-person transmission also plays a significant role in overcrowded settings. Diagnosis is usually made on a clinical basis, as laboratory confirmation requires culture of the organism. Mild cases of cholera are indistinguishable from common AWD but severe cases of cholera are uniquely dangerous in children with fluid losses that may be catastrophic. "Plan C" of the WHO diarrhea management protocols should be followed (see above) as outlined above. If an affected child also has severe malnutrition, especially with edema, then the treatment protocol is far more conservative and is best supervised in a specialty inpatient unit.

While aggressive fluid replenishment is the primary mode of treatment, oral antibiotic usage is also appropriate for cases of moderate to severe cases of cholera, in that they may reduce the volume and duration of diarrhea and even the period of bacterial shedding [18]. Unfortunately, in cholera endemic areas (Africa, South and Southeast Asia, etc.), multidrug resistance is also common. Ciprofloxacin, in particular, is associated with especially high rates of resistance. Ideally, antibiotic choice should be guided by drug sensitivity testing in a given area. Since that information may not be available early in an outbreak, empiric therapy with doxycycline (4–6 mg/kg single dose) is regarded as complementary therapy by Medicins Sans Frontieres when dehydration has been addressed, vomiting has diminished, and oral therapy can be used [19]. Another empiric choice may be azithromycin (20 mg/kg single dose) however aggressive fluid management to address critical dehydration is far more likely to be lifesaving than the specific antibiotic in most settings. Cholera may initially look like a number of other causes of severe AWD diarrhea in young children; however, the death of even a single child over age 5 due to a diarrheal illness must be reported and should raise the suspicion of an impending cholera epidemic.

In a refugee camp setting it may be necessary to set up specialized inpatient units for severe diarrhea or cholera in order to stockpile IV fluids and supplies and to efficiently handle the volume of patients. Young children, in particular, may require IV therapy and very close nursing supervision. The units also provide the opportunity to institute strict infection control measures and to train medical staff and to educate caregivers on sanitation, hygiene, and nutritional practices.

There are currently two cholera vaccines (Shanchol and Euvichol) available for broad public health use on a scheduled basis in endemic areas as well as for emergency vaccination once there is an outbreak. Generally, *two* doses of vaccine given a minimum of 2 weeks apart are optimal for immune response; however, there is increasing data that even one dose given at the onset of an outbreak may be beneficial [20].

Typhoid Fever

Typhoid fever caused by *Salmonella enterica* serotype Typhi/Paratyphi is one of the other major causes of epidemic diseases of children in refugee camps and other crowded environments. Transmission is primarily via the fecal-oral route with contamination of water and food sources spreading disease quickly. Enteric fever (which includes paratyphoid fever) is often a nonspecific illness especially in children under 5 years old. It may be characterized initially by fever lasting several days (often peaking in the second week), chills, and abdominal pain. Other symptoms could include malaise, headache, cough, and possible changes in bowel habits with diarrhea more frequently seen than constipation in children [21]. However, a change in bowel habits is not a reliable feature of typhoid fever regardless of age as most afflicted children have normal stools. Splenomegaly, abdominal tenderness, and distention may be noted on exam along with the classic fever-pulse dissociation, which is relative bradycardia in the setting of high fever. A characteristic exanthem sometimes seen early in the course of illness consists of discrete "rose spots" on the trunk and abdomen and represent areas of bacterial embolization [22]. The differential diagnoses for the enteric fever syndrome would include other multisystemic infections such as malaria, dengue, non-typhoid salmonella infections, leptospirosis, rickettsial infections, and amebiasis.

If not treated with appropriate antibiotics, the course of the disease may last several days with complications including confusion/delirium, coma, intestinal perforation, sepsis, and death. Of enteric fever patients, 1–4% become chronic carriers of the disease and will develop fecal shedding which can persist for more than a year. This group continues to represent a fertile reservoir for causing recurrent epidemics [22].

The diagnosis of enteric fever is challenging even under optimal circumstances but is especially difficult in low resource settings. Blood, stool, and bone marrow cultures may reveal the presence of the organism early in the course of the illness but are not highly sensitive commonly available. The Widal test, which measures long-lasting agglutinating antibodies and not necessarily acute infection, is of limited value in endemic areas where many people may have been exposed to the disease during their lifetime [22]. The clinical picture of enteric fever may look like malaria, though if malaria tests are negative then the diagnosis of enteric fever is often made on clinical grounds alone [21, 22]. In a child with more than 3 days of fever of unknown cause and variable abdominal symptoms (pain, distention), empiric therapy with antibiotics to cover enteric fever is indicated. Unfortunately, in areas endemic for enteric fever, the organism may already be multidrug resistant making empiric selection of the best drug problematic. Fluoroquinolone resistance is now widespread especially in South Asia where up to 80% of isolates are resistant, parenteral fluoroquinolone therapy may still be acceptable empiric therapy outside of South Asia. Azithromycin and ceftriaxone remain the best first-line therapies in seriously ill children with enteric fever, but resistance to those agents is starting to appear [23].

In this era of increasing drug resistance, broad public health mandates to prevent enteric fever are crucial, including ensuring safe water supplies, appropriate hygiene and sanitation measures, food safety, and most importantly, vaccination. In endemic areas, the WHO recommends typhoid conjugate vaccine be a part of all national vaccination programs starting at 6 months of age.

Diarrhea Complicated by Malnutrition (and Vice Versa)

Recurrent diarrhea in a child frequently leads to malnutrition through catabolism, reduced oral intake, and a net loss of vital calories and micronutrients. Conversely, malnutrition, due to effects on the intestinal mucosal barrier causing malabsorption of vital macro and micronutrients and on the immune response, can lead to increased susceptibility and recurrent bouts of diarrhea. This bidirectional relationship between diarrhea and malnutrition can lead to repeated episodes of illness and eventually to stunting, failure to thrive, and death [2]. That is why attention to the nutritional needs of a child is so crucial before, during, and after bouts of acute diarrhea. Breastfeeding throughout the course of diarrhea is a key recommendation especially in low resource areas [2]. Exclusive breastfeeding has also been shown to protect against future episodes of diarrhea supporting the WHO recommendation of breastfeeding only for all infants until age 6 months. Inadequate breastfeeding has been shown to increase diarrhea-related morbidity and mortality, hospitalization, and all-cause mortality. One comprehensive review of the literature showed that for those aged 0–5 months who were not exclusively breastfed compared to those who were, the relative risk (RR) of diarrhea-related mortality was 10.52. In those aged 6–23 months old, the relative risk of those who received no breastfeeding was 2.8 compared to those who received any breastfeeding [23].

In children with severe acute malnutrition (SAM), managing significant diarrhea is particularly challenging. Their volume status is precarious, vascular permeability and homeostasis are disturbed, and especially in edematous malnutrition, physical exam evaluation of dehydration is difficult. If available, oral ReSoMal may be an alternative to low osmolality ORS for fluid replacement purposes in the setting of SAM and ongoing diarrhea. This commercially available product has a lower concentration of sodium, higher concentration of potassium, and adds magnesium, copper, and zinc, not present in ORS. MSF recommends that the use of ReSoMal is reserved for treatment of complicated SAM with frequent stools without hypovolemic shock but does not recommend its use in children with cholera or uncomplicated SAM [24]. Oral or NG/OG feeding is always preferable to intravenous fluid administration in malnourished children due to their precarious intravascular volume status and risk of pulmonary edema. Broad-spectrum antibiotics (amoxicillin PO: 50 mg/kg 2 times a day for 5 days) are recommended in all children with SAM, and nutritional therapy should be provided in inpatient feeding centers for careful monitoring.

Persistent Diarrhea in a Low Resource Setting

Persistent diarrhea is defined as watery stools three or more times a day that lasts for more than 14 days. As noted above, malnutrition plays a significant role in causing and/or perpetuating diarrhea. There are several pathophysiologic mechanisms that may play a role in a child developing persistent diarrhea. Perpetuation of the original intestinal infection that triggered the initial acute episode (such as shigella which is well known to persist in the GI tract), structural changes in the gut lining limiting nutrient and micronutrient absorption, and impaired immune status are all important contributors. HIV infection in a child always needs to be considered in cases of chronic diarrhea. One manifestation of the altered immune state in these children is failure to clear cryptosporidium infection which may then result in chronic loose stools.

Children under 2 years old may be disproportionately affected by persistent diarrhea compared with older children. Stunting of growth, failure to thrive, susceptibility to other infections such as respiratory illnesses, and death may result [2].

Common infectious causes of persistent diarrhea may be viral, bacterial, parasitic, or mixed pathogen and may be the same agents that cause acute diarrhea. Examples include rotavirus, adenovirus, norovirus, shigella, enteropathogenic *E. coli*, campylobacter, and cryptosporidium. Persistent diarrhea also raises the possibility of chronic giardiasis, amebiasis, Cyclospora, and Strongyloides infection. Bloody diarrhea persisting for more than 2 weeks could be due to shigella or campylobacter and should be treated with appropriate antibiotics as with acute disease. The empiric antibiotic therapy in a child with persistent bloody diarrhea where cultures cannot be done should include two appropriate trials of antibiotics aimed at shigella, changing antibiotics every 2–3 days if bloody diarrhea persists [11]. If no clinical response is noted then using metronidazole might be a reasonable option for addressing amebiasis and giardiasis. In addition, if laboratory testing is available, stool cultures and microscopy for parasites (*E. histolytica*, giardia, and Strongyloides especially) should be done. Identifying a specific pathogen as the cause of persistent diarrhea may be difficult even in the best resource settings. Regardless of the cause, management is the same as it would be for a child with acute diarrhea: assess and treat for significant dehydration and possible sepsis (see section "Dehydration Triage and Management"). Death from dehydration is still the primary cause of death in a child with persistent diarrhea. Address the fluid needs and administration according to the WHO endorsed Plans A (for mild), B (for moderate), or C (for severe dehydration). Ensuring adequate nutrition throughout the illness is crucial with the continuation of breastfeeding being the next key intervention especially for ages 0–6 months.

Anti-helminth therapy with albendazole (200 mg single dose for <2 years old, 400 mg as single dose for >2 years old) is safe in children who may harbor intestinal roundworms, such as ascaris, pinworm, hookworm, and Strongyloides, and should be given on a regularly scheduled 6-month schedule. However, nematodes are rarely a cause of diarrhea but may aggravate anemia or undernutrition.

Zinc and vitamin A administration should be used in all cases of persistent or chronic diarrhea. Regular follow-up of the child, either in the clinic setting or through well-trained community health workers, is essential to track the response to therapy and to provide long-term evaluation of the child's nutritional status, growth, and development.

Other Gastrointestinal Problems

Acute Vomiting

Regardless of the underlying cause, repeated vomiting in a child is a significant concern as it may rapidly lead to dehydration. Acute vomiting may be a part of intestinal infection due to viral gastroenteritis, bacterial contamination of food sources, part of a secondary illness (e.g., malaria, enteric fever, sepsis, meningitis, urinary, or other infection), metabolic abnormalities (e.g., DKA, renal failure, adrenal crisis), toxic ingestion, motion sickness, underlying neurological or psychological factors, and many other causes beyond the purview of this discussion. Structural intestinal issues such as pyloric stenosis and intussusception need to be considered, especially if there is a worrisome pattern of recurrence. Common or benign vomiting is usually self-limited. Basic management of vomiting beyond initial observation includes continued small volume feeding with frequent sips of water or breast milk, but most importantly instructing the mother when to come to the clinic for assistance if vomiting persists. Prolonged vomiting (e.g., >12 h in a neonate, >24 h in children younger than 2 years old, >48 h in older children [25]) is certainly a reason to seek urgent medical attention.

The chief concern of ongoing vomiting, as with diarrhea, is the risk of dehydration. Signs of volume depletion that a caregiver should look for include lack of tears with crying, a dry mouth, a dry diaper for >6 h or not urinating for 6–8 h in an older child, listlessness, or profound lethargy. Avoiding full strength fruit juices is advisable because of the high sugar content. If any signs of dehydration are present, ORS is the optimal choice for volume and electrolyte repletion, and it reduces the incidence of further vomiting. However, for home use initially, frequent small volumes of water, milk, or dilute juice, are acceptable. If the fluids are quickly vomited, then small volume fluids should be tried again after 10–20 min. If vomiting persists and signs of dehydration develop, then further medical assistance is needed, and enteral or parental rehydration be considered. Anti-emetics, especially ondansetron, may be considered except in cases of suspected increased intracranial pressure or evidence of intestinal obstruction [25].

Abdominal Pain in Children

The comprehensive evaluation and management of a child presenting with abdominal pain in a low resource area are beyond the scope of this manual. However, the skill to recognize the child who has serious or life-threatening causes of abdominal pain is essential. Certain signs and symptoms may help distinguish between common benign causes (gastroenteritis or other viral processes, constipation, colic, etc.) and conditions which require further evaluation and testing. Urgent transfer may be necessary to address those situations requiring surgical consultation or at the very least, for closer monitoring and skilled nursing care. For any child less than 2 months old the presence of poor feeding, convulsions, temperature >37.5 or <35.5, lethargy, labored or rapid breathing (>60 breaths/min) with or without abdominal findings is sufficient to justify parenteral antibiotics (ampicillin plus gentamicin, or ceftriaxone alone) and immediate transfer to a hospital setting. For children greater than 2 months of age, the following danger signs should prompt further evaluation immediately [26]:

Some danger signs of abdominal pain in a young child (>2 months of age):

- association with vomiting for >12 h in an infant, or for >24 h in a child more than 12 months old with inadequate oral intake [25]
- signs of severe dehydration from diarrhea or vomiting or both (listlessness, lethargy, or coma)
- recurrent projectile vomiting or vomiting of bile or blood
- recurrent and progressive severe crampy abdominal pain in children ages 6–36 months old; consider intussusception as it is the most common abdominal emergency of childhood. Vomiting may be bilious (appears dark green whereas gastric fluid is all shades of yellow) and blood in the stool is commonly noted as well
- nonbilious, forceful vomiting after eating, especially in infants 3–12 weeks old. The child may look well between episodes and remains hungry after vomiting; consider pyloric stenosis
- any association with significant blunt trauma and abdominal pain; this will usually require immediate referral for appropriate imaging and management
- a palpable discrete and painful mass in the inguinal area in a highly irritable and uncomfortable child; this suggests an incarcerated inguinal hernia
- peritoneal signs or significant abdominal distension (surgical abdomen)
- once these more serious etiologies have been ruled out, a broad range of causative factors, including infections such as pharyngitis, pneumonia, and urinary tract infections can also manifest as abdominal pain in children. Finally, psychological or "functional" causes of abdominal pain, as well as abdominal migraine, need to be considered especially in populations of children exposed to violence, trauma, and numerous unpredictable circumstances.

References

1. Liu L. Child Health Epidemiology Reference Group of WHO and UNICEF. Global, regional, and national causes of child mortality: an updated systematic analysis for 2010 with time trends since 2000. Lancet. 2012;379(9832):2151–61.
2. Brown KH. Diarrhea and malnutrition. In: Symposium: nutrition and infection, prologue and progress since 1968. J Nutr. 2003;133:328s–32s. https://doi.org/10.1093/jn/133.1.328S.
3. Stormon M. Typhoid fever in children: diagnostic and therapeutic difficulties. PIDJ. 1997;16(7):713–4.
4. F-Diagram. Paths of disease transmission. Water1st International. https://water1st.org/problem/f-diagram/.
5. Aiello AE. Effect of hand washing on infectious disease risk in the community: a meta-analysis. Am J Pub Health. 2008;98(8):1372–81.
6. Luby SP. Effect of hand washing on child health: a randomized controlled trial. Lancet. 2005;366(9481):225–33.
7. Liu J. Use of quantitative molecular diagnostic methods to identify causes of diarrhea in children: a reanalysis of the GEMS case-control study. Lancet. 2016;388(10051):1291–301.
8. World Health Organization. The treatment of diarrhoea: a manual for physicians and other senior health workers. 4th rev. Geneva: WHO; 2005. https://apps.who.int/iris/bitstream/handle/10665/43209/9241593180.pdf?sequence=1.
9. National Institute for Health and Care Excellence. Acute diarrhoea in children: racecadotril as an adjunct to oral rehydration, Evidence summary (ESNM12). 2013. https://www.nice.org.uk/advice/esnm12/chapter/Product-overview.
10. Grousard V. Chapter 3: Gastrointestinal disorders. In: Shigellosis, treatment. Clinical guidelines diagnosis and treatment manual. Geneva: Medicins Sans Frontieres; 2018. https://medicalguidelines.msf.org/viewport/CG/english/chapter-3-gastrointestinal-disorders-16689160.html.
11. O'Reilly C. Diarrheal diseases. In: Townes D, editor. Health in humanitarian emergencies. Cambridge: Cambridge University Press; 2018. p. 310–35.
12. WHO. Integrated Management of Childhood Illnesses chart booklet. Geneva: WHO; 2014. p. 1–80. Available at: https://www.who.int/maternal_child_adolescent/documents/IMCI_chartbooklet/en/.
13. Lukacik M. A meta-analysis of the effects of oral zinc in the treatment of acute and persistent diarrhea. Pediatrics. 2008;121(2):326–36. https://doi.org/10.1542/peds.2007-0921.
14. Lazzerini M. Oral zinc for treating diarrhea in children. Cochrane Database Syst Rev. 2016;12:CD00536. https://doi.org/10.1002/14651858,CD005436.pub5. https://www.cochrane.org/CD005436/INFECTN_oral-zinc-supplementation-treating-diarrhoea-children.
15. Bhandari N. Effectiveness of zinc supplementation plus oral rehydration salts compared with oral rehydration salts alone as a treatment of acute diarrhea in a primary care setting: a cluster randomized trial. Pediatrics. 2008;121(5):e1279.
16. Imdad A, Herzer K, Mayo-Wilson E, Yakoob MY, Bhutta ZA. Vitamin A supplementation for preventing morbidity and mortality in children from 6 months to 5 years of age. Cochrane Database Syst Rev. 2010;(12):CD008524. https://doi.org/10.1002/14651858.CD008524.pub2.
17. Nelson E. Antibiotics for both moderate and severe cholera. N Engl J Med. 2011;364:5–7.
18. Olson D. Cholera case management. Management of a cholera epidemic. Geneva: Medicins Sans Frontieres; 2018. ISBN: 978-2-37585-023-7.
19. Ferreras E. Single-dose cholera vaccine in response to an outbreak in Zambia. NEJM. 2018;378(6):577–9.
20. Britto C. An appraisal of the clinical features of pediatric enteric fever, meta-analysis. Clin Infect Dis. 2017;64(11):1604–11.
21. O'Reilly C. Typhoid fever. In: Townes DA, Gerber M, Anderson M, editors. Health in humanitarian emergencies. Cambridge: University Press; 2018. p. 325–9.

22. Grouzard V. Enteric fever treatment. Clinical guidelines-diagnosis and treatment manual. Geneva: Medicins Sans Frontieres; 2018. https://medicalguidelines.msf.org/viewport/CG/english/shigellosis-16689596.html.
23. Lamberti LM, Fischer Walker CL, Noiman A, et al. Breastfeeding and the risk for diarrhea morbidity and mortality. BMC Public Health. 2011;11:S15. https://doi.org/10.1186/1471-2458-11-S3-S15.
24. Balkan S. Severe acute malnutrition. Clinical guidelines-diagnosis and treatment manual. Geneva: Medicins Sans Frontieres; 2018. https://medicalguidelines.msf.org/viewport/CG/english/severe-acute-malnutrition-16689141.html.
25. Di Lorenzo C. Approach to the infant or child with nausea and vomiting. UpToDate, literature review through Oct 2019. Walters Kluwer Publisher, Netherlands. Available from: https//www.uptodate.com/content/approach-to-the-child-with-nausea-and-vomiting.
26. Neuman M. Causes of acute abdominal pain in children and adolescents. UpToDate, literature review through Nov 2019. Walters Kluwer Publisher. Available from: https//www.uptodate.com//content/causes-of-abdominal-pain-in-children-and-adolescents.

Philip Bruce Murray, MD, DTM&H was trained as a general internist at the University of California, San Francisco. He has practiced in academic settings, on a Native American reservation, and in private practice in rural communities in California and Oregon. Since 2006 he has done volunteer work in multiple low resource settings including refugee camps in Uganda, Greece, and Bangladesh. He has written clinical protocols for both acute and noncommunicable chronic diseases for different international NGOs. He assisted in the Rohingya humanitarian disaster in Bangladesh in 2017, helping to develop early field clinics and opening a 24-bed field hospital for acute diarrheal illness. He was involved in the capacity building of Bangladeshi physicians teaching refugee medicine, tropical disease, and epidemic management on two subsequent trips in 2018. He now works for Josephine County, Oregon, as COVID-19 medical liaison and contact tracing coordinator.

Childhood Infectious Diseases in Pediatric Refugee Populations

25

Aurora Teresa Gadsden-Hevia

Prologue

Walking with my team in one of the informal tent settlements of Syrian refugees in Lebanon we were intercepted by a worried father. He wanted us to go into his tent and see his baby, a 1-year-old girl who had been having diarrhea and vomiting for the last 3 days and was now quite drowsy and dehydrated. There were two other children in the family who had diarrhea. While talking to the father we found out that it was very hard for them to go out of the settlement to look for medical assistance because of police blockades and transportation difficulties. It had been raining and the scarce latrines were flooding, there were puddles and mud everywhere and it was difficult to walk around. Drinking water was brought by truck every 2 weeks and it was often dirty. At the end of our visit we had seen around 20 children with diarrhea and many adults were also reported sick.

When large groups of people are displaced, due to war, violence, food insecurity, poverty, or any other situation, living conditions become harsh and inadequate. In Lebanon, for example, there are no refugee camps; people are scattered around in informal test settlements. This makes it difficult for agencies and NGOs to assist the population with water and sanitation interventions. Because the number of tents are limited, many families live and sleep in the same spaces, which favors overcrowding. These are ideal conditions for viral, bacterial, and parasitic infections to spread easily and cause diseases, individual deaths, and ultimately outbreaks.

Communicable disease control is a challenge in most contexts where refugees live. Prevention and preparedness to recognize and manage an outbreak is essential. Infectious diseases can be brought by the refugees from their places of origin or from places they passed along their journeys. Refugees can acquire communicable disease in the host country, or they can be caused by the conditions encountered once the populations are settled.

A. T. Gadsden-Hevia (✉)
Doctors Without Borders/Médecins Sans Frontières (MSF), Toronto, ON, Canada

© Springer Nature Switzerland AG 2021
C. Harkensee et al. (eds.), *Child Refugee and Migrant Health*,
https://doi.org/10.1007/978-3-030-74906-4_25

In this chapter, we will talk about infectious diseases in the context of children of refugee populations.

Introduction

According to the UNCHR there are five diseases that have the most immediate impact on large-scale mortality, causing 60–80% of deaths among refugees [1]. They are:

1. Measles
2. Diarrheal diseases (see Gastrointestinal Diseases chapter)
3. Acute respiratory infections (see Respiratory chapter)
4. Malaria
5. Malnutrition (see Nutrition chapters)

In this chapter of the book we will go over some infections that have not been reviewed in depth in other chapters of the book. We will also talk about other infectious diseases that cause significant morbidity in children. Please note that all drug dosages provided in this chapter should be confirmed with local providers and national dosing guidelines.

Measles

Overview

Measles is a particularly important disease to discuss in the context of refugee populations since it is extremely contagious. It is one of the main killers in displaced populations and refugees. When people live in overcrowded and unhygienic conditions it spreads rapidly and in higher infectious doses, resulting in more severe clinical disease, especially in malnourished children. If we look at history, measles accounted for 53% of deaths in refugee children in eastern Sudan and 42% in Somalia in 1985, after this it was clear to everyone that this particular infection should always be addressed in refugee populations [2].

Know Your Bugs: The Infectious Agent

Measles is caused by a virus called *Measles morbillivirus* of the genus morbillivirus and the family *Paramyxoviridae*. The only host of measles virus is humans [2].

Epidemiology, Incidence, and Mortality

Measles is a widespread problem around the globe. It caused 140,000 deaths in 2018 [3]. When caring for displaced populations, it is important to understand their risk of measles in order to have a clear picture of where measles outbreaks are happening in the local communities.

In developed countries, there are occasional outbreaks which usually start from imported cases that infect people who are not vaccinated. In low-income countries, where measles is endemic, it causes recurrent large-scale epidemics with very high death tolls.

Transmission

Measles is one of the most contagious microbes in the world. Nine out of ten vulnerable people will become infected if exposed to the virus [4].

Transmission occurs person-to-person through infected respiratory droplets (nose and throat) that go from a patient with measles to a healthy person's mucosa (nose, eyes, and mouth). These droplets can become airborne when a sick person talks, sneezes, or coughs, and they can remain in the air for up to 2 h, so it can be transmitted in public spaces, even in the absence of contact with someone who is ill. This is why large outbreaks can occur in areas of crowding.

The incubation period is 6–21 days. Contagiousness is estimated to be from 5 days before the appearance of rash to 4 days afterward; however, a malnourished or immunocompromised child can transmit the infection for much longer. The period of maximum contagiousness is thought to be during the late prodrome phase when the patient is febrile and has respiratory symptoms [4].

Clinical Features

Stages of infection [5, 6]:

Incubation period	Prodrome	Enanthem (involvement of the mucosa)	Exanthem (rash)	Recovery
6–21 days	2–4 days	48 h prior to the onset of rash Lasts 12–72 h	2–4 days after onset of fever	
Virus enters the respiratory mucosa or conjunctivae, replicates locally, spreads to lymphatic tissues, and disseminates through the bloodstream (viremia).	Fever (as high as 40 °C), malaise and anorexia, conjunctivitis (with lacrimation or photophobia), coryza (runny nose), and cough.	Koplik spots: 1–3 mm whitish, grayish, or bluish elevations with an erythematous base, on the buccal mucosa opposite the molar teeth. Does not appear in all patients.	Erythematous, maculopapular rash. Spreads cephalocaudally and centrifugally. Lymphadenopathy and splenomegaly, high fever, respiratory signs, pharyngitis, non-purulent conjunctivitis.	Clinical improvement typically ensures within 48 h of the appearance of the rash. Cough may persist 1–2 weeks.

The Rash
- Blanching in early stages (the skin becomes white after you put pressure and then release), after it becomes non blanching (stays red, even if you put pressure).
- Begins on the face and spreads downwards: cephalocaudal.
- Goes from the center of the body, outwards, to involve the neck, upper trunk and extremities: centrifugal.
- Petechia (tiny hemorrhages that look like less than 1 mm red dots) may be seen and in severe cases rash appears hemorrhagic.
- Palms and soles are rarely involved (very important point if you are suspecting a different diagnosis).
- After 3–4 days the rash darkens to a brownish color and begins to fade. Followed by fine desquamation.
- Rash lasts 6–7 days and fades in the order it appeared (head to toe).

Complications

As other viruses do, the measles virus can cause inflammation in various organs such as the brain, the lungs, and the liver. It can also affect the immune system, making a child more susceptible to other infections. In fact, measles-associated immune suppression can last up to 3 years after the infection, increasing morbidity and mortality from other infections. One or more complications occur in 30% of cases.

- Gastrointestinal complications: The most common is diarrhea in 8% of cases, caused by intestinal inflammation. Together with gingivostomatitis (painful mouth ulcers) can cause difficulty eating and drinking and high water loss, which leads to dehydration, electrolyte imbalance, and worsening malnutrition. It can also cause hepatitis (elevated liver enzymes), mesenteric lymphadenitis, and appendicitis [6].
- Respiratory complications: the virus on its own can cause laryngotracheobronchitis (croup), bronchiolitis, and severe pneumonitis associated with respiratory distress. Pneumonia is present in 6% of cases and it is the main cause of mortality. Bacterial superinfection is also likely and occurs in 5% of cases. Bronchiectasis has also been reported, which predisposes the child to recurrent respiratory infections [6].
- Otitis media occurs in 5–10% of cases [6].
- Coinfections:
  - Viruses: parainfluenza virus, adenovirus, cytomegalovirus, enterovirus, influenza, and respiratory syncytial virus.
  - Bacteria: *Staphylococcus aureus*, *Streptococcus pneumoniae*, *Haemophilus influenzae*, and *Steptococcus pyogenes*. Tuberculosis reactivations [7].

- Neurologic: encephalitis, acute disseminated encephalomyelitis, and subacute sclerosing panencephalitis [6].
  - Encephalitis: Occurs in 1 per 1000 cases. It can appear from day 1 to 14 of the rash. Characterized by persistent fever, headache, vomiting, stiff neck, meningeal irritation, drowsiness, irritability, seizures, and coma. Twenty-five percent will have neuro-developmental sequelae. Cerebrospinal fluid will show elevated lymphocytes, proteins, and normal glucose.
  - Acute disseminated encephalomyelitis (1 per 1000 cases): caused by post-infectious autoimmune response. Presents during the recovery phase, usually 2 weeks after the rash. It can show as fever, headache, neck stiffness, seizures, and mental status changes. Any abnormal neurological finding should be suspected (sensory loss, muscle weakness, paraplegia, etc). CSF shows the same findings as encephalitis. It has 10–20% mortality. Residual neurological abnormalities are common, including behavior disorders, mental retardation, and epilepsy.
  - Subacute sclerosing panencephalitis: Is a fatal progressive degenerative disease. Appears 7–10 years after measles infection. More common if measles presented at an early age (<2 years of age). It can start with personality changes, somnolence, and evolve progressively to dementia, motor or sensory deficit, vegetative state, and death. Patients may live weeks to years but it is almost always fatal.
- Ocular: xerophthalmia, keratitis, Bitot's spots (dry conjunctival lesion), keratomalacia, corneal ulceration, and blindness, especially in children with malnutrition and vitamin A deficiency [7].
- Cardiac: myocarditis and pericarditis [7].
- Death: the case fatality rate in developing countries can vary from 4% to 10% [2].

Immunity and Vulnerability

Contracting and surviving measles infection provides lifelong immunity. Children born to mothers who were vaccinated before pregnancy have immunity until the age of 3–6 months, after this anti-measles antibodies begin to fade. Immunocompromised children such as those with severe malnutrition, HIV/AIDS, blood malignancies, or affected cell-mediated immunity due to medications can develop severe measles and all its complications [6]. Pregnant women are at risk for severe complications. There can also be the risk of low birth-weight, abortion, intrauterine fetal death, and congenital measles which can present as a broad spectrum of illness from mild to severe. In addition, Vitamin A deficiency due to malnutrition contributes to delayed recovery and to the high rate of post measles complications. Measles infection can also precipitate acute vitamin A deficiency and xerophthalmia [7].

Diagnosis

The first way to diagnose measles is with compatible clinical signs and symptoms, plus a history of recent exposure or travel to a place with high measles prevalence, especially in the absence of previous measles immunity. It can be confirmed with reverse transcriptase-polymerase chain reaction tests (RT-PCR) on respiratory secretions (throat swab is preferred), blood, bronchial lavage, or urine samples, detecting measles specific immunoglobulin M (IgM) and IgG in blood serum or through isolation of measles virus in cell culture [5].

Usually in the context of an outbreak, not every patient can be tested. Diagnosis is done with clinical signs and symptoms that are specified in by a case definition (see outbreaks section below). Depending on the situation, some patients will be tested—usually the first ones to be suspected to have measles [8].

Treatment

There is no specific antiviral treatment for measles but in order to avoid complications, the focus should be on the following management:

- Early recognition/triage of patients with clinical signs of severity.
- Supportive care: good nutrition, adequate fluid intake, and treatment for dehydration with oral rehydration solution or intravenous fluids.
- Vitamin A: can reduce morbidity and mortality rates as well as blindness due to kerato conjunctivitis. Administer orally once daily for 2 days at the following doses [9]:
  Less than 6 months: 50,000 IU
  6–11 months: 100,000 IU
  Older than 12 months: 200,000 IU
  Children with clinical signs and symptoms of vitamin A deficiency: give the third dose 4–6 weeks later
- Close follow-up and continual assessment to detect infections and sepsis in a timely manner. Antibiotics to treat associated bacterial infections. Antibiotic prophylaxis is not recommended.
- Immune globulin (IG) can be considered for exposed susceptible individuals who are severely immunocompromised and for pregnant women. It can be given within 6 days of exposure to prevent or modify the diseases. Recommended dose: IV 400 mg/kg, IM 0.5 mL/kg (maximum 15 mL) [5].

Vaccination

Measles vaccination resulted in a 73% drop in measles deaths between 2000 and 2018 worldwide. It prevented an estimated 23.2 million deaths. It can provide herd immunity, but to stop broad transmission 85–90% of the population must be vaccinated [10].

The measles vaccine is often incorporated with rubella and or mumps vaccines. It is equally safe and effective in single or combined form. Adding rubella to the measles vaccine increases the cost only slightly and allows for shared delivery and administration costs. It is a live attenuated vaccine. Antibodies will develop in 94% of immunized children. The second dose is to ensure that children who had no response with the first dose, do develop antibodies [2].

General recommendations for measles immunization:

- Children 6–11 months in epidemic situations: they should receive one dose of vaccine. This dose is not considered valid and two valid doses should be administered after the first birthday.
- Children older than 12 months: two doses of vaccine, separated by 28 days minimum.
- All nonimmunized people: should receive two doses of vaccine, separated by 28 days to ensure protection.
- Exposed susceptible individuals: if the vaccine is administered within 72 h of exposure, it will provide protection or disease modification in some cases. Consider an individual as susceptible if they have not received any doses of measles vaccine or they have only received one dose [7].

Measles Outbreaks

A measles outbreak is defined as a two or more laboratory-confirmed measles cases that are temporally related (with dates of rash onset occurring 7–23 days apart) and epidemiologically or virologically linked or both (being a known contact or being in the same physical setting as the case during their infectious period for any length of time).

The main preventive measure for a measles outbreak is routine measles vaccination for children, combined with mass immunization campaigns in countries with high case and death rates [2].

All suspected cases of measles should be reported to public health authorities according to each country's protocol. Communication with public health authorities is very important. Health care systems should have guidelines for infection control measures and rapid response protocols for measles cases, including a clear case definition (see chapter on outbreaks for more information).

All health care personnel should have evidence of measles immunity. Give two doses with 28-day interval if there is no evidence of vaccination.

In case of outbreaks prioritize hospital admission for patients with clinical warning signs. Non-severe cases should receive outpatient treatment and be isolated at home. All patients should receive vitamin A as recommended [11].

Infection control:

- Airborne transmission precautions (see Appendix on precautions) for 4 days after the onset of rash in healthy patients and for the duration of illness in immunocompromised patients.
- Susceptible individuals should not be in contact with suspected or confirmed cases.
- Exposed individuals should be placed on airborne precautions and excluded from social contact or work from day 5 through day 21 after exposure. Even those who were vaccinated within 72 h of exposure.
- Patients with febrile rash illness should be in a separate waiting area or placed immediately in an isolated room.
- Patients should wear appropriate masks to prevent generation of droplets, and staff should wear respirators to filter airborne particles.
- If the patient goes home, he/she should remain in isolation at home for 4 days after rash onset.
- A room occupied by a suspected case should not be used for 2 h after the patient's departure [11].

Other Viral Infections Associated with Skin Rashes

There are many infectious diseases that present with skin erythema or other lesions. They can be caused by bacteria, rickettsias (a special kind of bacteria), fungi, and parasites. Many of them are associated with specific regions of the world. A thorough description of all of them is beyond the scope of this chapter; here we will focus only on the most common viral rashes of childhood [5, 12].

	Transmission	Signs and symptoms	Treatment and precautions	Complications	Vaccine
Chickenpox/ Varicella Varicella–Zoster virus (VZV)	Breathing droplets from naso-pharyngeal secretion Direct contact with vesicle fluid Incubation period: 10–21 days	Fever, malaise, pharyngitis, loss of appetite. Rash: appears in successive crops, pruritic, macules–papules–pustules–crusts. Lesions in different stages on face, trunk, and extremities. New vesicle formation stops within 4 days. Crusts fall within 1–2 weeks and leave hypopigmentation.	– Antihistamines for pruritus. – Antipyretics. At-risk hosts: Acyclovir Oral: 20 mg/kg/dose in 4 doses for 5 days. IV: 1500 mg/m^2 or 30 mg/kg/day in 3 doses. Precautions: In hospital: Isolation – Standard – Contact – Airborne	– Skin and soft tissue bacterial infection: cellulitis, myositis, necrotizing fasciitis, and toxic shock syndrome. – Encephalitis: acute cerebellum ataxia, diffuse encephalitis. – Pneumonitis and pneumonia – Hepatitis – Reye syndrome associated with salicylates.	Vaccine: Live attenuated virus vaccine 2 doses: Minimum age 12 months, Second dose minimum interval 1–3 months. Outbreaks: Common.
Hand-foot-mouth disease Multiple Enterovirus serotypes, most common Coxsackievirus	Fecal—oral route. Contact with vesicle fluid or oral and respiratory secretions. Virus stays in stools for 6 weeks to several months, in respiratory tract up to 30 days. Incubation period: 3–5 days.	– Infants and children <7 years. – Mouth and throat pain and mild fever – Oral enanthem: erythematous macules that progress to vesicles that rupture and form painful ulcers. – Exanthem: Non pruritic, usually not painful. Macular, maculopapular, or vesicular on hands, feet, buttocks, upper thighs, and arms.	– Good oral intake and hydration. – Pain and fever control. No specific antiviral therapy available. Precautions in hospital: – Standard – Contact	– Dehydration due to refusal to drink. – Palmar and plantar desquamation 1–3 weeks after. – Nail dystrophy or shedding of nails 1–2 months after. – Rhombencephalitis, acute flaccid paralysis, aseptic meningitis. – Pulmonary edema and hemorrhage. – Myocarditis – Pancreatitis – Conjunctival ulceration – Fetal loss	No vaccine. Good hand hygiene in the home (especially when changing diapers). Outbreaks: Common.

	Transmission	Signs and symptoms	Treatment and precautions	Complications	Vaccine
Roseola infantum (Exanthem subitum or sixth disease) Human Herpesvirus 6 (HHV-6) Other: HHV-7, enteroviruses, adenovirus es, and parainfluenza virus type 1	HHV-6: transmission not clear, possibly through saliva from mother to infant and perinatal. Shedding is thought to be lifelong. Incubation period: not certain, but thought to be 9–10 days.	– Children <2 years. – High fever (up to 40 °C) for 3–5 days, palpebral conjunctivitis, edematous eyelids, inflamed tympanic membrane, coryza, cough, vomiting, diarrhea, cervical, post-auricular, and/or occipital lymph nodes. – Fever suddenly disappears and a blanching macular or maculopapular rash develops. Starts on neck and trunk and spreads to face and extremities (can be confused with drug allergy).	– Good oral intake and hydration. – Fever control Precautions: Hand hygiene. Children are not to be excluded from normal activities. Not considered contagious.	– Complications are rare. – Seizures. – Aseptic meningitis. – Encephalitis. – Thrombocytopenic purpura.	No vaccine widely available. Outbreaks: Unlikely.
Rubella Rubella virus	Inhalation of respiratory droplets and aerosols. Shedding: 1–2 weeks before symptoms and stops 7 days after rash appears. Incubation period: 14–18 days.	– Low–grade fever and lymphadenopathy (Characteristic: posterior cervical, posterior auricular, and suboccipital) 1–5 days before the rash. – Rash: pinpoint, pink maculopapules. Appears on the face and spreads down and becomes generalized in 24 h. Due to the risk of congenital rubella and international efforts for vaccination coverage rubella should be confirmed by measuring IgM antibodies.	Supportive. Precautions: – Standard – Contact – Droplet For 7 days after the onset of the rash. *Avoid contact with women of child-bering age and pregnant women.	– Post-infectious encephalitis. – Congenital rubella syndrome (not described in this chapter, more information on: https://www.who.int/news-room/fact-sheets/detail/rubella)	Vaccine: Usually in combination with measles. Schedule 2 doses. In children >12 months, with an interval of at least 28 days between doses. Outbreaks: Likely in unvaccinated population.

Erythema infectious or fifth disease Parvovirus B19	Inhalation or mucosal contact with respiratory droplets and saliva. Vertical transmission during pregnancy and through blood products. Incubation period: 4–21 days.	– Fever, malaise, myalgias, watery eyes, headache, nausea, diarrhea. – Rash: appears 2–5 days later, distinctive malar erythema with pallor around the mouth (slapped cheek rash). Sometimes followed by a pruritic, symmetric, macular, lace-like rash on trunk that spreads peripherally to arms, buttocks, and thighs.	Supportive. Precautions: – Standard – Droplet (if immunocompromised children) Children with rash are no longer contagious, no need to be isolated or excluded from normal activities.	– Arthralgia and chronic arthritis. – Papular purpuric gloves and socks syndrome, in teenagers. – Transient aplastic crisis – Myocarditis – Pregnant women: miscarriage, intrauterine fetal death, hydrops fetalis.	Vaccine: No Outbreaks: common in school-aged children.

Diarrhoeal Diseases

Displaced children are at great risk of infectious diarrheal diseases. In this chapter, we will focus on the organisms that can cause severe diarrhea with high morbidity and mortality rates in refugee children. Less severe causes of diarrhea such as amebiasis and giardiasis will be reviewed elsewhere.

Rotavirus
- Virus.
- Leading cause of diarrhea in children <5 years [13].
- Incubation period: 1–3 days.
- Transmission: fecal-oral route between people. Ingestion of contaminated water or food and contact with contaminated surfaces or objects.
- Clinical features:
  - Acute onset fever, usually high
  - Projectile vomiting
  - Profuse watery diarrhea that leads to rapid dehydration
- Complications: dehydration, electrolyte abnormalities, acidosis.
- Diagnosis: clinical, antigen-detection immunoassay, or RT-PCR on stool for surveillance purposes or research.
- Treatment: self-limited, oral rehydration therapy, and fever control.
- In hospital: standard precautions, contact precautions for children with diapers or incontinence for the duration of the illness.
- Surfaces should be washed with soap and water; bleach can also be used.
- Outbreaks common in child care centers and pediatric wards.
- Vaccine available: 4 oral, live attenuated [14].

Shigella
- Bacteria, gram-negative bacilli. *Shigella dysenteriae* serotype 1 (Sd1) produces shiga toxin and causes more severe illness.
- Most frequent cause of dysentery.
- Incubation period: 1–7 days.
- Transmission: humans are the only host. Fecal-oral route, contaminated objects, food and water, and sexual contact. Houseflies are also a vector.
- Causes large scale and prolonged dysentery epidemics. It is highly contagious because the infective dose is very low (ingesting 10 organisms is enough). Risk factors: overcrowded areas with poor sanitation and water supplies.
- Clinical features:
  - Ranges from watery or loose stools with minimal constitutional symptoms to high fever, abdominal cramps or tenderness, tenesmus, and mucoid bloody stools.
  - Sd1 causes more severe illness in children <5 years, especially neonates, malnourished children, and children recovering from measles [15].
- Complications: dehydration, electrolyte abnormalities, generalized seizures, sepsis, pseudomembranous colitis, toxic megacolon, intestinal perforation, rectal prolapse, hemolysis, and hemolytic-uremic syndrome (HUS) [5].
- Diagnosis: Culture of feces or rectal swab specimens or PCR assays. Determining antibiotic susceptibility is essential in areas where Shigella is endemic and in case of an outbreak.
- Treatment: mild infection is self-limited oral rehydration salts, zinc supplementation. No antibiotics and anti-motility agents should be given. If severe disease or risk factors:
  - Essential to investigate regional resistance to antimicrobials.
  - Due to high resistance ampicillin, Trimethroprim/sulfametoxazol (co-trimoxazol) and nalidixic acid are no longer recommended.
  - First-line: Ciprofloxacin (irrespective of age) 15 mg/kg/dose 2 times a day for 3 days.
  - Second-line: Ceftriaxone 50–100 mg/kg/dose IM/IV once a day for 2–5 days or Azithromycin 20 mg/kg/dose once a day for 1–5 days (resistance is rapidly developed) [15].
- Case fatality rate is 15% in hospitalized children.
- Outbreaks:
  - Cases of dysentery and deaths due to bloody diarrhea should always be recorded and reported every week in order to rapidly detect and increase in cases.
  - At least one laboratory within the country should be able to isolate and identify Shigella, including Sd1, and perform antimicrobial susceptibility testing.
  - Establish rapid preventive measures and health education: water and sanitation (hand hygiene, clean water, adequate food preparation, appropriate disposal of human waste), support breastfeeding, control of flies.
  - Clear case definition and accessible care facilities.
  - Isolate patients on in an independent area of the care facility, use standard and contact precautions [15].
- No vaccine available.

E. coli

- There are five types of diarrhea producing *Escherichia coli*: Shiga toxin-producing (STEC), enteropathogenic (EPEC), enterotoxigenic (ETEC), enteroinvasive (EIEC), and enteroaggregative (EAEC) [12].
- STEC, serotype O157-H7 are the organisms associated with outbreaks in at-risk populations, we will focus only on this type. Although other types of *E. coli* can cause important diarrhea in children.
- Transmission: food or contaminated water, fecal-oral route, contact with infected animals, and contaminated objects [16].
- Incubation period: 3–8 days.
- Clinical features: begins with non-bloody diarrhea, that becomes bloody after 2–3 days. Severe abdominal pain, low-grade fever. Can mimic intussusception, appendicitis, ischemic colitis.
- Complications: hemorrhagic colitis, hemolytic-uremic syndrome, coagulopathy [5].
- Diagnosis: Stool culture and PCR assays. Rapid enzyme immunoassays and immunochromatographic assays for detection of shiga toxin in stool.
- Treatment: oral rehydration salts. Anti-motility agents should not be given. Antimicrobials are not recommended in case of STEC. In case of outbreaks, it is essential to differentiate between shigella and STEC. Strict hand hygiene measures while taking care of children with dysentery [15].
- Precautions in hospitalized patients: standard and contact.
- No vaccine available.

Salmonella
- Bacteria, gram-negative bacilli.
- Two kinds of *Salmonella* infection:
  - Gastroenteritis caused by nontyphoidal *Salmonella* (serovars *Typhimurium, Enteritidis,* and all other non *Typhi* or *Paratyphi* serovars):
    Diarrhea, abdominal cramps, and fever. Affects distal small intestine and colon.
    Bacteremia and focal infection, such as meningitis, brain abscess, and osteomyelitis.
    More common in infants and children with hemoglobinopathies (Sickle cell) and immunocompromising conditions.
    Reservoirs include humans, birds, mammals, reptiles, and amphibians (turtles). Food vehicles like poultry, beef, eggs, and dairy, as well as fruits, vegetables, peanut butter, powdered infant formula, cereal, and bakery products. Contaminated water and contact with infected animals can be another mode of transmission [12].
    Incubation period: 6–72 h.
  - Enteric fever caused by *Salmonella* serovars *Typhi, Paratyphi* A, B, and C [8].
    Fever, headache, malaise, anorexia, lethargy, abdominal discomfort and tenderness, hepatomegaly, splenomegaly, dactylitis, rose spots, and changes in mental status.
    Either diarrhea (stool tends to have pea soup appearance) or constipation.
    There can be bacteremia, invasive infection with severe clinical symptoms, and meningitis.
    Characteristic: Relative bradycardia (slower heart rate than expected for a given temperature).
    Only human hosts, usually chronic carriers that contaminate food and water.
    Incubation period: 7–14 days.
- Diagnosis: Culture of stool, blood, urine, bile, and other tissues. Test to detect salmonella antigens such as enzyme immunoassay, latex agglutination, and monoclonal antibodies. Gene-bases PCR [5].
- Treatment:
  - Antibiotics are not indicated for asymptomatic or mild infections (prolongs duration of fecal excretion).
  - Antibiotics for children with a high risk of invasive disease.
  - Recommended agents depend on local resistance patterns. Amoxicillin, ampicillin, and trimethoprim-sulfamethoxazole used to be the treatments of choice but resistance is common thus fluoroquinolones or azithromycin can be used.
  - If resistant to fluoroquinolones (usually in Southeast Asia) empiric treatment can be started with ceftriaxone.
- Precautions: in hospitalized patients use standard and contact precautions for diapered and incontinent children for the duration of illness.
- Outbreaks are rare in children, except for *Salmonella* serovar *Typhi* or *Paratyphi*.
- Vaccines: only for *S. Typhi*, there are 3: live oral Ty21a, injectable typhoid conjugate vaccine (Vi polysaccharide antigen), injectable unconjugated polysaccharide vaccine. For more information [8].

Campylobacter
- Bacteria, comma-shaped, gram-negative bacilli. Twenty-five species, most common. *C. jejuni* and *C. coli.* Reservoirs can be domestic and wild birds and animals.
- Transmission due to contaminated food and water, unpasteurized milk or contact with feces of infected animals or people.
- One of the main causes of diarrhea in children <5 years.
- Incubation period: 2–5 days. Excretion of bacteria continues for 2–3 weeks [12].
- Clinical features:
  - Diarrhea, abdominal pain (can be severe, mimicking appendicitis or intussusception), malaise, and fever. Stool can contain visible or occult blood.
  - In neonates and young infants, bloody diarrhea without fever is common.
  - Fever can be high and can result in febrile seizures.
- Complications:
  - Prolonged, relapsing, or extraintestinal infection in immunocompromised children.
  - Acute idiopathic polyneuritis: Guillain-Barré syndrome.
  - Reiter syndrome (arthritis, urethritis, and bilateral conjunctivitis).
  - Myocarditis, pericarditis, and erythema nodosum.
  - Outbreaks are rare but can be a cause of healthcare-associated diarrhea, especially in neonates [5].
- Diagnosis: culture from feces, antigenic enzyme immunoassay, and multiplex nucleic acid amplification tests.
- Treatment:
  - Rehydration salts.
  - Azithromycin (10 mg/kg/day, for 3 days) or erythromycin (40 mg/kg/day, divided in 4 doses, for 5 days). They shorten the duration of illness and excretion of susceptible organisms and prevents relapse.
- Precautions: In hospitalized patients, standard and contact precautions are recommended for children with diapers or incontinence for the duration of illness.
- No vaccine available.

Cholera
- Bacteria *Vibrio cholerae*. Gram-negative comma-shaped rod. Humans are the only host but free-living bacteria can stay in bodies of water [17].
- Only toxin-producing serogroups O1 and O139 cause epidemic cholera.
- Endemic area: area where bacteriologically confirmed cholera cases, resulting from local transmission, have been detected in the last 3 years.
- There have been massive outbreaks around the world, associated with inadequate access to clean water and sanitation [18].
- Incubation period 12 h to 5 days.
- Contaminated food and water, particularly raw or undercooked shellfish, raw or partially dried fish, or moist grains or vegetables.
- Bacteria can be present in asymptomatic people from 1 to 10 days, infecting others.
- Clinical features:
  - Severe acute watery diarrhea that can kill within hours.
  - Stool has rice-water appearance, white-tinged, and contains small flecks of mucus.
  - No fever, no abdominal pain [5].
- Complications: Hypovolemic shock, hypokalemia, metabolic acidosis, hypoglycemia.
- Diagnosis: rapid diagnostic test (WHO has authorized this type of test only for detection purposes), PCR, or culture on stool samples.
- Treatment:
  - Prompt administration of oral rehydration salts or isotonic intravenous fluids.
  - Breastfeeding should be promoted.
  - Zinc supplement.
  - Antibiotics decrease duration and volume of diarrhea and shedding of viable bacteria. Choice of therapy depends on the severity of disease, age, and patterns of antibiotic resistance. Possible options [17]:
    Doxycycline 4–6 mg/kg, single dose. Not recommended for children <8 years.
    Ciprofloxacin 15 mg/kg, 2 times a day for 3 days.
    Azithromycin 20 mg/kg, single dose.
    Erythromycin 12.5 mg/kg, 4 times a day for 3 days.
    Tetracycline 12.5 mg/kg, 4 times a day for 3 days [17].
- A surveillance system is very important in a humanitarian crisis such as displacement of populations and overcrowded refugee camps. One or more positive tests should trigger a cholera alert.
- Outbreak management:
  - Surveillance system.
  - Information for population: disinfection of drinking water (chlorination or boiling), thorough cooking of food, appropriate hand hygiene after defecating and before preparing or eating food, safe disposal of feces, identification of symptoms, location of treatment sites, and adequate funeral practices.
  - Ensure access to clean water and appropriate sanitation.
  - Rapid detection and treatment: trained health personnel, clear disease definition, appropriate treatment centers, and protection equipment.
  - All patients: standard and contact precautions for the duration of the illness [19].
- Vaccine: there are three oral, WHO-approved vaccines that require two doses [20].

Malaria

Overview

Malaria or Paludismo is a life-threatening disease caused by a parasite that spreads to people through the bite of the female *Anopheles* mosquitoes. It can be preventable and curable if treated on time.

Know Your Bugs: The Infectious Agent

Malaria is caused by the parasite *Plasmodium*, there are five species:

- *Plasmodium falciparum:* The most deadly. Causes 99.7% of malaria in Africa, 50% in Southeast Asia, 71% in the Eastern Mediterranean region, and 65% in the Western Pacific.
- *Plasmodium vivax:* Second most deadly. It is found in central and south America (75% of cases), India, and Southeast Asia.
- The less dangerous *Plasmodium ovale, Plasmodium malariae, Plasmodium kowlesi* (comes from monkeys, rarely affects humans) [5].

Epidemiology, Incidence, and Mortality

Children under 5 years are the most vulnerable group, accounting for 67% of deaths of malaria worldwide. According to the WHO 2019 Malaria Report, in 2018 there were an estimated 228 million cases of malaria (405,000 deaths) of which 93% occurred in the African region (and 94% of deaths), followed by the South East Asia region with 3.4% and Eastern Mediterranean region with 2.1%. The six countries most affected were: Nigeria (25%), the Democratic Republic of the Congo (12%), Uganda (5%), Côte d'Ivoire (4%), Mozambique (4%), and Niger (4%). For specific information by country review the WHO World Malaria report 2019 [21].

Transmission

In most cases, malaria is transmitted by the bites of female Anopheles mosquitoes. They bite between dusk and dawn. They like to lay their eggs in water, that is why malaria transmission is higher during the rainy season in tropical countries. It can also be transmitted from the mother to the fetus during pregnancy and through blood transfusions that contain parasites [12].

Immunity and Vulnerability

The people most at risk of contracting malaria and developing severe disease are infants, children under 5 years, pregnant women, and people with HIV/AIDS and anatomical or functional asplenia, (children with sickle cell anemia), as well as nonimmune migrants, mobile populations, and travelers who have never been in contact with the disease. In areas with intense transmission partial immunity is developed over years of exposure and can reduce the risk of severe diseases; however, if a person leaves the area, immunity will be lost [21].

Clinical Features

If working with refugees in a malaria-endemic area, always think of malaria if a child comes with fever. This also applies to newborn babies born to mothers with a positive malaria test. The sooner a child starts treatment, the better the outcome. In susceptible people, if treatment is delayed death can occur within hours [22].

There are two clinical presentations:

1. Uncomplicated malaria: confirmed parasitic diagnosis plus general malaise, high fever, chills, rigor, sweats, headache, anorexia, nausea, vomiting, diarrhea, abdominal pain, arthralgia, myalgia, and pallor from anemia.
2. Severe malaria: confirmed parasitic diagnosis plus organ dysfunction with one or more of the following clinical or laboratory signs [22]:

Clinical	Laboratory
• Severe pallor • Altered consciousness (Glasgow <11) or long-lasting coma (>30 min) without an identifiable cause (Cerebral malaria) • Prostration (inability to sit up or drink) • Malarial retinopathy • >2 seizures in 24 h (focal or generalized) • Respiratory distress, deep breathing (sign of acidosis) • Shock (hyperthermia/hypothermia, hypotension, tachycardia, slow capillary refill time) • Jaundice (yellow conjunctiva and/or palms) • Hemoglobinuria (dark/red urine) • Signs of bleeding on the skin (petechia, bruises), conjunctiva, nose, gums, stool • Acute renal failure (urine output <1 mL/kg/h) despite adequate hydration	• Hemoglobin <5 g/dL, hematocrit <15% • Hypoglycemia • Metabolic acidosis (bicarbonate <15 mmol/L) • Hyperlactataemia (lactate >5 mol/L) • Urine positive for blood • Hyperparasitaemia (>10% of Red blood cells or 500,000 parasites/mcl) • Thrombocytopenia • Renal failure • Pulmonary edema (confirmed with X-ray) • Disseminated intravascular coagulation

Associated infection such as sepsis, pneumonia, and meningitis should always be considered and rapidly treated, since clinic and laboratory signs are impossible to differentiate.

Malaria in Newborns

Congenital malaria presents in the first 7 days of life. It can be acquired vertically (from mother to child through the placenta) or at the time of birth (mother without malaria). Neonatal malaria presents from day 8 to 28. It can be acquired from mosquito bites or infected blood. Clinical signs and symptoms can be indistinguishable from neonatal sepsis [22].

Complications

- Severe anemia
- Renal failure
- Shock
- Disseminated intravascular coagulation
- Cerebral edema and increased intracranial pressure
- Neurological sequel
- Hypersplenism: with danger of splenic rupture
- Relapse of infection: for as long as 3–5 years after primary infection, attributed to latent hepatic stages (hypnozoites) with *P. vivax* and *P. ovale*, or as long as decades with *P. malariae*
- Associated bacterial infection
- Pregnancy: maternal anemia, fetal loss, premature delivery, intrauterine growth retardation, delivery of low birth-weight infants, early neonatal death [22]

Diagnosis

- Microscopy: thick blood film to detect and count parasites (even if scarce) and thin blood film to detect species and determine the degree of parasitemia. If no parasites are seen, but there are clinical signs, microscopy should be repeated every 12–24 h for at least 3 days [5].
- Rapid diagnostic test (RDT) for antigen-detection. This test should be confirmed with microscopy because low-level parasitemia may not be detected. There are different brands that detect different species. You should refer to each test's manufacturer guidelines [5].

Treatment

Malaria treatment is based on the infecting species, possible drug resistance, and severity of the disease.

The recommended management by WHO is as follows [9]:

Severe Malaria:

- If child is unconscious, protect the airway and minimize risk for aspiration pneumonia: open airway, place in recovery positions, and place nasogastric tube.
- Check for hypoglycemia and correct.
- Treat seizures with rectal or IV diazepam. Do not give prophylactic anticonvulsants.
- Antipyretics for fever (paracetamol or ibuprofen).
- Check for dehydration and treat appropriately and after it is corrected, ensure proper IV fluids or nasogastric feeding.
- Ensure close follow-up, vital signs, alertness, and urine output.
- Treat complications: hypoxia, hypoglycemia, severe anemia, seizures, and associated or suspected infection.
- Antimalarial treatment [9]:
  - Rectal artesunate should be given to all children before referral from a health center to a hospital.
  - Parenteral artesunate is the drug of choice for severe *P. falciparum* malaria. If not available use parenteral artemether or quinine, until the child can take oral medication or for a minimum of 24 h.
  - Artesunate: 2.4 mg/kg IV or IM on admission, then at 12 and 24 h, then daily until the child can take oral medication but for a minimum of 24 h even if the child can tolerate oral medication earlier.
  - Quinine: loading dose of quinine dihydrochloride salt at 20 mg/kg by infusion in 10 mL/kg of IV fluid over 2–4 h. Then, 8 h after the start of the loading dose, give 10 mg/kg quinine salt in IV fluid over 2 h, and repeat every 8 h until the child can take oral medication. The infusion rate should not exceed a total of 5 mg/kg/h of quinine dihydrochloride salt. Never as a bolus injection. It can be given as a diluted divided IM injection. Loading dose split into two as 10 mg/kg of quinine salt into the anterior aspect of each thigh. Then, continue with 10 mg/kg every 8 h until oral medication is tolerated.
  - Artemether: 3.2 mg/kg IM on admission, then 1.6 mg/kg daily until the child can take oral medication.
  - After 24 h and when the child can tolerate oral medication, complete treatment with a full course of Artemisin-based combination therapy. See uncomplicated malaria.

Uncomplicated Malaria:

- Treat with a first-line antimalarial agent. Refer to national guidelines [9].
- Treat for 3 days with one of the following artemisin-based combination therapies:

Combination	Presentation	Dose
Artemether–lumefantrine	Tablets 20 mg artemether, 120 mg of lumefantrine	5–<15 kg: 1 tablet twice a day 15–24 kg: 2 tablets twice a day for 3 days >25 kg: 3 tablets twice a day for 3 days

Artesunate plus amodiaquine	Tablets containing 25/67.5 mg, 50/135 mg, or 100/270 mg of artesunate/amodiaquine	4 mg/kg/day artesunate and 10 mg/kg/day amodiaquine:
		  3–<10 kg: 1 tablet (25/67.5 mg) twice a day for 3 days
		  10–18 kg: 1 tablet (50/135 mg) twice a day for 3 days

Artesunate plus sulfadoxine–pyrimethamine	Separate tablets of 50 mg artesunate and 500 mg sulfadoxine–25 mg pyrimethamine	4 mg/kg/day artesunate once a day and 25 mg/kg sulfadoxine—1.25 mg/kg pyrimethamine on day 1.
		Artesunate:
		  3–<10 kg: half tablet once daily for 3 days
		  ≥10 kg: one tablet once daily for 3 days
		Sulfadoxine–pyrimethamine:
		  3–<10 kg: half tablet once on day 1
		  ≥10 kg: one tablet once on day 1

Artesunate plus mefloquine	Separate tablets of 50 mg artesunate and 250 mg mefloquine base	4 mg/kg/day artesunate once a day for 3 days and 25 mg/kg of mefloquine divided into two or three doses.

Dihydroartemisinin plus piperaquine	Tablets containing 40 mg dihydroartemisinin and 320 mg piperaquine	4 mg/kg/day dihydroartemisinin and 18 mg/kg/day piperaquine once a day for 3 days.
		  5–<7 kg: half tablet (20/160 mg) once a day for 3 days
		  7–<13 kg: one tablet (20/160 mg) once a day for 3 days
		  13–<24 kg: one tablet (320/40 mg) once a day for 3 days

- Children with HIV infection: if on treatment with zidovudine or efavirenz should avoid amodiaquine-containing artemisinin-based combination therapy, and those on cotrimoxazole (trimethoprim plus sulfamethoxazole) prophylaxis should avoid sulfadoxine–pyrimethamine.
- Uncomplicated *P. vivax, ovale,* and *malariae* malaria: still responsive to 3 days' treatment with chloroquine, followed by primaquine for 14 days.
- For *P. vivax*:
  - Give a 3-day course of artemisinin-based combination therapy as recommended for *P. falciparum* (with the exception of artesunate plus sulfadoxine–pyrimethamine) combined with primaquine at 0.25 mg base/kg, taken with food once daily for 14 days.

- Give oral chloroquine at a total dose of 25 mg base/kg, combined with primaquine: initial dose of 10 mg base/kg, followed by 10 mg/kg on the second day and 5 mg/kg on the third day plus Primaquine at 0.25 mg base/kg, taken with food once daily for 14 days.
- Chloroquine-resistant vivax malaria should be treated with amodiaquine, mefloquine, or dihydroartemisinin plus piperaquine as the drugs of choice [9].

Prevention

1. Reduce the number of bites [16]:
   - Reducing mosquitoes: indoor residual spraying with insecticides once or twice a year. This should be implemented at a high coverage level.
   - Avoiding mosquitoes: if a refugee area can be selected, special care should be taken to avoid proximity to vector breeding sites, such as ponds, streams, or swamps. Attempt to get rid of unnecessary collections of water or using larvicides.
   - Reducing contact with mosquitoes: sleeping under an insecticide-treated net provides a physical barrier from bites and also kills mosquitoes. This also needs to be consistent within the population in order to work.
2. Kill the parasite before the person develops the disease (drug prophylaxis): suppresses the blood stage of malaria infection. It can be given continuously or intermittently. This program can be difficult to implement but can have a big impact.
   - IPT (intermittent preventive treatment): administration of a curative dose of an effective antimalarial drug (Sulfadoxine–pyrimethamine (SP)).
     - Pregnant women: IPTp at each antenatal care visit, starting in the second trimester, at least twice during pregnancy.
     - Infants: IPTi: one dose of SP at each contact through the expanded program on immunizations (EPI), usually 10 weeks, 14 weeks, and 9 months of age [23, 24].
     - Children: IPTc: seasonal malaria chemoprevention.

HIV/AIDS

This is a very complex topic that cannot be covered to its full extent in this chapter; therefore, we will only talk about essential information for first contact with a child in whom HIV is suspected. For children already diagnosed, please refer to national guidelines.

Overview

An estimated 1.8 million children aged 0–14 were living with HIV at the end of 2019, 150,000 children were newly infected and 95,000 died of AIDS-related illnesses. Infants and children have an immature immune system and are less able to suppress HIV viral replication. Because of this, without prompt diagnosis and treatment 50% will die by the age of 2 and 80% by the age of 5.

Countries in Sub-Saharan Africa have been the hardest hit by the global HIV epidemic, but there can be infected people in every country. Each country's HIV prevalence should be reviewed in order to organize services for displaced or refugee populations.

HIV infection is a serious problem in refugee populations during humanitarian crises for a number of reasons. HIV/AIDS positive people may be subject to violation of human rights. Health care systems are unable to provide appropriate testing and treatment. Antenatal care may not be easily available and therefore there may be no testing available and no prevention of mother-to-child transmission (PMTCT) programs. Drugs and follow-up may not be easily available. There is no epidemiological evidence that refugee or displaced persons have a higher risk of contracting or transmitting AIDS; however, host countries may engage in discriminatory measures such as mass testing. The risk is the same as for other populations; however, sexual abuse and sex work may be increased and there may be less availability of condoms. Culturally appropriate programs to prevent HIV transmission should be implemented [16].

Transmission

- In children 90% of HIV infections are acquired through mother to child transmission during pregnancy, labor, and delivery, or later through breastfeeding.
- Transfusion with contaminated blood.
- Sexual abuse.
- Injury with contaminated objects such as razors, needles, or non-sterile surgical instruments.
- In adolescents risk factors are the same as adults [25].

Prevention of Mother to Child Transmission (PMTCT)

All pregnant women should be tested for HIV at the beginning of antenatal care and in the third trimester. Partners should also get tested. All HIV testing (child or adult) must be confidential, be accompanied by counseling, and conducted only with informed consent so that it is both informed and voluntary. HIV serological antibody test (ELISA or rapid tests) should be used [25].

All HIV positive pregnant women need to be properly evaluated (CD4, viral load if possible, screening for TB and sexually transmitted diseases) and proper treatment started. She should continue treatment after delivery and during breast-feeding. Counseling is essential to avoid loss to follow up [25].

Babies born to HIV positive mothers or abandoned babies with a positive rapid HIV test should be started on Nevirapine (NVP) once a day for 6 weeks (according to national guidelines). At 6 weeks NVP can be stopped, and cotrimoxazole syrup started (which should continue until a confirmed negative HIV test is obtained). Exclusive breastfeeding for at least 6 months is recommended [9].

The best way to diagnose HIV in infants is to look for evidence of the virus in the blood, rather than looking for antibodies or antigens (because they may be acquired from the mother, lasting for up to 18 months). This may require sending a blood sample (whole blood, serum, or dried blood spots on paper) to a specialized labora-tory that can perform this test [9, 25]:

- HIV RNA or DNA PCR testing (which detects viral DNA) should be performed at 6 weeks, and if positive, perform a confirmatory PCR.
- If breastfeeding stops, perform a rapid test 6 weeks after cessation. If positive, do a confirmatory PCR.
- If breastfeeding at 9 months, perform a rapid test. If positive, do a confirmatory PCR. If negative and continues to breastfeed, do a rapid test 6 weeks after breast-feeding cessation and if positive, do a PCR test.
- If exclusively formula-fed do a confirmatory rapid test at 18 months.
- If clinical features of HIV at any age a PCR test should be done.

Clinical Features

Clinical presentation of HIV infection in children is highly variable. They can show severe signs and symptoms in the first year of life (rapid progression, 25–30%); they can slowly develop symptoms early in life, then follow a downhill course and die at the age of 3–5 years (50–60%); or, they can be long-term survivors, who live beyond 8 years of age (5–25%).

Signs that indicate possible HIV infection include [12]:

- Recurrent infection: >3 severe episodes of a bacterial infection (pneumonia, meningitis, sepsis, cellulitis, chronic otitis media, tuberculosis) in the past 12 months.
- Persistent diarrhea (>14 days).
- Severe acute malnutrition that does not respond to therapy or persistent failure to thrive.
- Oral candidiasis or thrush: especially if it lasts >30 days despite antifungal treat-ment, recurs, extends beyond the tongue, or presents as oesophageal candidiasis.
- Chronic parotitis: unilateral or bilateral parotid swelling ≥ 14 days, with or without associated pain or fever.
- Generalized lymphadenopathy with no apparent cause.

- Hepatomegaly with no apparent cause.
- Persistent and/or recurrent fever.
- Progressive neurological impairment, microcephaly, developmental delay, hypertonia, or mental confusion.
- Herpes zoster (shingles).
- HIV dermatitis: erythematous papular rash. Typical skin rashes include extensive fungal infections of the skin, nails, and scalp and extensive molluscum contagiosum.
- Chronic suppurative lung disease.
- Lung infection consistent with Pneumocystis jiroveci (PCP).
- Lymphocytic interstitial pneumonia.
- Kaposi sarcoma.
- Acquired recto-vaginal fistula (in girls).

For clinical staging see national guidelines or WHO Pocketbook of Hospital Care for Children: guidelines for the management of common childhood illnesses–second ed. 2013 [9].

Diagnosis

- All testing should be done after age-appropriate counseling.
- Children with HIV positive parents and with HIV siblings should be tested.
- Adolescents with risk factors should always be offered testing.
- Children younger than 18 months should be tested with a PCR and confirmed with a second one if positive.
- For children above 18 months two positive rapid HIV tests confirm the diagnosis [9, 25].

Treatment

All HIV positive children under 5 years should be started on antiretroviral drugs (ARV) immediately. If over 5, start ARV in CD4 count is less than 500 cells/mcl or with severe or advanced disease [25]. Once started children must take their medicine regularly. Supply must be assured for all children. Advocacy for pediatric formulations to facilitate treatment should continue. Adolescents should be accompanied and counseled in specific adolescent clinics. Children with HIV should be immunized unless specific contraindications. For specific guidelines on treatment options and follow up see national guidelines or WHO Pocketbook of Hospital Care for Children: guidelines for the management of common childhood illnesses–second ed. 2013 [9].

Appendix: Precautions for Infection Control

Infections may be passed from one person to another, especially in hospital settings. Patients can transmit the infection to other patients, health care personal and even the hospital environment. Depending on the way a microbe is transmitted it needs different preventions or precaution methods. They are described here.

Type of precaution	
Standard	• All patients no matter what disease they have. • Respect the 5 moments of hand hygiene. • Gloves, gowns and eye protection if in contact with blood or body secretions. • Follow respiratory hygiene/cough etiquette principles. • Ensure appropriate patient placement according to isolation needs. • Properly handle and clean and disinfect patient care equipment and instruments/devices. • Clean and disinfect the environment appropriately. • Handle textiles and laundry carefully. • Follow safe infection practices. Wear a surgical mask when performing lumbar punctures. • Ensure healthcare worker safety including proper handling of needles and other sharps.
Contact	• Use contact precautions for patients with known or suspected infections that represent an increased risk for contact transmission. • Standard precautions PLUS: • Put on gloves before room entry. Discard gloves before room exit. • Put on gown before room entry. Discard gown before room exit. • Do not wear the same gown and gloves for the care of more than one person. • Use dedicated or disposable equipment. Clean and disinfect reusable equipment before use on another person.
Droplet	• Use droplet precautions for patients known or suspected to be infected with pathogens transmitted by respiratory droplets that are generated by a patient who is coughing, sneezing, or talking. • Standard precautions PLUS: • Use an appropriate mask to cover nose and mouth. • Use eye protection. • Remove face protection after leaving the room.
Airborne	• Use airborne precautions for patients known or suspected to be infected with pathogens transmitted by the airborne route (e.g., tuberculosis, measles, chickenpox, disseminated herpes zoster). • Standard precautions PLUS: • Put on a fit-tested N-95 or higher level respirator before room entry. • Remove respirator after exiting the room and closing the door. • Door to room must remain closed.

5 Moments for Hand Hygiene:

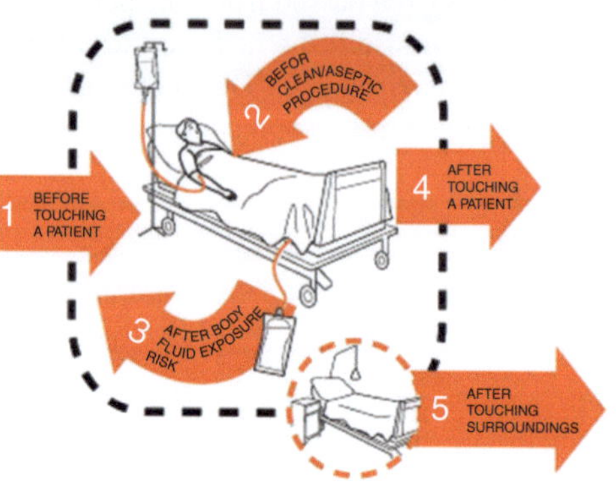

More Information:

- 5 Moments for Hand Hygiene: https://www.who.int/gpsc/5may/background/5moments/en/.
- Tools on infection prevention and control: https://www.who.int/infection-prevention/tools/en/.
- Infection control CDC: https://www.cdc.gov/infectioncontrol/basics/transmission-based-precautions.html.

References

1. UNHCR. Refugee health EC/1995/SC.2/CRP.29. 1995. Available from: https://www.unhcr.org/excom/scaf/3ae68bf424/refugee-health.html.
2. Médecins Sans Frontières. Management of a measles epidemic. 2013. Available from: https://medicalguidelines.msf.org/viewport/mme/english/management-of-a-measles-epidemic-30542833.html.
3. World Health Organization. More than 140,000 die from measles as cases surge worldwide. 5 Dec 2019. Available from: https://www.who.int/news/item/05-12-2019-more-than-140-000-die-from-measles-as-cases-surge-worldwide.
4. CDC Center for Disease Control and Prevention. Measles (Rubeola) for healthcare providers. CDC Center for Disease Control and Prevention. Available from: https://www.cdc.gov/measles/hcp/index.html.
5. American Academy of Pediatrics. Red Book 2018: report of the committee on infectious diseases. Elk Grove Village: American Academy of Pediatrics; 2018.
6. Gans H, Maldonado Y. Measles: clinical manifestations, diagnosis, treatment, and prevention. Up to Date. 2019. Available from: https://www-uptodate-com.pbidi.unam.mx:2443/contents/measles-clinical-manifestations-diagnosis-treatment-and-prevention?search=sarampion&source=search_result&selectedTitle=1~150&usage_type=default&display_rank=1.
7. Cherry J. Measles in textbook of pediatric infectious diseases. Philadelphia, PA: Elsevier; 2017.

8. UNHCR. Epidemic preparedness and response in refugee camp settings guidance for public health officers. Geneva: UNHCR; 2011. Available from: https://www.unhcr.org/protection/health/4f707f509/epidemic-preparednes-response-refugee-camp-settings-guidance-public-health.html.

9. World Health Organization. WHO pocket book of hospital care for children: guidelines for the management of common childhood illnesses. 2nd ed. 2013. Available from: https://www.who.int/maternal_child_adolescent/documents/child_hospital_care/en/.

10. World Health Organization. Measles fact sheet. 2019. Available from: https://www.who.int/news-room/fact-sheets/detail/measles#:~:text=During%202000%E2%80%93%202018%2C%20measles%20vaccination,2000*%20to%20142%2C000%20in%202018.

11. World Health Organization. Guide for clinical case management and infection prevention and control during a measles outbreak. Geneva: World Health Organization; 2020. Available from: https://apps.who.int/iris/handle/10665/331599.

12. Cherry JD, Harrison GJ, Hotez PJ, Kaplan SL, Steinbach WJ. In: Cherry JD, Harrison GJ, Kaplan SL, Steinbach WJ, Hotez PJ, editors. Feigin and Cherry's textbook of pediatric infectious diseases, vol. 1. Philadelphia, PA: Elsevier; 2019.

13. UNICEF, World Health Organization. Diarrhoea: why children are still dying and what can be done. New York: UNICEF, World Health Organization; 2009.

14. World Health Organization. Rotavirus, immunization, vaccines and biologicals. Available from: https://www.who.int/immunization/diseases/rotavirus/en/.

15. World Health Organization. Guidelines for the control of shigellosis, including epidemics due to Shigella dysenteriae type 1. Geneva: World Health Organization; 2005. Available from: https://apps.who.int/iris/bitstream/handle/10665/43252/924159330X.pdf?sequence=1.

16. Médecins Sans Frontières. Refugee health, an approach to emergency situations. London: MacMillan; 1997. Available from: https://www.humanitarianlibrary.org/sites/default/files/2014/07/rh.pdf.

17. Médecins Sans Frontières. Management of a cholera epidemic. 2018th ed. Available from: https://medicalguidelines.msf.org/viewport/CHOL/english/management-of-a-cholera-epidemic-23444438.html.

18. World Health Organization. Health topics, cholera. Available from: https://www.who.int/immunization/diseases/rotavirus/en/.

19. Organisation mondiale de la santé. Managing epidemics: key facts about major deadly diseases. 2018. Available from: https://apps.who.int/iris/handle/10665/272442.

20. World Health Organization. Cholera vaccines. Available from: https://www.who.int/cholera/vaccines/en/.

21. World Health Organization. World malaria report 2020: 20 years of global progress and challenges. Geneva: World Health Organization; 2020. Available from: file:///Users/usuario/Downloads/9789240015791-eng.pdf.

22. Médecins Sans Frontières. Pediatric guidelines. Geneva: Médecins Sans Frontières; 2017.

23. World Health Organization. WHO policy recommendation on intermittent preventive treatment during infancy with sulphadoxine-pyrimethamine (IPTi-SP) for Plasmodium falciparum malaria control in Africa. 2010. Available from: WHO policy recommendation on intermittent preventive treatment during infancy with sulphadoxine-pyrimethamine (IPTi-SP) for Plasmodium falciparum malaria control in Africa.

24. WHO Global Malaria Programme (GMP), Department of Immunization, Vaccines & Biologicals (IVB) and UNICEF. Intermittent preventive treatment for infants using sulfadoxinepyrimethamine (SP-IPTi) for malaria control in Africa: implementation field guide. 2011. Available from: WHO Global Malaria Programme (GMP), Department of Immunization, Vaccines & Biologicals (IVB) and UNICEF.

25. Médecins Sans Frontières (Association), South Africa. MSF HIV/TB clinical guide for primary care 2018. 2018.

Teresa Gadsden completed a Pediatric and Infectious diseases fellowship in Mexico's Children Hospital "Federico Gómez" 2009–2012 and 2015–2017, Mexico City, as well as training in tropical medicine in Hospital Cayetano Heredia 2016, Lima, Peru as part of the Infectious diseases fellowship. She completed a bacteriology course at National Polytecnic University 2016, Mexico City and is certified by the International Society of Travel Medicine, Washington, DC, 2019. She worked for Doctors Without Borders since 2012 in Niger, Democratic Republic of Congo, Haiti, Lebanon, and Guinea Bissau. In Lebanon, she designed and conducted an assessment of living conditions, health habits, and healthcare-seeking behavior of Syrian refugees in the Bekaa valley. She serves as a volunteer advisor, pediatrician, and infectious diseases specialist for MSF telemedicine since 2016. She is currently working as a clinical case coordinator in MSF telemedicine and as pediatrician, infectious disease specialist, and travel medicine doctor in a private clinic and Hospital Español in Mexico City.

Care and Interventions for Displaced Adolescents

Naomi N. Duke and Marlene Goodfriend

Care of Adolescents Prior to Resettlement

Adolescence is defined as the period between 10–19 years of age, a time of rapid developmental changes including physical, cognitive, psychological, and social [1]. The adolescent is not a child and not an adult. The adolescent is defining himself/herself as an individual in the world separate from family. To do this the adolescent requires support and direction from families and the sociocultural environment. In times of displacement from one's home and familiar surroundings, there is disruption of the usual support and care from family, social, educational, and religious institutions and the medical system. Physical separation from family, such as the case with unaccompanied minors and adolescents placed in detention and holding facilities, causes increasing stress and despair and risk to ongoing development.

During the immediate phase, usually first 4 weeks, of a displacement, interventions are aimed at providing basic needs (food, water, shelter, clothing, medical care) and keeping families together. Unaccompanied minors require connection with protection agencies responsible for providing care of this vulnerable group, i.e., ICRC and UNICEF. It is important to know what agencies are present in the specific context and what they can provide. Other interventions in the immediate period include normalizing responses to the displacement and recommending calming interventions such as deep breathing and progressive muscle relaxation. Connection to others and ability to calm oneself can be protective against the later development of post-traumatic stress disorder [2]. These interventions are further explained in the manual *Psychological first aid: Guide for field workers* [3]. Every field worker in an emergency situation should become familiar with this guideline

N. N. Duke (✉)
Duke University School of Medicine, Durham, NC, USA
e-mail: naomi.duke@duke.edu

M. Goodfriend
Medecins Sans Frontieres, Jacksonville, FL, USA

© Springer Nature Switzerland AG 2021
C. Harkensee et al. (eds.), *Child Refugee and Migrant Health*,
https://doi.org/10.1007/978-3-030-74906-4_26

(see Chap. 8 of this manual). With all beneficiaries, it is important to ask what they need, and what will help them. Adolescents will tell you! Often adolescents have ideas on what would be distracting and calming for themselves in the early stages of a displacement. Particularly with adolescents, it is important to advise against over-exposure to media that replays the conflict they recently fled or other atrocities. See Fig. 26.1.

In the intermediate-later period, post displacement interventions should be specifically tailored to the adolescent age group. The absence of familiar and necessary supports can have severe consequences for the developmental progress of the adolescent. Many refugee settings include a large number of adolescents, often unaccompanied minors. Their special needs require attention through intervention programs targeting health, social, psychological, and educational needs. During times of displacement, the adolescent is vulnerable to influences that can have a negative impact on development. All adolescents, particularly unaccompanied adolescents, are at risk for trafficking. Adolescents are exploited in refugee camps in different ways, including sexual abuse, uncompensated work, and enticement to illegal activities. They are introduced to alcohol and drugs. Due to having little to do, substance use is a tempting activity along with indiscriminate sexual behaviors and delinquent behaviors such as theft. Psychoeducation programs for adolescents need to include information on these risks, and how to avoid them and promote positive coping skills such as talking together, singing, dancing, drawing, and writing.

In refugee camps, vulnerable groups are frequently defined as women, children, the elderly, and disabled. Adolescents are not included in this list. A first step in intervening with displaced adolescents is to recognize the specific needs of this age group. Their health needs especially sexual reproductive health concerns require special attention. If possible, the medical clinic should include an adolescent-friendly space. Adolescents do not want to sit in a clinic with crying babies, and young children. Females are usually more comfortable with female providers, and in some cultures a medical examination by a member of the opposite sex is not permissible. Another challenge is developing activities suitable for females and males. Frequently the boys are organized into sports activities (Photo 26.1) and there is nothing available for the girls.

Example In a camp for Eritrean refugees, boys participated in football. A football tournament was organized with prizes. The girls protested and asked for sports activities for themselves. They also asked for other activities, and the NGO initiated

Fig. 26.1 Immediate phase interventions

- Basic needs
- Keeping families together
- Protection of unaccompanied minors
- Calming interventions
- Avoid media exposure

Photo 26.1 Boys playing football in a refugee camp

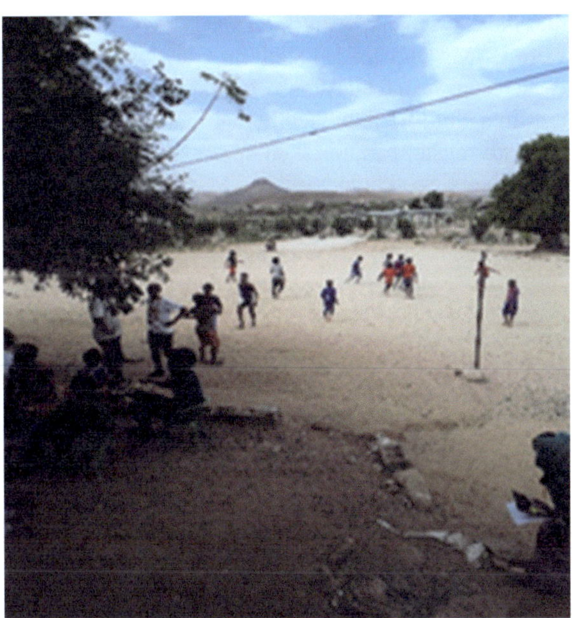

discussion groups for teenage girls that concluded with a coffee ceremony, a popular cultural activity.

There can be a lack of space in refugee camps, including crowded living quarters, and absence of areas for socialization and hanging out. There are often child-friendly spaces where young children can play and safe spaces for breastfeeding mothers, but nothing for adolescents.

Example A community center in a refugee camp in Shire, Ethiopia had a room where teenagers could be together, play music, and dance. It was a space of their own and the adolescents enjoyed being there. One author visited this setting and the teenagers performed a dance typical of their culture. They obviously were happy doing this and appreciated the compliments on their wonderful dancing.

Whereas recognition of adolescents as a specific and vulnerable group is the first step in developing interventions, the second step is to sit down with groups of adolescents and ask them, what do you need? Listen to them.

Example During focus group discussions with adolescents in a refugee camp, an NGO learned that they wanted recreation such as movies and a place to dance and listen to music. One said, "Music is as important as food." They complained that the teachers in camp schools were impatient and did not answer questions about the assignments. Some stopped attending school because of this. In a meeting with adolescents that were members of the camp's Child Parliament, the NGO learned that there was inadequate food for UAMs (unaccompanied minors) and that there were UAMs who needed clothing.

In response to focus group discussions with adolescents, the NGO developed activities in a child-friendly facility that included space for adolescents to watch movies, listen to music, participate in sports and crafts, and learn to play cultural musical instruments. See Photo 26.2. The NGO advocated with agencies overseeing the camp about inadequate food and clothing for the UAMs and problems in the schools.

Health concerns including sexual and reproductive health, and mental health problems become apparent during the middle-later phases of a displacement. Health facilities require staff capability in addressing birth control, protected sex, sexually transmitted diseases, and unwanted pregnancies as well as other medical problems. Health education for girls should include information about the physical changes of puberty and what to expect with menstruation. This is an opportunity to dispel myths, such as menstruation being a curse or a sign of impurity. Adolescents, and in fact all women, require information on how to procure feminine hygiene products, which can be difficult to find in a camp setting. Adolescents of both sexes should be asked about feeling safe using latrines during nighttime visits. Especially if areas are poorly lit, male and female adolescents are vulnerable to sexual violence. Poorly lit latrines and occurrences of sexual violence are issues to address through advocacy.

Moderate-severe mental health problems become more apparent in the middle-later phases of a displacement. Experiencing a humanitarian disaster and consequent displacement can result in symptoms of post-traumatic stress disorder,

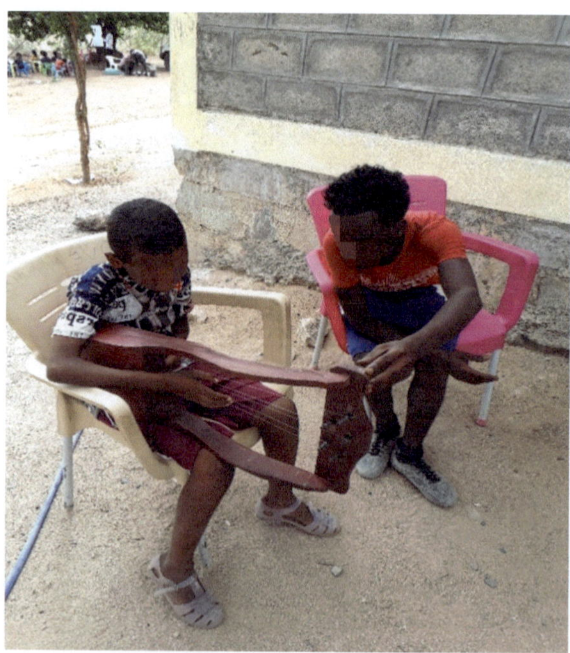

Photo 26.2 Adolescents practicing music on cultural instruments

moderate-severe depression and anxiety, and substance use. Chronic disorders such as schizophrenia and bipolar disorder can become apparent during late adolescence. Adolescents can present with an array of symptoms including sad mood, withdrawal, symptoms of psychosis, somatic complaints, flashbacks, and poor functioning. Adolescent suicide attempts frequently occur and one attempt can set off a copycat epidemic. Psychoeducation for adolescents should include awareness of signs and symptoms of mental distress. Adolescents require information that there is help available for emotional distress and how to access this. It is necessary for doing fieldwork to know which organizations offer mental health care including assessment, counseling, and treatment with psychiatric medication. Before establishing linkage with an organization for mental health care, it is important to visit the potential referral source and assess the physical facility, availability of providers trained in interventions for adolescents, and overall quality of care. See Fig. 26.2 for interventions for adolescents during the middle-later phases of displacement.

Adolescents who are separated from families and placed in detention centers or government holding facilities experience continual disruption in their lives. Challenges include ongoing crowded living conditions, inadequate food, water, and sanitation, inattention to medical problems, and absence of opportunity for education and social activities. This is coupled with the emotional distress of being physically apart from family. The separation from family is frequently unexpected and done abruptly without explanation. This has severe repercussions for mental health and development, especially for the preteen adolescent.

Whereas a single organization cannot be responsible for all interventions, workers need to be aware of special needs and vulnerabilities of adolescents in refugee camps and detention centers. In order to intervene effectively with this group, the first steps involve assessing the provision of basic needs and asking and listening to how the adolescent is feeling and what he/she needs. If one organization cannot deliver needed services, know what other organizations are present and what they provide. Advocacy is an important and necessary component of insuring care for adolescents (and all vulnerable populations) in refugee camps and detention centers.

Fig. 26.2 Middle-later phase interventions

- Ask and listen
- Ongoing provision of basic needs
- Adolescent focused medical care
- Schooling and vocational training
- Psychoeducation about risks and support of positive coping skills
- Culturally appropriate psychosocial activities
- Mental health care
- Advocacy

Care of Adolescents Throughout Resettlement

Upon arrival or release from confinement (if applicable) in the host country, providers must strive to understand the range of experiences youths have encountered and will encounter, all of which impact an adolescent's health and well-being going forward. As referenced earlier, displaced adolescents are vulnerable to trafficking and other serious crimes. Some adolescents are traumatized and stigmatized on multiple levels, including carrying a brand of refugee or asylum-seeking status in a new country, experiencing poor mental health as a result of adversities encountered in home communities and on the journey to a new country, and for some youth, being unaccompanied. The ability to support displaced adolescents to settle and thrive in a host country depends not only on where they have been but also on the conditions to which they have arrived. Being in a host country may give rise to a number of new challenges for adolescents in this new phase of life, including encountering barriers to accessing social services and health benefits, facing food insecurity and housing instability, and living in fear of deportation or separation from trusted adults without notice or preparation. The remainder of this chapter discusses the importance of understanding where youth have been, using a framework for interviewing and assessing adolescents during the resettlement process, as a means to help them move forward and to envision a hopeful future.

Adolescent Development Through the Lens of Migration and Displacement

In Western cultures, the developmental phases of adolescence are generally organized according to chronologic age with characteristic features: early (10–13 years of age, rapid physical change, and limited decision-making capacity); middle (14–17 years of age, rise in importance of peer networks which may present the stage for increased risk-taking); and late (18-mid 20s, improved abstract thinking, and maturation of decision-making capacity) phases [4]. During all phases of adolescence, the importance of emotional health comes to the forefront, as this period may be further complicated by rises in experiences of depression and anxiety.

While there is wide variation in how adolescence is defined across cultures, periods marked by changes in brain development, physiology (puberty), and emotional maturity are common for all adolescents. As such, displaced adolescents may experience similar challenges and opportunities along the continuum of development. For example, there may be commonalities in friction points between youth and their parents/adult guardians, including disagreement about curfews and decisions about dress or other adornments, desires of family/host members for youth to spend more time at home, concerns by adults about the influence of peers and a desire to know the value systems of peer groups, negotiation in prioritizing family values and goals, respect of elders and keeping cultural traditions, and desires of the adolescent to have more freedom. Frequently, the resettled adolescent adapts to a new culture and language faster than their parents do. This can lead to conflict and even estrangement between the adolescent and their family.

Experiences of migration and displacement also create unique contextual demands that may hinder or reshape normative development [5]. Thus, it is critical that providers be able to recognize the bounds of normative development unique to each adolescent in order to support youth well-being. For example, experiences of abuse, exploitation, and trauma may present severe threats to identity development and self-esteem. As such, providers are advised to organize care using a trauma-informed lens (see National Child Traumatic Stress Network, Refugee Services Toolkit [6]).

Inclusion of a trauma-informed lens when working with adolescents post-migration requires the provider to address a number of contextual factors, past and present. The provider must be able to assess traumas related to the adolescent's country of origin (e.g., witness or experience of violence, persecution, violation of human rights), the migration journey (e.g., violation of human rights, exploitation, loss), arrival in a new country (e.g., racism, discrimination, loss), and while remaining in the host country (e.g., racism, discrimination, loss, stresses of acculturation, finding a sense of identity). There may also be a multigenerational component to trauma, which will necessitate assessment of family members whenever possible. A trauma-informed lens also requires identifying youths' contexts for resilience, including connections to trusted adults, a sense of community (school and neighborhood), and cultivating a positive future orientation.

Health Screening and Anticipatory Guidance

Effective engagement of adolescents necessitates creating nonjudgmental and safe environments in which youth can discuss experiences, hopes, and fears, access accurate information, and clarify their feelings and choices. In many Western cultures, it is general practice to perform behavioral screens and to discuss sensitive topics with the adolescent alone. However, in all interactions, it is important that the adolescent be given the choice to have a parent/trusted caregiver present. When working with adolescent minors alone, health providers and youth advocates must be familiar with laws and regulations related to youth consent and confidentiality (see WHO "Making Health Services Adolescent Friendly" [7]). While adolescent one-on-one conversations are built upon a standard of privacy, there are exceptions to this premise, including in contexts of self-harm, current abuse and neglect of the youth, and adolescent risk of harm to another. As previously noted, providers must be aware of adolescent preference and cultural requisites related to seeing male and female providers. It is also critical that providers use the language preference of the adolescent and family. Depending on the timing of the clinical encounter in the resettlement process, youth may have some mastery of the primary language of the host country, while the primary caregiver remains more comfortable with the language of their home country. In situations in which the adolescent and parent/other adult caregiver are seen together (at least initially) and their language preferences differ, having an appropriate medical interpreter to facilitate communication with the caregiver is necessary. Youth should not be used as translators for their parents/other adult caregivers. Visit summaries and any other care-related documents must be available in the primary language of the adolescent and parents/adult caregivers.

A number of mnemonics and questioning frameworks exist for screening and providing anticipatory guidance for adolescents. A common mnemonic used by adolescent health providers is *HEEADSSS*, which stands for Home, Education, Eating, Activities, Drugs, Safety, Sexuality, and Symptoms of Depression/Suicidality. An alternate mnemonic includes rearrangement of the letters and an additional **S** at the beginning of the screen to remind providers to start discussions by focusing on an adolescent's strengths before spending time on contexts of risk ("What are you most proud of about yourself? What do you love about yourself? What would your family say your best qualities are? How about your friends?"; see SSHADESS psychosocial screen [8]). See Table 26.1 for examples of themes using the *HEEADSSS* mnemonic. The themes presented in Table 26.1 are meant to guide

Table 26.1 Example HEEADSSS themes

H: Consider household members and family dynamics that may include ongoing fears related to forced separations and the threat of parental detainment and deportation, as well as current levels of housing stability.
E: Identify previous learning opportunities, as well as experiences with compulsory education requirements in the host country. Identify previous experiences and current expectations related to work.
E: Evaluate the adequacy and consistency of meals. Determine whether the adolescent has been able to locate familiar foods that satisfy cultural needs and preferences. Ask about concerns related to weight or body changes, in the past, during the journey, and since resettlement.
A: Assess the level of engagement of the adolescent in home, school, and community contexts. Inquire about where time is spent and ask about peer groups. Discussion about cultural traditions and/or adolescent rites of passage may advance insight into the adolescent's previous level of function prior to the migration experience and current level of function in their immediate context. Identify sources of joy and activities that give a sense of meaning and purpose.
D: Screen for past substance use and exposures, and the potential for current perceived pressures as a means to find peer groups or to self-medicate due to stressors.
S: Recognize that arrival in the host country does not always relieve past threats, and location in the new space may bring new threat experiences. Ask the adolescent about current places where they feel safe and places where they do not feel safe. Ask about previous and current experiences of victimization, including being bullied and excluded because of differences. Inquire about fears related to policing and the justice system of the host country.
S: Normalize adolescence as a time when individuals begin having feelings of attraction towards others or have desires for a personal, romantic relationship. Open the door to discussion about gender identity and related experiences in the adolescent's country of origin or countries of exposure during the migration journey, and in the new country. Screen for safety in relationships. Ask about physical contact, including sexual activity, and knowledge of/access to contraception and barrier protection.
S: Assess for past and present struggles with feelings of sadness and self-harm behaviors. Identify sources of strength that buffer against sadness and keep the young person centered.

questions and are not meant to be exhaustive. More than one encounter is necessary to gain an understanding of the many facets of the young person's story. The themes enable an open-ended question format to support dialogue and the development of a trusting relationship over time. Additional screeners may facilitate a deeper understanding of experiences and their emotional impact (see Table 26.2). In some cultures, it is more acceptable to approach behavioral and emotional health using language of stress and signs of distress, than using language focused on diagnosis. For example, engaging in discussion of physical health manifestations (e.g., chronic headaches, fatigue), sleep problems, social withdrawal, or acting out as representing stress or burden on the body's ability to achieve balance or a sense of wholeness, may be better received than focusing on a diagnostic label. In this context, it is sometimes helpful to pose questions that reference past successes with navigating difficult times, such as "During difficult times, what did you think about or tell yourself to get through? Are there memories that you try to hold onto? What are ways that have helped you keep yourself safe and feel whole?" Coping skills may be positive (e.g., talking to a friend; listening to music; exercise) or negative (e.g., drinking alcohol or use of other drugs). Both should be acknowledged and further discussed.

Physical health screening includes assessment of nutritional status, physical development and signs of trauma, assessment of immunization status, and consideration of laboratory assessment—a tiered approach based on country of origin/exposure, time in refugee camps or detention centers, and requirements of the host country (see Table 26.3). Common dietary deficiencies, including vitamin D, calcium, and iron, may be exacerbated by dietary inadequacies related to the displacement experience.

There are a number of topics to discuss related to anticipatory guidance for adolescents (see Table 26.4). For displaced adolescents (and in some sense for all adolescents), the discussion must be guided by cultural humility and helping the adolescent to know and embrace their value. For adolescents, opportunities for thoughtful and creative expression may provide additional support for coping and thriving, including physical activity, school-based art therapy and play, culturally sensitive cognitive behavioral therapies, biofeedback and mindfulness training, and community-based cultural events.

In sum, clinical providers and child health advocates can support optimal health and development for displaced adolescents (and their caregivers) in a multitude of settings without prescribed borders. Providers may promote recovery and resilience by taking the time to listen to adolescents, helping them to develop and nurture their voices, applying a trauma-informed lens in the care setting, and offering a safe and respectful environment for care. Providers should use culturally sensitive assessments, provide continuity of care, develop trusting and collaborative relationships, and strive to help young people to find the tools necessary to build a life in their new home.

Table 26.2 Psychosocial screeners tested among refugee populations

Name of screener	Website link	Notes
Adverse Childhood Experiences—International Questionnaire (ACE-IQ)	Available through World Health Organization (WHO): https://www.who.int/violence_injury_prevention/violence/activities/adverse_childhood_experiences/en/	Intended to measure types of adversities in all countries and the link between adversity and risk behaviors later in life. Appropriate for ages 18 years and above.
Patient Health Questionnaire-9 Modified for Adolescents (PHQ-A)	Available through the Reach Institute, Guidelines for Adolescent Depression in Primary Care (GLAD-PC): https://www.thereachinstitute.org/images/pdfs/glad-pc-toolkit-2018.pdf The GLAD-PC toolkit contains other psychosocial screens, communication aids, and intervention recommendations for the care of adolescents in the primary care setting.	Depression screen. Appropriate for ages 12 years and above. Multiple language translations.
Pediatric Symptom Checklist (PSC-17, PSC-35)	Available through American Academy of Pediatrics (AAP) Bright Futures: https://brightfutures.aap.org/materials-and-tools/tool-and-resource-kit/Pages/Developmental-Behavioral-Psychosocial-Screening-and-Assessment-Forms.aspx	Psychosocial screen. Appropriate for ages 11 years and above. Parent-completed and youth self-report versions. Multiple language translations.
Refugee Health Screener (RHS-15)	Created by pathways to wellness. Introduction and strategies for operationalizing available through Refugee Health Technical Assistance Center: https://refugeehealthta.org/webinars/mental-health-screening-and-care/ English version for informational purposes only: http://refugeehealthta.org/wp-content/uploads/2012/09/RHS15_Packet_PathwaysToWellness-1.pdf	Mental health screen, highly sensitive and specific for anxiety, depression, post-traumatic stress disorder. Appropriate for ages 14 years and above. Multiple language translations with community participation.

Table 26.3 Physical exam, immunizations, and laboratory assessment

Physical examination	Notes
Height, weight, body mass index	May give insight into the nutritional status and metabolic risk.
Blood pressure, heart rate	Stress and trauma may manifest as elevations in blood pressure and resting heart rate.
Vision and hearing screens	May reflect trauma, or absence of preventive care.
Dental screening	May give insight into nutritional status, toxic exposures, and absence of preventive care.
Skin	Scarification, tattooing, cultural adornment may signify cultural transitions.
Cardiovascular	Rheumatic heart disease remains the most common cause of acquired heart disease in the developing world.
Musculoskeletal	May reflect congenital deficiencies, trauma-related injuries, evidence of nutrient deficiencies, and structural changes most evident during growth (scoliosis).
Breast and genitourinary	Provides pubertal assessment and screening for female genital cutting, or evidence of abuse.
Psych/behavioral	Stress and trauma may manifest as flat or anxious affect or limited engagement.
Vaccine preventable illness	
Routine adolescent immunizations	Tdap, MCV4, HPV9 https://www.cdc.gov/vaccines/schedules/hcp/imz/child-adolescent.html
Additional considerations	MMR, HBV, varicella, HAV, IPV https://www.cdc.gov/vaccines/schedules/hcp/imz/child-adolescent.html
Guidance on laboratory assessment	
AAP Immigrant Health Toolkit	https://www.aap.org/en-us/Documents/cocp_toolkit_full.pdf
US Centers for Disease Control and Prevention Refugee Health Guidelines	https://www.cdc.gov/immigrantrefugeehealth/guidelines/refugee-guidelines.html
WHO Refugee and Migrant Health	https://www.who.int/health-topics/refugee-and-migrant-health#tab=tab_1

Advocacy Before and After Resettlement

Advocacy is an important activity at any stage of care for displaced adolescents. Advocacy can be focused on mobilizing agencies for services as well as raising awareness with in national organizations, such as the AAP and government bodies, of conditions, especially in refugee settings and detention centers. Further, providers and child health workers in host countries are in a unique position to advocate for these youth by partnering with community groups that serve refugee populations, acting as a resource for legislators, local and national news outlets about discriminatory and traumatic practices, and using professional platforms (e.g., AAP, SAHM, NCTSN) to advocate for best practices in the care of displaced adolescents and their families.

Table 26.4 Framework for adolescent anticipatory guidance

Anticipatory guidance topics
• Understanding normal physical growth and development, puberty and related body changes
• Maintaining a sense of self and developing strategies to find one's voice
• Preparation and expectation for healthy adulthood; future orientation and goal planning
• Intersections between cultural expectations, gendered roles, norms and values of home and host communities-countries, including marriage (partnering) and fertility planning, school engagement, and career development
• Upcoming developmental milestones, anticipated transitions related to the host country and associated safety, including school attendance and graduation, driving, and voting
• Identifying healthy peer and romantic relationships
• Importance of having at least one trusted adult in whom can talk to about anything
• Reproductive safety and access to a range of services, and the interface with cultural beliefs, attitudes, and expectations; provision of accurate information about reproductive health issues, including contraception and barrier protection
• Identifying community assets and opportunities to engage with cultural traditions
• Review of safety contacts, in case of migration-related threats
Approach to provision of anticipatory guidance
In general
• Cultural humility: Be flexible and humble enough to recognize position as that of the learner when engaging youth and families about cultural beliefs and migration experiences
• Support by screening for basic needs
• Work with community partners to support access to benefits and services
• Provide reassurances of not being involved with immigration, customs enforcement
For adolescents
• Operate from a lens affirming the value of the young person
• Use a strengths-based approach: seek to understand ethnic and racial identity as assets that may foster resilience
• Take time to engage and to develop trust
• Do more listening
• Take time to understand cultural considerations and the desire of the adolescent to maintain and/or transition from cultural practices that may be different from those of the host country; this necessitates careful navigation with caregivers and cultural elders to facilitate support of a youth's independence and the development of a diverse identity

References

1. World Health Organization (WHO). Adolescent health. https://www.who.int/maternal_child_adolescent/adolescence/universal-health-coverage/en/.
2. Hobfoll SE, et al. Five essential elements of immediate and mid-term mass trauma intervention: empirical evidence. Psychiatry. 2007;70(4):283–315. https://www.researchgate.net/publication/5668133_Five_Essential_Elements_of_Immediate_and_Mid-Term_Mass_Trauma_Intervention_Empirical_Evidence.
3. Psychological first aid: guide for field workers. WHO. 2011. https://www.who.int/mental_health/publications/guide_field_workers/en/.
4. Society for Adolescent Health and Medicine. https://www.adolescenthealth.org/Home.aspx.

5. Ko LK, Perreira KM. It turned my world upside down: Latino youths' perspectives on immigration. J Adolesc Res. 2010;25(3):465–93. https://www.ncbi.nlm.nih.gov/pmc/articles/PMC3169195/pdf/nihms307191.pdf.
6. National Child Traumatic Stress Network. Refugee Services Toolkit. https://www.nctsn.org/resources/refugee-services-core-stressor-assessment-tool.
7. World Health Organization (WHO). Making health services adolescent friendly. https://www.who.int/maternal_child_adolescent/documents/adolescent_friendly_services/en/.
8. Ginsburg K, American Academy of Pediatrics (AAP). SSHADESS psychosocial screen. https://www.aap.org/en-us/professional-resources/Reaching-Teens/Documents/Private/SSHADESS_handout.pdf.

Naomi Duke, MD, PhD is an Associate Professor, board certified in Internal Medicine, Pediatrics, and Adolescent Medicine. During her two decades of experience in clinical practice in academic and community settings, she has witnessed the persistence of health inequities across generations via intersectionality of race and ethnic identity, gender, class, and immigration status. Her research focuses on advancing knowledge and advocacy efforts around the relevance of childhood adversity and social context for later disparities in health outcomes, including morbidity and mortality related to stress physiology, perceptions of physical and emotional wellbeing, and health-related behaviors. Her background in medicine, sociology, and public health uniquely positions her to inform health services delivery and research programming addressing interactions between socio-cultural context and adolescent and young adult health.

Marlene Goodfriend, MD is trained as a pediatrician and as a psychiatrist. She has worked with vulnerable populations both in the United States and in the resource poor world for more than 40 years. Recently she completed 9 years of work as a mental health advisor with the humanitarian organization Médecins Sans Frontières. Throughout her career, she has participated in the care of refugee children and their families in the United States, the Middle East, Southeast Asia, and sub-Saharan Africa including in conflict/post-conflict settings and refugee camps. She has developed psychosocial programs, trained colleagues, and delivered patient care. What has touched her deeply is the resilience of the children and families who experience the most dire circumstances and their openness and receptivity to our help.

Reproductive Health

Martha C. Carlough

General Overview

According to the World Health Organization, Reproductive Health is *"a state of complete physical, mental and social well-being and not merely the absence of disease or infirmity, in all matters relating to the reproductive system and to its functions and processes"* [1]. This implies that all people, including refugee and migrant children and adolescents, should have the freedom to decide if, when, and how often to reproduce and to be able to do so safely [1]. Reproductive health includes planning for safe, healthy, and desired pregnancy and birth as well as the prevention of pregnancy through contraception, prevention, and treatment of sexually transmitted infections (including HIV/AIDS) and prevention of gender-based and sexual violence.

In migrant and refugee contexts, children and adolescents are among the most at risk of challenges to their reproductive health and safety and yet these needs often go unmet. The breakdown of family units and unsafe physical situations during migration as well as in camps, urban resettlement areas, and conflict zones increase the potential for sexual violence. This is often against a backdrop of preexisting gender inequities and rapidly changing social norms for younger people [2]. As a sense of loss or hopelessness increases in adolescents, risk-taking sexual behaviors may also increase for both boys and girls. Adolescent boys may face particular pressures including recruitment into armed conflict, human trafficking, and involvement in sexual violence. Unaccompanied boys may be forced into transactional sex, increasing risks of sexually transmitted infections. Girls have the same risks and the

M. C. Carlough (✉)
Department of Family Medicine, University of North Carolina—Chapel Hill, Chapel Hill, NC, USA

Office of Global Health Education, University of North Carolina—Chapel Hill, Chapel Hill, NC, USA
e-mail: Martha_carlough@med.unc.edu

© Springer Nature Switzerland AG 2021
C. Harkensee et al. (eds.), *Child Refugee and Migrant Health*,
https://doi.org/10.1007/978-3-030-74906-4_27

additional risk of unplanned pregnancies and unsafe abortion. Girls are also challenged to manage menstrual hygiene with a lack of privacy, sanitation, and disposal areas.

Many adolescent girls come from societies where it is common—and often encouraged—to marry and bear children at younger ages, and they may actively desire to have children; to form a family of their own after loss. There may in fact be societal pressures to reproduce in post-conflict situations to replenish populations.

Female genital cutting (FGC), defined by the World Health Organization as *"all procedures that involve partial or total removal of the external female genitalia, or other injury to the female genital organs for non-medical reasons,"* is still practiced to some extent in more than 30 countries though the prevalence is highest in a much smaller number of countries, including Djibouti, Somalia, Mali, Guinea, Egypt, Sierra Leone, and Sudan [3]. The majority of girls undergo FGC before 15 years of age. The extent of cutting may vary from ceremonial nicking or tattooing of skin to infibulation or the complete removal of the labia minora and majora and severe narrowing of the vaginal orifice. There are both short-term and long-term physical and mental health consequences of FGC including hemorrhage, infection, infertility, obstructed labor during delivery, fistula formation, PTSD, and depression. Although there is a growing human rights movement towards abolishing FGC, and it is illegal to perform FGC in many countries including the USA where it also is a reportable child abuse, up to 3 million girls worldwide still undergo FGC each year. Clinicians and mental health professionals need to be prepared to care for girls who are at risk of or who have undergone FGC at all stages of resettlement and to provide protection and support, good medical care, and avoid further traumatization by being unfamiliar with or unaware of the consequences of FGC [4]. Further details on classification of FGC and care for girls and women who have undergone FGC can be found in *WHO Guidelines on the management of health complications from female genital mutilation* listed in *Additional Resources*.

A significant proportion of deaths among women of reproductive age in camps are due to complications of pregnancy and childbirth. Adolescent girls are at higher risk of these complications and may be even less likely to seek help. Reasons for delayed care include lack of familiarity with health care services, denial about pregnancy, and fear of others' responses to their pregnancy (including perpetrators of sexual violence). Morbidities including malnutrition and micronutrient deficiencies, preterm birth, perinatal mortality, and intrauterine growth retardation are all more common in refugee situations [5, 6]. Often countries with conflict or instability have high maternal mortality and limited reproductive health services at baseline, and these services may be further disrupted in humanitarian emergencies. It is essential that appropriate, accessible resources to meet these needs are provided.

Attention to reproductive health care, including safe maternity care, was not historically considered part of core initial services in humanitarian emergency response. This has changed in recent years. The Sphere Handbook for Minimum Standards of in Humanitarian Response now includes reproductive health care as an essential service and many collaborative projects are focused on these areas (see *Additional*

Resources) [7]. There is a clear need to provide health information for independent decision-making and adolescent-friendly reproductive health services, including maternity care. In addition, organizations must be diligent in both preventing situations that exacerbate gender-based violence and in caring for children and adolescents who have been victimized. It is also critical that services are offered in a respectful, positive manner with attention to confidentiality and consent [8].

Systematic Approaches to the Most Common Reproductive Health Issues

Preventing and Managing the Consequences of Gender-Based Violence

Gender-based violence is defined by the UN High Commissioner for Refugees as violence directed against a person on the basis of gender or sex. Numerous studies have demonstrated that the stresses of poverty, war, and blurred public and private lives in camps increase the risks of gender-based violence. An International Red Cross study of three large refugee camps Iraq, Sudan, and Kenya demonstrated that up to 40% of women and girls who sought health care did so because of gender-based violence [9]. Efforts to prevent gender-based violence and provide early, widely available, and confidential care are critical.

Minimum standards of safety and protection include planning for the layout of toilets and washing facilities as well as food and water distribution areas to maximize safety. Toilets and showers should have doors that lock from the inside and be in lighted, visible areas close to the center of camps. Adolescents who are not in family units should have their own registration cards and female workers should be involved in the distribution of food and other supplies. Particular attention should be paid to providing protection and support to girls most at risk, including those who are unaccompanied, single heads of household, or those with disabilities. Safe public spaces for girls and boys to gather should be available, and community-based programs to increase social skills and to promote equitable gender norms should be offered. As much as possible, recommendations such as these must be included in planning for the prevention and response to gender-based violence.

Safe, confidential, and clearly marked spaces in clinics should be established for holistic care of victims of gender-based violence. A code of conduct for workers, list of patient rights (including the rights of children), and clear protocols should be posted. Health care workers should all be trained in supportive communication, trauma-based care, and protecting confidentiality, and children should be allowed to choose the gender of the health care worker who will care for them. Special attention should also be given to providing consultation and care by a health worker who comfortably speaks the same language as the victim and is aware of cultural and social issues.

Girls and boys who have experienced sexual violence should be able to receive health care immediately to avert preventable consequences including unwanted pregnancy, sexually transmitted infections (including HIV), and further psychological trauma. Legal support to survivors should also be offered, including protection from retaliations or threats such as by clearly separating perpetrators.

> **Gender-Based Violence: Key Actions for Health Care Workers**
> - Be prepared to offer trauma-based care, including documentation of any wounds or bruises
> - Provide care of wounds and prevention of tetanus and hepatitis
> - Provide emergency contraception within 120 h of the incident (refer to international or national protocols for recommended treatment)
> - Provide pregnancy testing and pregnancy options information including safe abortion referral to the full extent of the law
> - Provide presumptive treatment of sexually transmitted infections (per international or national protocols)
> - Provide postexposure prophylaxis for the prevention of HIV within 72 h of incident (per international or national protocols)
> - Offer referrals for additional services as needed, including emergency care for life-threatening injuries as well as legal, psychological, security, and community services

Preventing and Managing Sexually Transmitted Infections (STIs)

Sexually transmitted infections are caused by a myriad of bacteria, viruses, and parasites but relatively few pathogens are responsible for the majority of infections. Syphilis, gonorrhea, chlamydia, and trichomoniasis are all curable, and Hepatitis B virus (HBV), Herpes, human immunodeficiency virus (HIV), and human papillomavirus (HPV) can be mitigated with appropriate treatment. Sexually transmitted infections often occur without symptoms and so may be easily spread further, through untreated sexual partners and some through maternal to child transmission. Undiagnosed and untreated STIs can result in lifelong complications for adolescents including pelvic inflammatory disease and infertility, cervical cancer, and neurologic sequelae of tertiary syphilis. Some STIs, particularly those associated with genital ulcers, increase the risk of acquiring HIV significantly.

Adolescents can avoid sexually transmitted infections by delaying sexual activity, decreasing the number of sex partners and by consistently using condoms. It is important for those working with migrant and refugee adolescents to be prepared to provide confidential counseling on all options. Support for delaying initiation of sexual activity by creating safe space and enjoyable ways for adolescents to socialize and develop platonic friendships may be particularly important for girls who are not only at risk of more severe consequences of STIs but pregnancy. Limiting the number of sex partners also obviously reduces risk though often risk of infection may originate from a partner with a history of many sexual partners.

Condoms are the most reliable method for preventing sexually transmitted infections. When used consistently and correctly, male latex condoms are a very effective method of protection against STIs. Female condoms are also an option but are often less available and often less familiar. Condoms should be made available in accessible, private areas in humanitarian emergency situations so that anyone who may need them has access. This may include toilet and washing areas and clinics but also drop-in centers, schools, community service offices, and other places where adolescents may gather. Health workers should be prepared to demonstrate correct use of condoms to both boys and girls and health education should include negotiation with partners for consent and expected condom use. Unfortunately, sexually transmitted infections may still occur despite condom use, and genital ulcers and warts can be transmitted through contact by areas not covered by condoms. Finally, it is wise to remember that STIs in children are always a reason to consider child abuse and gender-based violence.

To Use a Condom Correctly
- Store condoms in a cool, dry place (avoid having in direct sunlight or carrying in wallets) and do not use with oil-based lubricants
- Put on the condom before any penetrative intercourse.
- Withdraw the penis after ejaculation while the penis is still erect to avoid the condom slipping off inside the vagina.
- Dispose of condom properly and use a new condom for each new act of intercourse
- If a condom breaks or slips, seek care for potential exposure to STI or pregnancy

HIV awareness and prevention deserve special emphasis in emergency situations and for adolescents most at risk. Accessible information about preventing HIV to all persons and widely available testing and counseling linked to antiretroviral (ARV) initiation is important. Priority groups for testing include pregnant girls and women (and their partners), children with severe acute malnutrition, and adolescents being tested and treated for other STIs. Inter-Agency supply kits, developed and distributed by UNFPA in crisis situations, only contain basic supplies for reproductive health. Post-exposure prophylaxis (PEP) antiretroviral medications for emergency use are included for care following rape or other episodes of unprotected intercourse, but insufficient for providing ongoing treatment for HIV. Treatment regimens for HIV/AIDS will vary based on national protocols but early initiation of combined highly active antiretroviral therapy (HAART) is important. And of course, safe and sterile medical procedures and blood transfusions reduce the risk of HIV transmission and other infections. Infection prevention protocols must be practiced carefully in low resource situations such as refugee camps and urban clinics. Refer to Chap. 25 for more information on HIV prevention and treatment.

In resource-limited settings, syndromic management of STIs is important for management and supported by the World Health Organization and many national government health systems. Syndromic management is based on the identification of consistent groups of symptoms which guide algorithm-based treatment choices without laboratory testing for the most common STIs. This simple same-day treatment approach avoids the need for multiple visits, which may further compromise confidentiality for adolescents. For example, chlamydia, gonorrhea, primary syphilis, and trichomoniasis are all generally curable with single-dose regimens of antibiotics (although resistance of gonorrhea to multiple antibiotics is increasing). For herpes, HIV, and HBV effective antiviral medications can significantly modulate the disease processes. There are pitfalls of syndromic management and misdiagnosis, and certain situations, including pregnancy, may necessitate other medication regimens. A helpful resource available electronically detailing the WHO syndromic management guidelines is *Sexually Transmitted and other Reproductive Tract Infections: A guide to essential practice* (listed in *Additional Resources*).

Although vaccination programs for STIs are often a later stage intervention in humanitarian emergency settings, vaccines for both HBV and HPV are available. Global coverage of infant HBV is approximately 85%, and HPV vaccine programs are now found in approximately 50% of countries in the world. Where the HPV vaccine is available, a two or three-dose series (three for children who have HIV or are otherwise immune-compromised) is recommended between 9–14 years of age.

Family Planning

Reproductive health needs, including the need for family planning, do not disappear when adolescents are forced to leave their homes or communities. In fact, they may increase when adolescents flee their homes and communities in an emergency, where they may not be able to bring contraceptives with them or understand how to obtain them in new situations. Displacement may increase the need for contraception, while at the same time increase barriers to access—particularly for adolescents. As previously mentioned, the disruption of family and social support structures can pose more challenges for adolescents who may be more at risk of exposure to early sexual activity and unsafe sexual practices. Youth-friendly family planning services need to be integrated into the early stages of humanitarian response to ensure that, in addition to condoms, a variety of birth-control methods are available. Services should include emergency contraception, oral contraceptive pills, injectable contraceptives, and (if feasible) intrauterine devices and implants. In addition, these services need to be located near schools or community gathering areas, allow for drop-in visits, and offer easily accessible health education materials. All providers involved in youth-friendly services must have a common understanding that reproductive health services are basic health services and available to all. It may be helpful, with informed choice, to encourage adolescents to consider longer acting and reversible contraceptive methods requiring fewer clinic visits. As soon as possible in the humanitarian response, comprehensive services should be developed with community education, client follow-up, and maintenance of a contraceptive supply chain system. It is also helpful to collaborate with national family planning programs if possible and to consider local cultural issues which may make some family planning methods more or less acceptable.

All health workers should be aware that adolescents requesting contraceptives have a right to receive these services, regardless of age or marital status. Adolescents requesting family planning services should be asked about STI symptoms, and family planning should be discussed with those presenting for STI clinics and other health care needs. For adolescent girls who already have children, encouraging birth spacing of at least 18 months is preferable.

> **Family Planning: Key Actions for Health Care Workers**
> - Make sure condoms are widely available to adolescents and can be obtained privately and without asking permission
> - Sexual health education should be integrated into community education and school curricula
> - Sites of youth-friendly family planning services should be clearly marked and widely known
> - Proactively discuss family planning with adolescents of both genders presenting for health care, including care for STIs
> - Provide emergency contraception within 120 h of incident
> - Health care workers should be prepared to discuss and offer all methods of family planning, starting with the method the adolescent is most interested in
> - Long-acting and reversible methods should be encouraged
> - Healthy timing and spacing of pregnancies should be encouraged

Care During Pregnancy and Childbirth

As children make up almost half of the refugee population globally, adolescent pregnancy and birth is a critical part of the care of refugee and migrant children. More than 15 million adolescent girls give birth every year, the majority of these in low- and middle-income countries and in poor, less educated and rural populations. In addition, almost 4 million girls undergo unsafe abortions every year. Although adolescent fertility has declined globally in the last two decades it remains high in much of sub-Saharan Africa and parts of the Middle East. Adolescent pregnancy is associated with increased risk of hypertensive disorders of pregnancy (i.e., preeclampsia/eclampsia), maternal undernutrition and micronutrient deficiencies, systemic infections (including malaria), preterm and low birth weight births, stillbirth, and neonatal death. Delayed access to operative delivery in situations of obstructed labor, which are more common in adolescent girls with immature pelvic bone development, may result in uterine rupture and obstetric fistula formation. Girls who have undergone female genital cutting, particularly infibulation during which external genitalia are excised and the vaginal orifice is significantly decreased, are at even higher risk. A careful examination by a trained health worker familiar with female genital cutting during prenatal care allows for appropriate birth planning.

Pregnancy is a leading cause of death among 15–19-year-old girls, most often occurring during abortions or during childbirth. Adolescent girls are twice as likely to die than women over 20 years of age, and very young adolescents (under 15) are five times as likely to die. Social consequences of the early child-bearing area also broad, including stigma, rejection by her community or her family, and limitations on future education and employment. Unaccompanied girls are at even higher risk and may be more vulnerable to exploitation and sexual violence.

Life-saving maternal interventions must be a part of the earliest stages of humanitarian response, particularly when locally available health services may not be available or functional. This should initially focus on clean and safe delivery services with a skilled birth attendant, available 24 h a day. Services for adolescents should be confidential, respecting their rights and privacy, and must be provided regardless of age or marital status. As much as possible, delivery at a health facility should be encouraged, but pregnant girls should also be provided with a simple clean delivery package (see Key Actions below) to be used either in the facility or at home. If skilled birth attendants are available in the community, they should be identified early as they may serve as a trusted link to adolescent mothers.

In addition to managing normal labor and delivery, health care workers must be prepared to provide basic emergency services, including administration of intravenous antibiotics, uterotonic medications to prevent postpartum hemorrhage (oxytocin, misoprostol), magnesium sulfate and antihypertensive medications, removal of retained products, manual removal of placenta, assisted vaginal delivery, and maternal and newborn resuscitation. Comprehensive emergency obstetric care further includes surgical care (laparotomy and cesarean section), anesthesia, and safe blood transfusion. Post-abortion care, including manual vacuum aspiration is a life-saving intervention and should be available as soon as possible, either in the refugee camp or on referral including management of bleeding, treatment for infection, and tetanus prophylaxis (with both tetanus vaccination and tetanus immunoglobulin if available and indicated).

In the post-emergency phase of response, additional interventions should be introduced including community-based antenatal and postpartum care, maternity waiting homes for pregnant girls at risk, breastfeeding support, neonatal care, and mental health support groups for mothers [10].

Pregnant adolescents are particularly at risk of malnutrition and micronutrient deficiencies in refugee situations. Underlying nutritional problems, including iron deficiency anemia, iodine deficiency, and Vitamin A and D deficiencies are exacerbated in emergencies. Populations which may usually have access to oil and fish to supply fatty acids may no longer have access to a range of food supplies. Pregnant adolescents should be provided with blanket access to balanced protein and energy supplements throughout pregnancy, postpartum, and while breastfeeding. They should also be given daily prenatal vitamins or multiple micronutrient tablets (MMN), iodinated salt, as well as Vitamin A supplementation (100,000 IU) when postpartum. In situations where a vegetarian-based diet is common, additional B12 vitamins may be needed. All pregnant or breastfeeding adolescents with acute global malnutrition should be admitted for therapeutic feeding and supportive care, if possible.

Every maternal death in refugee situations, including deaths to girls or women who were referred for care and died at other facilities, should be investigated. This review process allows opportunity to learn from often preventable delays or missed opportunities to provide the best quality care possible and to improve systems for the future. Maternal death investigations should be undertaken in a collaborative, system-based environment as a learning exercise.

Care During Pregnancy and Childbirth: Key Actions
- Identify all visibly pregnant adolescents and provide them with clean delivery kits (containing soap, plastic gloves, a sheet of plastic, a new razor blade, and clean string for cord care)
- As early as possible in a crisis, ensure basic emergency obstetric care, including clean and safe delivery, is available at all times. Encourage delivery at health facility with a skilled attendant
- Ensure that comprehensive emergency obstetric care, including anesthesia, surgery, and blood transfusion services are available by referral. If comprehensive services are not available, move quickly to develop on-site comprehensive obstetric capacity.
- Organize a safe referral and transport system for maternal and neonatal emergencies, which includes care for unsafe abortion
- Provide adolescent-friendly prenatal care including nutrition support, screening for STIs and HIV, presumptive treatment for malaria and soil-transmitted helminths according to national protocols, HAART for HIV/AIDS if applicable and tetanus immunization (two doses 1 month apart in first pregnancy for girls immunized as infants OR a complete series of five doses per national protocol if not previously immunized)
- Provide postpartum care including breastfeeding support and family planning options
- *Investigate and document every maternal death*

References

1. World Health Organization. Definition of reproductive health. 2020. https://www.who.int/westernpacific/health-topics/reproductive-health. Accessed 27 Jul 2020.
2. International Rescue Committee. Private violence, public concern: intimate partner violence in humanitarian settings. https://www.rescue.org/report/private-violence-public-concern-intimate-partner-violence-humanitarian-settings. Published 1 Jan 2015. Accessed 27 Jul 2020.
3. World Health Organization. WHO guidelines on the management of health complications from female genital mutilation. Geneva: WHO; 2016. https://www.who.int/reproductivehealth/topics/fgm/management-health-complications-fgm/en/. Accessed 14 Sept 2020.

4. Goldberg H, Stupp P, Okoroh E, Besera G, Goodman D, Danel I. Female genital mutilation/cutting in the United States: updated estimates of women and girls at risk, 2012. Public Health Rep. 2016;131(2):340–7. https://doi.org/10.1177/003335491613100218.
5. Pimentel VM, Eckardt MJ. More than interpreters needed. Obstet Gynecol Surv. 2014;69(8):490–500.
6. Bollini P, Pampallona S, Wanner P, Kupelnick B. Pregnancy outcome of migrant women and integration policy: a systematic review of the international literature. Soc Sci Med. 2009;68(3):452–61.
7. Sphere Project. Sphere handbook: humanitarian charter and minimum standards in disaster response. 2018. https://spherestandards.org/. Accessed 27 Jul 2020.
8. Marcell AV, Burstein GR, Adolescence CO. Sexual and reproductive health care services in the pediatric setting. Pediatrics. 2017;140(5) https://doi.org/10.1542/peds.2017-2858.
9. Ivanova O, Rai M, Kemigisha E. A systematic review of sexual and reproductive health knowledge, experiences and access to services among refugee, migrant and displaced girls and young women in Africa. Int J Environ Res Public Health. 2018;15(8) https://doi.org/10.3390/ijerph15081583.
10. Medecins Sans Frontieres. Refugee health—an approach to emergency situations. London: MacMillan Educational Ltd.; 1997.

Additional Resources

Inter-Agency Standing Committee (IASC). Guideline: integrating gender-based violence interventions in humanitarian action. Aug 2015. https://gbvguidelines.org/en/.
Inter-Agency Working Group on Reproductive Health in Crises. Inter-agency reproductive health kits for crisis situations. 4th ed. Jan 2008. Available from: http://www.iawg.net/resources/rhkits.html.
Inter-Agency Working Group on Reproductive Health in Crisis. Adolescent sexual and reproductive health toolkit for humanitarian settings. Aug 2016. Available from: https://iawg.net/resources/adolescent-sexual-reproductive-health-toolkit-humanitarian-settings.
World Health Organization. Sexually transmitted and other reproductive tract infections. A guide to essential practice. 2005. Available from: http://www.who.int/reproductivehealth/publications/rtis/9241592656/en/index.html.
World Health Organization. Pregnancy, childbirth, postpartum and newborn care. A guide to essential practice. 2015. Available from: https://www.who.int/maternal_child_adolescent/documents/imca-essential-practice-guide/en/.
World Health Organization. WHO guidelines on the management of health complications from female genital mutilation. 2016. Available from: https://www.who.int/reproductivehealth/topics/fgm/management-health-complications-fgm/en/.

Martha C. Carlough, MD, MPH is a family physician with additional training in both clinical and public health aspects of Maternal and Child Health and over 25 years' experience in global health and development work. Dr. Carlough currently serves as Director of the Office of Global Health Education within the Institute for Global Health and Infectious Diseases as well as Professor in the Department of Family Medicine at the University of North Carolina School of Medicine. A recognized expert in the field of international safe motherhood and family medicine, she has worked specifically in areas including emergency obstetric and newborn care, skilled birth attendant training, family planning, prevention of maternal to child HIV transmission, community level nutrition and health surveillance, and care of refugees and displaced persons both globally and in the USA. She is passionate about safe and gentle childbirth worldwide and enjoys teaching and working in a wide variety of situations.

Newborn Care

Ante Wind and Daniel Martinez Garcia

Overview

In 2018, 2.5 million infants died worldwide within the first month of life. Of those, 75% died within the first week of life. Neonatal deaths represent 47% of the total deaths of children under 5 years old. This figure does not even include the additional 2.5 million annual stillbirths that occur globally [1].

Risk of neonatal death is particularly high in refugee and migrant settings. Limited access to care, population movements, breakdown of essential medical services, safety concerns, and curfews may lead to inadequate prenatal care and unsafe deliveries. Furthermore, there may be limited treatment modalities, a lack of neonatal-friendly drug formulations and medical equipment, and minimal availability of staff skilled in newborn care. Hygiene standards are often difficult to maintain due to lack of access to soap and clean water, crowding, and shared living spaces. All of these factors, plus the inherent vulnerability of newborns, negatively influence newborn survival [2].

Preterm birth, asphyxia, infections, and congenital birth defects are the most common causes of neonatal death. Luckily, even in low resource settings, many of these can be addressed with simple measures such as reliable prenatal and perinatal care, diligent hygiene control, thermoregulation, maintaining normal blood glucose levels, and support of breastfeeding. Through detail-oriented, conscientious neonatal care we can have a major impact on overall child mortality rates.

In this chapter, we will first present you with the practical information you need to get your bearings when starting to care for newborns in refugee or migrant

A. Wind (✉)
Unity Health Care, Washington, DC, USA

D. M. Garcia
Médecins Sans Frontières (MSF), Geneva, Switzerland

EveryWhereSchools (EWS), Geneva, Switzerland

© Springer Nature Switzerland AG 2021
C. Harkensee et al. (eds.), *Child Refugee and Migrant Health*,
https://doi.org/10.1007/978-3-030-74906-4_28

settings. This is followed by an explanation of levels of care and coordination between organizations. This chapter concludes with specific guidance about how to manage the most common neonatal pathologies.

Practical Information

Levels of Care

Capacity for the provision of newborn care varies widely site by site. Level of care standards exists to provide recommended management of newborns according to the setting. It is helpful to be familiar with these terms so that you will know what to expect in your context. These levels of care include the *essential*, the *intermediate*, and the *comprehensive packages of care*.

These varying levels of newborn care can be provided in different physical spaces: in the home, in the clinic, or in the hospital. Depending on the context and local capacities, you can adapt these levels of care by including or removing elements. In the following section, each of these neonatal packages of care will be explained in more detail.

Collaboration and Continuity of Care

Your organization may not be the only actor providing the range of services from prenatal to postnatal care for the mother and newborn. Other actors may include the local ministry of health, existing national and international development actors, national and international NGOs, and of course the local community, including traditional or local birth attendants. Close collaboration with other actors to minimize gaps and provide high quality of care from the prenatal to the postnatal period and from the community up through the hospital level will help improve neonatal outcomes.

Neonatal and maternal health are inextricably linked. Preventative management via appropriate care of both the neonate and the mother is vital to reducing neonatal mortality and morbidity [2]. Newborn care consists of a continuum of care starting with general health education, family planning to avoid undesired and teenage pregnancies, prenatal care, and nutritional support during pregnancy. It also includes access to skilled birth attendants and essential newborn care at birth. It continues through to the appropriate postnatal care of both the mother and child until at least the first month of life. Ideally, maternal/obstetric care should not be separated from neonatal care.

Exclusive Breastfeeding

An important component of a preventative care strategy includes exclusive breastfeeding for the first 6 months of life, starting within the first hour after delivery. Breastfeeding promotes mother and child bonding, ensures safe and affordable nutrition and hydration, decreases risk for infections in the neonatal period and beyond, and may have a positive impact on neurodevelopmental outcomes. Additionally, there are benefits for the mother including decreased postpartum bleeding, increased birth spacing, and decreased postpartum depression [3].

Helping Babies Breathe

One of the most significant initiatives in newborn care has been the Helping Babies Breathe (HBB) program. Up to 10% of newborns may need assistance to initiate breathing after delivery via stimulation, clearance of the airway, or ventilatory support. HBB is an evidence-based education program for traditional or local birth attendants, midwives, nurses, and doctors that teaches the basic skills needed to perform newborn resuscitation during the first minute of life, the "golden minute." HBB materials are free online and training-of-trainer courses are available. As long as the correct supplies are available, this method can be used in the household, community setting, and primary or secondary healthcare facility [4].

Quality of Care

Optimizing access to basic obstetrical and neonatal care is pivotal to decreasing maternal mortality and improving neonatal outcomes. This includes ensuring pregnant women are aware of local obstetric services available, that she has the means to reach these services, or, at a minimum have a skilled birth attendant in the home, and that adequate care is provided by the birth attendant.

Once the baby is delivered, a strong focus on hygiene, thermoregulation, maintaining normal blood glucose levels, and supporting breastfeeding and/or age-appropriate feeding is all that is needed for the vast majority of newborns, including most premature infants, to survive. Directing your efforts on providing the best quality of care that you can in these four areas, including utilizing skilled birth attendants, will go a long way to improving outcomes [2].

Take time with your medical team to evaluate how well each of these factors are being addressed. If there are limitations, consider all potential root causes to better understand these gaps. Are they due to barriers caused by security concerns, geographical distance, or cost? Lack of critical equipment or medications? Inadequate or insufficient staff training? Ineffective communication with the mothers or with maternity care providers? Structural factors of the physical space/neonatal unit? Social, economic, or cultural factors? Try not to make assumptions, dig deeper, and get the whole team (including the parents) involved to improve the quality of care.

Prevention of Mother to Child Transmission of HIV (PMTCT)

The risk of vertical transmission of HIV can be reduced to almost zero if the mother is appropriately managed. The "Prevention of Mother to Child Transmission of

HIV" (PMTCT) program starts in the prenatal period with HIV screening for the mother and provision of counseling and anti-retroviral drugs (ARVs). Most areas with known high HIV prevalence will already have PMTCT programs. If there is no program, this should be discussed within your organization and with the local health authorities. Refer to "Useful additional resources" at the end of the chapter for sources that provide more detailed information on HIV management for exposed newborns [5].

Data Collection, Reporting, and Analysis

Remember the importance of high-quality data. All newborns should be registered. Name, date of birth, origin, birth weight, gestational age (if possible), diagnoses (if appropriate), and vaccination status should all be noted. Outcomes, meaning stillbirth, discharge, transfer, or death, must also be recorded. Refer to the *Roadmap to Accelerate Progress for Every Newborn in Humanitarian Settings 2020–2024* for other indicators to follow [6]. Maintaining an accurate register is a challenge and requires diligent effort from the entire healthcare team. Regularly review and analyze the data and outcomes with the team. When the entire team is involved with the data collection, analysis, and reporting, the team members will better understand why data collection is relevant to their work rather than an additional burden. Sharing improvement in indicators over time can be very encouraging to teams working in resource-limited settings.

Death

Despite your best efforts, you will be faced with maternal deaths, stillbirths, and neonatal deaths. Counsel the parents, ensure that they know that it is not their fault. Encourage the mother to attend postnatal care appointments where she can be supported in case of postnatal depression, and, when appropriate, consider discussing family planning options. Additionally, the parents should be provided a record of newborn death (often necessary for legal purposes).

Management: Levels of Care

Antenatal Care

Newborn outcomes and maternal mortality improve when appropriate antenatal care is delivered. This includes linking anti-natal care programs with existing educational and family planning programs. Do not forget to address the teenage population. Pregnant women should be screened for preeclampsia, and infections such as HIV, syphilis, other sexually transmitted infections (STIs), and asymptomatic bacteriuria. They should receive education about the importance of good nutrition for themselves, breastfeeding for their infant, family planning, and safe delivery in a health facility and with a skilled birth attendant. They should also be screened for anemia and provided with iron, Vit D, and iodine supplementation when appropriate. Additional micronutrients can be provided when available. Additionally, pregnant women should receive folate, tetanus vaccinations, and, if living in a malaria-endemic region, mosquito nets, malaria prophylaxis, and screening and treatment for malaria. Women at risk for preterm delivery less than 34 weeks should receive antenatal steroids [2, 7].

Essential Newborn Care in the Community

The *essential package of newborn care* refers to the care that every newborn should receive regardless of where they are born; at home, in an outpatient clinic, or in a hospital setting. It is the minimal standard. It includes delayed cord clamping, thermal care, infection prevention, early initiation of breastfeeding, vitamin K and ophthalmic antibiotic administration, assessment of danger signs, and postnatal care [8].

Although mothers should be encouraged to give birth in a health facility, in some cases this is not culturally acceptable or logistically possible, in which case local birth attendants or community health workers can assist the birth in the household. The provision of high-quality newborn care in the community starts with training for these birth attendants. All birth attendants should receive the "Helping Babies Breathe" and the "Helping Babies Survive: Essential Care for Every Baby" trainings and, if possible, the basic material to perform these resuscitations [8].

Additionally, birth kits should be provided to every expectant mother. These kits provide essential supplies needed for a safe and clean delivery. The kits vary per organization. If neither your organization nor any partner organizations are providing birth kits, refer to the Healthy Newborn Network toolkit for information about what to include in a newborn health kit [2].

Routine Care

Routine care should be provided to every newborn, regardless of where they are born; at home or in a hospital setting. Please refer to the next section for technical guidance on routine care.

Essential Newborn Care in Health Clinics or Hospital Settings

Outpatient health clinics should be able to provide routine care. Infants who progress well and have no significant risk factors are usually kept with the mother until discharge from the clinic no earlier than 24 h after delivery [9].

If there are danger signs or risk factors such as prematurity or low birth weight, then the child should be admitted to a newborn unit [9]. If there is no newborn unit, then you should identify where newborns with complications or prematurity are being sent and how well the referral process is working. If no referral is possible, assess if these newborns are stable enough to stay with their mothers in the maternity ward or in a pediatric unit. Make sure that referral criteria are clear and evaluate the capacity of referral vehicles to maintain the warmth of the baby and a hygienic environment.

Intermediate Package of Newborn Care

The *intermediate package of newborn care* refers to a slightly higher level of care that can be provided in a low resource hospital setting [8]. It comprises all the elements of *essential newborn care* plus the availability of skilled staff and the essential medications to manage the most common neonatal complications such as asphyxia, prematurity, sepsis, other common infections, and jaundice.

If you are working in or managing a newborn unit then take some time to consider the following aspects of care.

Ensure that admission and discharge criteria to the newborn unit exist. If there are none, then refer to the resources at the end of this chapter to help you create them.

Upon arrival, assess available human resources. Are there doctors, clinical officers, nurses, or midwives familiar with newborn care? If not, is staff training ongoing? Is there enough staff? (Ideal ratios of staff per patient are as follows: doctors 1:20, nurses 1:5–10, nurse assistants 1:5–10) [2]. Optimize communication between the health providers taking care of the mothers and the midwives, doctors, or nurses caring for the newborn. The history of prenatal care and maternal health and complications should be known to the team providing the newborn care. A simple, checklist-based sign-out sheet can be created for better communication between the maternity and newborn units.

Within the newborn unit, ideally you should have four separate spaces: (1) critically ill newborns born in the same health facility, (2) stable sick newborns born in the same health facility, (3) premature but otherwise well infants receiving kangaroo parent care, and (4) ill newborns admitted from outside of the health facility.

Consider the physical space housing the newborns. Evaluate the electric capacity, insulation, room temperature, minimizing visitors, space for mothers, and access to clean water. There should be a handwashing point at the entrance. There should be one bed per patient. Mother must be provided a place to sleep: they may share a bed with the newborn or may be provided a separate bed beside the crib. Beds and cots should not be made of wood as these are difficult to clean. Critically ill children should not share a treatment space. In other words, they should not be touching. See Fig. 28.1 as an example of a low-cost method to minimize contamination. Mothers should have a dedicated space to shower and wash their clothes. Breastfeeding counseling, education, and support should be offered every day in these units.

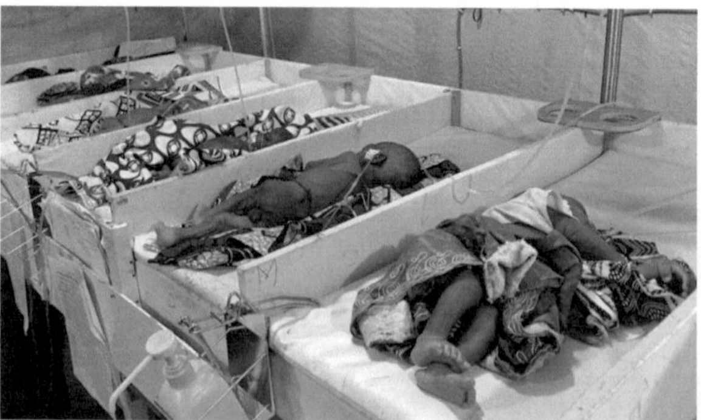

Fig. 28.1 Example of a simple approach to prevent patient–patient contamination in a crowded critical care/resuscitation area. (Permission obtained from Ante Wind)

What medical resources are available? You will need medications, IV fluids, glucose, etc. formulated especially for newborns. A glucometer is important. Ideally, you may also have a warming lamp or blanket, a digital weight scale, a digital thermometer, a phototherapy light, oximeter, and a bedside hemoglobin machine. The Healthy Newborn Network toolkit noted at the end of this chapter contains lists of the specific medications and supplies needed to run a newborn unit. In addition, the *"Toolkit for setting up special newborn units, stabilization units, and newborn care corners"* by UNICEF can provide some background information useful when setting up a newborn unit [10].

Comprehensive Package of Newborn Care

The *comprehensive package of newborn care* includes a higher level of care including provision of the skilled human resources, medications, and equipment needed to provide case management of complex neonatal care, ventilatory support, and simple neonatal surgery [8]. This is not commonly seen in humanitarian and resource-limited settings and is beyond the scope of this book. However, two points are worth commenting on.

Incubators are often available in facilities providing a higher level of care. Maintaining the cleanliness and maintenance of incubators in low resource settings is a major challenge. Incubators that cannot be adequately cleaned and/or maintained between newborns, or during prolonged hospitalizations, put the neonate at higher risk for a hospital-acquired infection and critical incidents such as burns. The risk-to-benefit ratio should be evaluated. Often skin to skin may be the better option.

Bubble CPAP is a low cost, relatively simple way to provide extra respiratory support to newborns suffering from respiratory distress syndrome. In this method, blended and humidified oxygen is delivered via nasal prongs or mask. Pressure in the system is maintained by placing the distal end of the tubing in water. The level of the water determines the pressure delivered to the airways, and the ability of the pressurized oxygen to "bubble" out prevents too much pressure from being delivered.

Bubble CPAP in low resource settings has been shown to decrease the risk of respiratory failure but is not without risks [10]. This technique requires the use of specific bubble CPAP equipment, a rigorous and well-planned implementation involving intensive training of medical staff, excellent hygiene conditions, low staff turnover, high level of supervision and patient monitoring, and continuous evaluation to ensure that the correct patients are being placed on CPAP and that outcomes are being improved by its use. These prerequisites are often not present in refugee or migrant settings. If you do decide to implement CPAP, do so in collaboration with experts in bubble CPAP familiar with implementation in a low resource setting. Do not attempt to build homemade CPAP systems.

Management: Technical Guidance

Only a general overview of the management of the most common situations and pathologies will be provided in the sections that follow. Please refer to the WHO Recommendations on Newborn Health and the Healthy Newborn Network website including their Newborn Health in Humanitarian Settings Field Guide Newborn Care Charts for more detailed technical guidance [9, 11].

Routine Care

Prior to birth, the following items should be available and ready for use: 1–2 clean and dry cloths, a hat, a cord clamp or ties, clean scissors/blade/scalpel, a bulb or penguin suction device, 2 face masks of differing sizes, a clock or watch, a ventilation bag/mask, and a stethoscope. The mother's perineum should be washed, and the birth attendant should wash their hands and wear sterile gloves. Upon delivery, the birth attendant should dry, warm, and stimulate the baby by rubbing his or her back firmly. As long as the baby is crying or breathing, the baby should then be placed in the mother's arms. Suctioning the mouth after delivery is no longer recommended, unless the child is not breathing and there is meconium or visible obstructive mucous [4]. For both vaginal and caesarian delivery, if there is no need for urgent ventilatory support, cord clamping should be delayed by 1–3 min, even for premature and HIV-exposed newborns. This provides extra hemoglobin to augment iron reserves in the infant for up to 6–8 months of life and decreases the incidence of anemia thus ameliorating the impact of iron deficiency and malaria to which newborns in low resource settings are often prone [12].

After delivery, every newborn should receive vitamin K, cord care with chlorhexidine, antibiotic eye ointment (per national protocol), a complete physical exam, and, if a scale is available, the newborn should be weighed. Breastfeeding should be encouraged within the first hour of life. The newborn should also receive vaccinations per the national protocol (OPV, BCG, Hep B are commonly given). Chlorhexidine digluconate 7.1% (4% base) is now recommended for 7 days of cord care for any infant born in a setting of high neonatal mortality (>30/1000 live births) [2]. Any neonate born less than 2000 g should be placed skin to skin with their caretaker to avoid hypothermia [8]. Defer bathing until 24 h of life due to the risk of hypothermia.

As part of routine care, neonates should also be screened for danger signs and risks for sepsis. Danger signs include poor feeding, convulsions, decreased movement or activity, fast breathing or chest indrawing, feeling too hot or cold (temperature <35.5 or >37.5 if a thermometer is available), birth weight less than 2.5 kg, jaundice on the first day of life, or jaundice on palms and soles at any time [2, 9].

Risks for sepsis will be described in further detail below.

All neonates should be screened for possible HIV exposure. If the mother has HIV then, within hours of delivery, the infant should receive prophylactic ARVs. At discharge, the newborn and mother should be referred to the PMTCT program for testing, follow-up, and management.

Ensure that every mother has support at home, and if she does not, consider which programs might be available to help provide her with support. The mother should be given a record of the newborn birth [2].

When the child is born at home, there should be a point of contact with a health care worker within 24 h. Follow-up visits should be made on day 3, between days 7–14, and at 6 weeks in order to monitor weight gain and discuss concerns [9]. The mother can come to the clinic or a home health agent/community health worker can come to the home.

Prematurity and Low Birth Weight

According to the World Health Organization (WHO), "preterm birth is the leading cause of perinatal and neonatal mortality and morbidity (globally). Preterm infants are particularly vulnerable to complications due to impaired respiration, difficulty feeding, poor body temperature, and high risk of infection" [13].

Inadequate prenatal services in refugee or migrant contexts place the neonate at higher risk for premature and small for gestational age birth. Extreme prematurity is defined as <28 weeks, very preterm is 28–32 weeks, and moderate to late preterm is 32–37 weeks. Low birth weight (LBW) is defined as <2500 g and very low birth weight (VLBW) is defined as <2000 g [2].

Preventing premature delivery via appropriate antenatal care is really important. If premature delivery is inevitable, administer antenatal steroids to the mother for any pregnancy at less than 34 weeks gestation [13]. Steroids promote lung maturation and improve outcomes in premature neonates.

In addition to managing any specific complications such as sepsis or respiratory insufficiency, the primary methods of managing prematurity and low birth weight include avoiding hypoglycemia, avoiding hypothermia, maintaining good hygiene practices, providing age-appropriate feeding, and avoiding apnea.

Hypothermia is defined as a temperature less than 35.5 °C. The best way to manage and avoid hypothermia is via Kangaroo Care (KC, also referred as Kangaroo Mother Care or KMC). KC is a method to keep stable newborns warm through continuous 24-hour skin to skin contact with the caretaker (usually the mother or father). In low- to middle-income countries KC has been associated with decreased mortality, decreased risk of severe infections, and decreased incidence of hypothermia in low birth weight neonates [13]. See the insert below for an explanation of the Kangaroo Care Method.

In cases where skin to skin care is not providing sufficient warmth or the caretaker is not available, a heat lamp can be used. Make sure that the team has read the user manual to avoid overheating or burning the newborn. Also remember to always check the blood glucose level in the hypothermic child [13].

Kangaroo Care Method

To position the newborn in the KC position, start by undressing the baby. The newborn should only wear socks, a diaper, and a hat. He/she should then be placed vertically between the caretaker's breasts with the head positioned to the side, the arms out to the side, and the hips in frog-leg position. A cloth should be secured around the newborn-parent dyad to keep the newborn in this position. The newborn can breastfeed on demand every 2–3 h if the mother or a wet nurse is available. This KC position should continue even after discharge until the baby's weight surpasses 2 kg [14].

This method is easy to set up but requires persistence to teach and to maintain. In some cultures, 24-h contact is not accepted. In that case, any number of hours spent in the skin to skin position is better than none [13]. If a father or other caretaker is available, encourage them to participate in KC as well to maximize the potential benefit for the newborn.

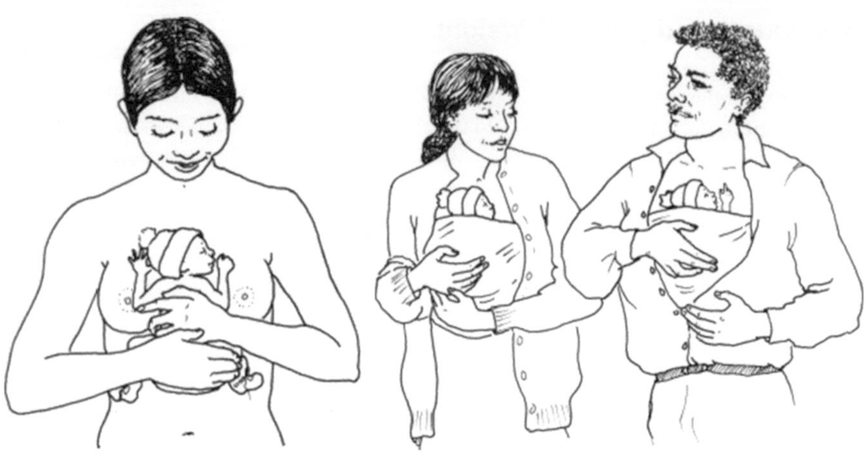

Permission obtained from WHO [14]

Resuscitation

All health care providers should be competent in basic neonatal resuscitation. As mentioned above, intervening during the "golden minute" is crucial to improving neonatal outcomes. Within the first minute of life, the newborn should be breathing spontaneously. If he/she is not, then positive pressure ventilation should be started. For a detailed explanation of neonatal resuscitation in low resource settings, please refer to the Helping Babies Breathe resources [4].

In brief, if after stimulation of the newborn, he/she is still not breathing, clamp the cord, open the airway, suction only if you see obstructing secretions, and initiate positive pressure ventilation within the first minute of life. The ventilation bag/mask does not need to be connected to oxygen when you initiate ventilations. Often just a few ventilations will stimulate spontaneous breathing. Effective ventilation can be monitored by seeing the chest rise and feeling the heartbeat at the umbilical cord stump. The heartbeat should be greater than 100 beats per minute. If it is not, ventilation should be continued. Oxygen can be initiated at this time [4]. If the heartbeat falls below 60 beats per minute, compressions should be started in conjunction with ventilation. Please see the APLS algorithm below (Fig. 28.2). For a detailed explanation of advanced resuscitative efforts please refer to current guidelines such as those from the AAP Neonatal Resuscitation Program, the European Resuscitation Council, or the Advanced Pediatric Life Saving website [15–17]. If the heart rate is greater than 100 beats per minute, check for spontaneous breathing. If there is spontaneous breathing, then monitor closely and continue to provide routine care [4]. Refer to Fig. 28.3.

If after 10 min of resuscitation there is no heartbeat, stop the resuscitation. If after 20 min of resuscitation, a heartbeat is still present but there is no spontaneous

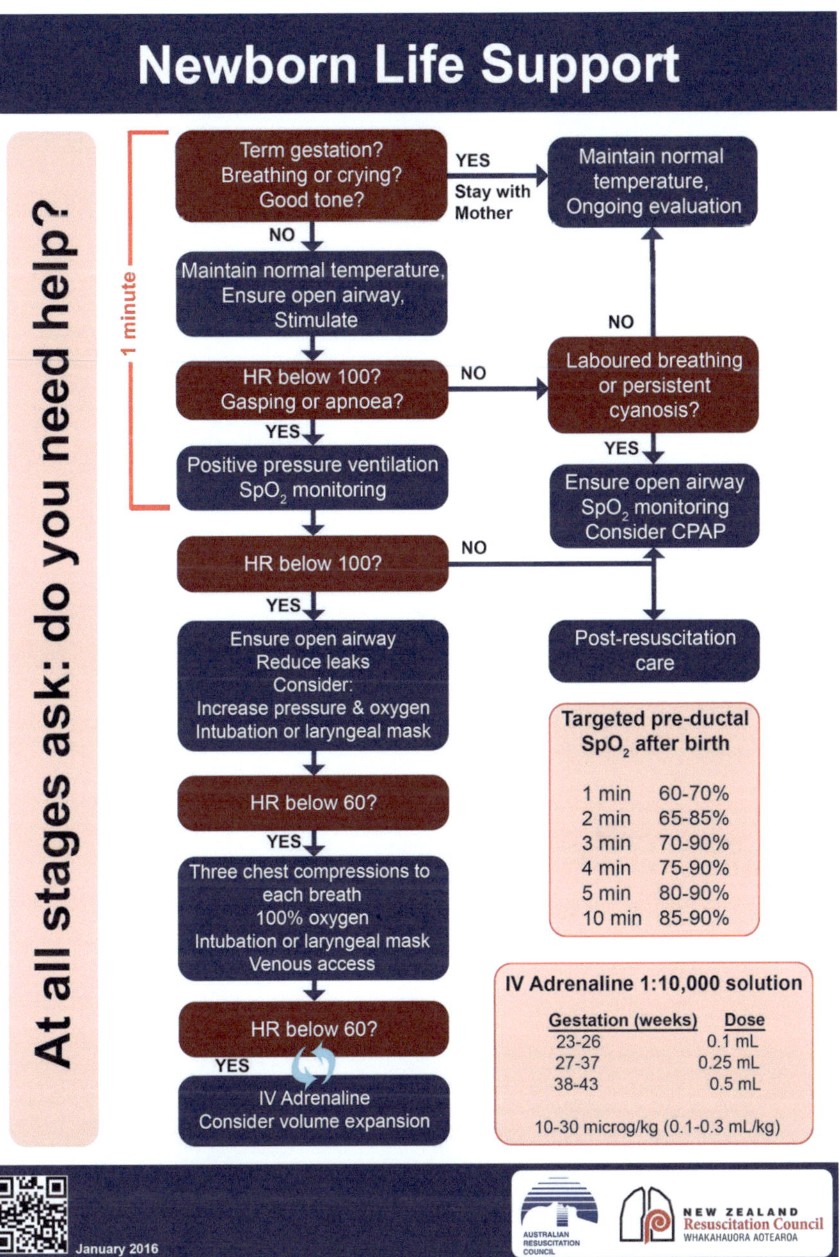

Fig. 28.2 Advanced resuscitation algorithm. (Permission obtained from APLS [18])

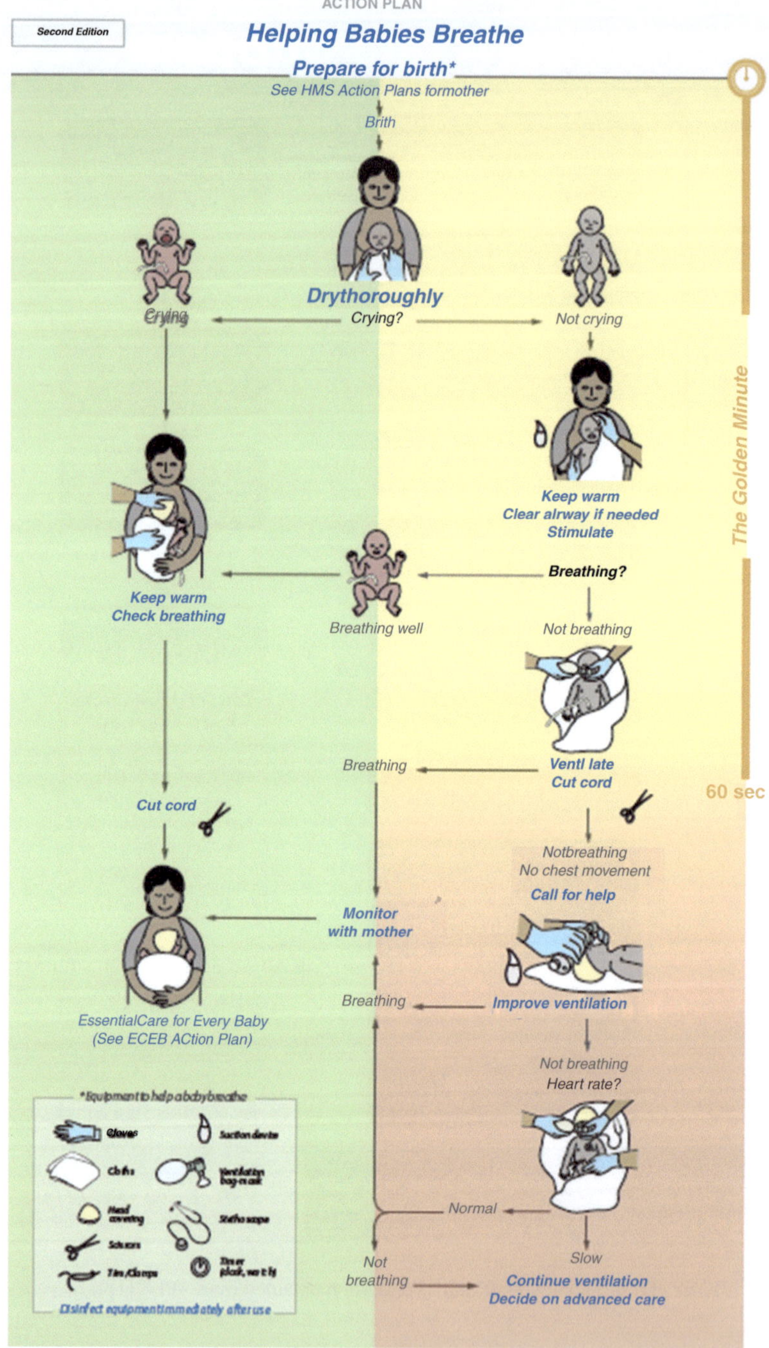

Fig. 28.3 Helping babies breathe resuscitation algorithm. (Permission obtained from the AAP [4])

breathing, resuscitation should be stopped (unless a higher level of care, including a ventilator, is an option) [9].

Critically Ill Neonates

Many of the most common pathologies present similarly in neonates. Sepsis, pneumonia, meningitis, omphalitis, osteomyelitis, and even tetanus can all present similarly in the initial stages. All may have a constellation of the following symptoms: hypotonia, hypoglycemia, poor feeding, hypothermia, and/or jaundice. If you are faced with a critically ill newborn and you do not yet know the etiology, focus on managing oxygenation, perfusion, hypoglycemia, and hypothermia, and then do your best to manage the specific etiology.

Provide positive pressure ventilation if needed. Start supplemental oxygen if the saturations are less than 92%. Maintain hydration via breastfeeding, cup/spoon/nasogastric feeding, or intravenous (IV) fluids. Check the blood glucose, hemoglobin, and test for malaria if appropriate. Treat any seizure activity with phenobarbital (after correcting any hypoglycemia). Administer antibiotics if there is any suspicion of infection (if all else fails, ampicillin and gentamycin are a good starting point until you gain some clarity on the exact etiology). Monitor closely with frequent vital signs and good nursing care. And always be vigilant about hygiene. Refer as soon as possible to a higher level of care if needed.

Neonatal Risk for Infection, Sepsis, Pneumonia, and Meningitis

Due to their immature immune systems, neonates are at high risk for infections. Maternal factors also influence this risk for infection, including maternal peripartum fever, chorioamnionitis, foul-smelling amniotic fluid, or prolonged rupture of membranes greater than 18 hours. A neonate with a twin with signs of sepsis should also be considered at risk since he/she has been exposed to the same maternal bacteria. A neonate with the above risk factors plus prematurity, low birth weight, the need for resuscitation, or home delivery is at even higher risk for infection [2, 9].

A newborn with risk factors for infection should be treated with 48 hours of antibiotics, regardless of symptoms. The newborn should then be reassessed. If at any point there are danger signs, consider treating for systemic infection with a full course of antibiotics [9].

Early sepsis, meningitis, or pneumonia are often due to maternal microbes (gram-negative bacteria) whereas later onset infections (>7 days) are more often due to environmental microbes (gram-positive bacteria) [8]. In malaria-endemic regions, always consider malaria as a possible etiology. Malaria should be screened for with a blood smear, not an antigen-based rapid diagnostic test as antigens can pass from the mother to the newborn causing a false-positive result [19]. Of note, in low resource settings without X-ray availability, neonatal pneumonia is hard to differentiate clinically from sepsis and the treatment is essentially the same.

Sepsis, meningitis, and pneumonia are also often quite difficult to differentiate. All may present with hypotonia, poor feeding, tachypnea, low or high temperatures, hypoglycemia, jaundice, or pallor. In meningitis, you may have irritability, seizures, or a bulging fontanelle. Nuchal rigidity is not often seen in neonates. A lumbar puncture is advisable to help differentiate the two, but it is often not feasible. However, once again management is similar; err on the side of caution and treat for meningitis if you have clinical suspicion as such. Refer to the technical guides for antibiotic management.

Remember that prevention is the best approach to neonatal sepsis. Neonatal infections can be prevented via health education programs, maternal vaccinations, good antenatal and perinatal care, antibiotics for prolonged rupture of membranes, maintenance of hygiene standards during delivery with skilled birth attendants, clean cord care, and early and effective breastfeeding initiation [2].

Perinatal Asphyxia

Perinatal asphyxia results from oxygen deprivation just prior to, during, or after delivery. Good prenatal care and skilled resuscitation can prevent many cases of neonatal asphyxia. Oxygen deprivation leads to metabolic acidosis, hypoxic ischemic encephalopathy, seizures, and multi-organ dysfunction. The newborn may present with hypotonia, bradycardia, poor reactivity, decreased muscle tone, and/or difficulty feeding.

The devastating outcomes of birth asphyxia can be minimized by reducing factors that lead to maternal deaths, ensuring good perinatal care, increasing early access to cesarean sections in case of fetal distress, and symptomatic management for those cases that could not be avoided. Optimize blood glucose levels, feeding, fluid balance (the infant may need a nasogastric tube if suck-swallow coordination is affected), normothermia, and mother-child bonding. Consider empiric antibiotics and treat any seizure activity. Encourage the mother to engage with the infant. Effective breastfeeding indicating good suck-swallow coordination is a good prognostic indicator.

Seizures

Neonatal seizures can be subtle. They can present with symmetric or asymmetric rhythmic movements, tonic posturing, apnea, eye deviation, repetitive hand movements, or chewing-like movements of the mouth. First, rule out hypoglycemia. If hypoglycemia has been ruled out or empirically treated and seizures continue, treat with phenobarbital. Phenobarbital should be continued until the newborn is seizure-free for 3 days [2]. Make sure to look for underlying causes such as meningitis or perinatal asphyxia. Treatment with pyridoxine or calcium is also indicated in certain situations [2].

Hypo- and Hyperglycemia

Hypoglycemia can be fatal and can have long-term neurodevelopmental consequences. Many neonatal morbidities like low (or high) birth weight, hypothermia, maternal gestational diabetes, poor feeding, and sepsis put newborns at high risk for hypoglycemia. Blood glucose should be above 45 mg/dL (2.5 mmol/L). Symptoms of hypoglycemia include jitteriness, hypotonia, apnea, poor feeding, bradycardia, and cyanosis. Most newborn units will have preestablished protocols to treat hypoglycemia. If not, a reasonable approach would be the following: if the neonate is asymptomatic, provide immediate breastfeeding (or 5 mL/kg of 10% glucose solution given orally), and if symptomatic, provide an IV bolus of 3 mL/kg D10% [8]. If you do not have IV access, consider using a nasogastric tube.

In sick, low birth weight or large for gestational age newborns, the glucose should be checked once prior to each feed until it is normal for three feeds. If you have to treat hypoglycemia, recheck the blood glucose level after 20 min to ensure it has normalized.

Of note, hyperglycemia is most often a stress response in a neonate or a sign of a critically ill child. Do not administer insulin. Manage comorbid conditions and maintain hydration. When the neonate improves, the blood glucose should normalize.

Feeding and IV Fluids

The WHO recommends 6 months of exclusive breastfeeding. In otherwise healthy newborns breastfeeding is simple, inexpensive, provides optimal nutrition, and decreases the risk of infection. You may find that there are cultural misconceptions that limit breastfeeding, for example, a belief that mothers cannot breastfeed if they become pregnant again.

In cases where the mother is deceased or unavailable, breastfeeding alternatives may be required. In this case, there are three options. First, if culturally acceptable, a wet nurse can be found. She should be tested for infectious diseases including TB and HIV and provided thorough education, health promotion, and nutritional support to ensure exclusive breastfeeding.

Secondly, infant formula can be used. Infant formula should only be given if there is a safe water source, reliable formula supply, adequate equipment for preparation, and a supportive caretaker who understands how to prepare the formula correctly and hygienically. Pay attention to the source of your infant formula to ensure its quality and nutritional value. Note that a 6-month supply of formula is about 20 kg of formula powder. Using a cup, not a bottle, as demonstrated in Fig. 28.4, will help maintain hygienic conditions [20].

The least preferred option is to use other milk products. Animal milk is not physiologically adapted for infants and must be mixed with water and sugar before use. Using animal milk (including powdered milk) is nutritionally suboptimal, has insufficient micronutrients, and has infectious risks. It should only be used as a last resort and temporary option while finding a better solution [20].

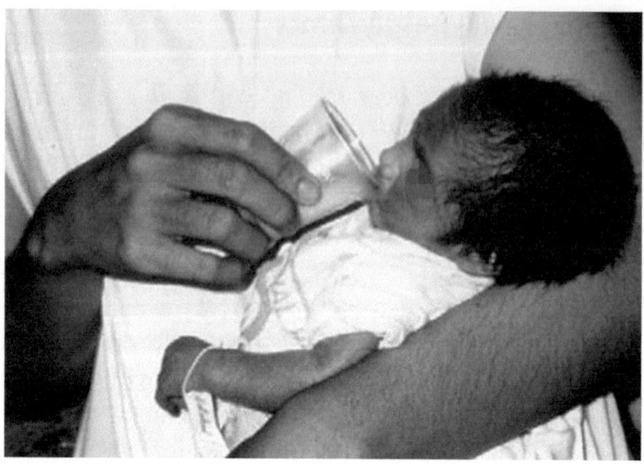

Fig. 28.4 Using a cup for infant feeding. (Permission obtained from WHO [20])

Premature infants less than 1500 g require closer management of their fluid intake. They are initially only fed a small aliquot of expressed or donor breastmilk via nasogastric tube, spoon or cup, and the remainder of their fluid needs are administered via an intravenous catheter. Day by day the feeds and total fluids are slowly increased. As the baby tolerates the feeds, the IV fluids are then slowly weaned. Please refer to the *WHO optimal feeding of low birth weight infants technical review* for detailed guidance [21].

Neonatal Conjunctivitis

Most cases of neonatal conjunctivitis can be prevented by testing and treating the mother for sexually transmitted infections and by administering prophylactic ophthalmic antibiotic ointment at birth.

Most often, eye discharge is due to an obstructed lacrimal duct which can be managed with warm compresses and lacrimal duct massage. If there is copious purulent discharge and eye redness, consider neonatal conjunctivitis. Neonatal conjunctivitis is most often caused by chlamydia or gonorrhea and requires systemic antibiotics. Gonococcal conjunctivitis tends to present within the first week and is treated with ceftriaxone. Chlamydia generally presents after day of life 5 and is treated with azithromycin or erythromycin. You may need to treat with both antibiotics if you cannot differentiate. Note that vertically transmitted herpes can also infect the eye. If the mother has active herpetic lesions, if the conjunctivitis looks atypical, or the infection does not respond to antibiotics this should be considered.

Omphalitis

Omphalitis is an infection of the tissue surrounding the umbilicus. Clinical signs include purulent, foul-smelling discharge from the umbilical stump, periumbilical erythema, and fevers. It occurs when bacteria are introduced into the freshly cut umbilical cord due to poor hygiene practices, overcrowding, shared housing, and lack of education on cord care. Antibiotic management should include good staphylococcal plus anaerobic coverage in severe cases. Additionally, apply chlorhexidine digluconate 7.1% 2–4 times daily [8].

Tetanus

Tetanus is a preventable, noncommunicable, life-threatening disease that presents at 3–21 days of life. Symptoms include difficulty feeding, progressing to muscle rigidity and seizure like muscle spasms, and eventually leading to whole-body rigidity and opisthotonos. Initially, they may present with symptoms similar to meningitis.

The best management is prevention. Always check the maternal vaccination status. Mothers should receive two tetanus vaccinations during their first pregnancy, 4 weeks apart, and then 1 dose every pregnancy thereafter until she has received 5 doses. Hygienic birth environment, sterile equipment, and cord care are equally important.

If a child does present with tetanus, the management consists of providing a soothing environment with minimal handling, and limited visual or auditory stimuli. Isolation is not mandatory as it can decrease surveillance. Always keep a ventilation bag/mask and suction nearby. Place a nasogastric tube to facilitate feeding. Give antibiotics for comorbid sepsis, tetanus immune globulin for neutralization of the tetanus toxin, metronidazole for toxin inhibition, morphine and diazepam emulsion (regular diazepam is contraindicated in newborns) for the management of muscle spasms, and tetanus vaccine to prevent future recurrence [8]. In resource-limited settings, the prognosis is poor. The rate of both mortality and long-term neurologic sequelae after tetanus infection are frequently above 50% [22].

Malaria

Any newborn with signs of infection in a malaria-endemic region should be tested for malaria. A blood smear is a gold standard for diagnosing congenital malaria. However, if you do not have a lab, or even if the blood smear is negative but you clinically suspect malaria, treat empirically. Congenital malaria should always be treated as severe malaria. Since dosing with oral artemisinin combination therapy (ACTs) is difficult, these newborns should be admitted and treated with IV artesunate if possible. If this is not possible then administer the ACT dose for a 5 kg child [19].

Syphilis

For neonates with intrauterine exposure to syphilis, the specific treatment regimen depends on whether the mother was treated, with which drug she was treated, and whether the infant is symptomatic [8]. Even asymptomatic neonates must be treated if maternal management was inadequate.

Jaundice

Jaundice in a newborn can be physiologic due to the immaturity of the liver, high red blood cell turnover, or insufficient feeding, or it can be pathologic due to hemolysis, sepsis, or congenital conditions. Risk factors for jaundice include prematurity, polycythemia, cephalohematoma, and poor feeding. Jaundice must be treated aggressively because at high levels bilirubin can cross the blood-brain barrier causing kernicterus with potentially devastating neurological consequences.

It is unlikely that you will have a laboratory or point of care method to measure the bilirubin level or to determine whether it is a conjugated or unconjugated hyperbilirubinemia. The clinical exam is useful as the higher the bilirubin level is, the further the jaundice descends down the body and to the extremities. If there is only facial jaundice (in dark skin, check by blanching the skin on the nose), the newborn does not need treatment. If the jaundice extends below the umbilicus, consider treatment. If the jaundice extends to the palms and soles, then the bilirubin is very high needs to be managed urgently.

Some health centers may have proper phototherapy, in which case you should ensure that all staff are fully trained in its use and that the equipment is properly maintained and cleaned. Be sure to cover the patient's eyes and genital area. Maximize the time spent under the light to decrease the bilirubin as quickly as possible but encourage frequent breastfeeding and adequate hydration as stooling and voiding will help excrete bilirubin as well.

If you do not have phototherapy, then cautiously encourage indirect sunlight exposure. In more stable settings you may consider setting up a simple phototherapy structure using commercially available window tinting, as demonstrated in Fig. 28.5. Please see referenced articles for detailed instruction. Note that if you use either indirect sunlight or filtered sunlight, the newborn should be checked hourly to monitor for hyperthermia, hypothermia, dehydration, or sunburn. Only previously studied window tinting such as Air Blue 80 or Gila Titanium should be used as other brands may transmit variable amounts of ultraviolet light, infrared radiation, and blue light [23].

Encourage good hydration via breastfeeding and, depending on the severity, consider starting maintenance IV fluids to decrease the bilirubin. If there are signs of kernicterus (obvious jaundice, somnolence or irritability, opisthotonos, or unusual cry) treat for meningitis, as kernicterus can mask the symptoms of meningitis. In these cases, initiate phototherapy, maintenance IV fluids, and if feasible, provide an exchange transfusion. In these severe cases, referral to a higher level of care would be prudent, if possible.

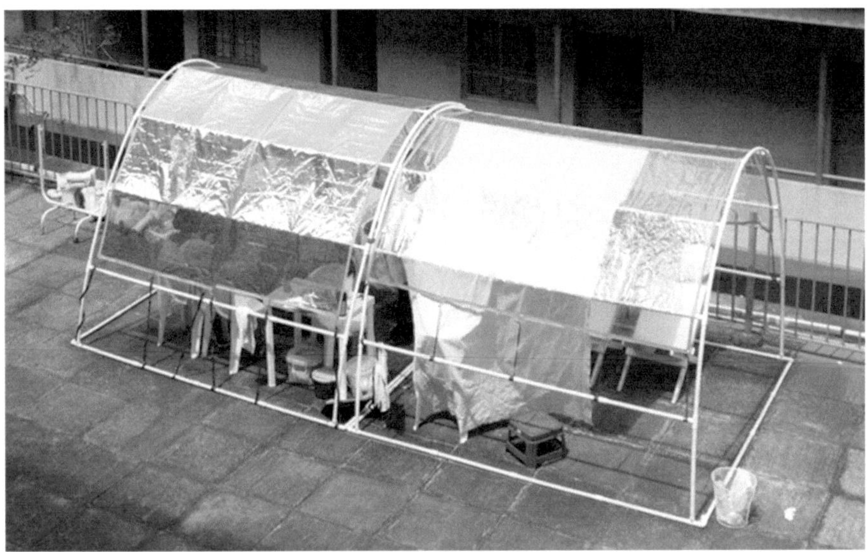

Fig. 28.5 Example of a filtered light structure using window tinting. (Permission obtained from Tina Slusher [23])

Maternal Health

As mentioned above, the health of the baby and the mother are inextricably linked. Pay attention to the mother as well as the baby. Ensure that she is receiving medical follow-up. Additionally, as elsewhere, mothers are at risk for postpartum depression and anxiety. If you notice these symptoms, address them early and link the mother linked to mental health services or, if unavailable, support within her own community. The death of the mother, and to a lesser extent of the father, significantly increases the risk of death of the child, particularly in the early years of life. It is paramount to consider the newborn health within the health of its family.

Personal Mental Health

Lastly, remember to take care of yourself. You may be faced with more deaths than you have ever experienced previously, and from conditions that would most likely be preventable or treatable in a high-resource setting. Before leaving to work in these difficult contexts, reflect on how you will deal with these challenges. Know that it is normal to feel culpable. It is normal to grieve for the baby and the family. Some people like to write about their experience in a journal, exercise, or share their worries with family and friends. It may help to talk to others who have had similar experiences. If you feel overwhelmed, speak to your supervisor and ask about what type of mental health support is available to you.

Useful additional resources

Healthy Newborn Network [11]
Helping Babies Breathe [4]
Kangaroo care: a practical guide [14]
Neonatal resuscitation program [15]
Prevention of mother to child transmission of HIV protocol [5]
Roadmap to accelerate progress for every newborn in humanitarian settings 2020–2024 [6]

References

1. Newborns: reducing mortality. 2019. Available from: https://www.who.int/news-room/fact-sheets/detail/newborns-reducing-mortality.
2. Interagency Working Group on Reproductive Health in Crises. Newborn health in humanitarian settings: fieldguide. New York: WHO, UNICEF, Save the Children; 2018.
3. American Academy of Pediatrics Section on Breastfeeding. Breastfeeding and the use of human milk. Pediatrics. 2012;129(3):e827–41.
4. Helping babies breathe provider guide 2016. 2nd ed. Elk Grove Village, IL: American Academy of Pediatrics; 2016.
5. MSF International AIDS Working Group. Prevention of mother-to-child transmission (PMTCT) of HIV protocol. Geneva: Médecins Sans Frontères; 2017.
6. Roadmap to accelerate progress for every newborn in humanitarian settings 2020–2024. Save the Children, UNICEF, WHO, UNHCR; 2020.
7. WHO recommendations on antenatal care for a positive pregnancy experience. Geneva: WHO; 2016.
8. Bottineau MC, Spector J. Neonatology. In: Kravitz AS, van Tulleken X, editors. Oxford handbook of humanitarian medicine. 1st ed. Oxford: Oxford University Press; 2019. p. ADD. (Oxford handbooks).
9. WHO recommendations on newborn health: guidelines approved by the WHO Guidelines Review Committee. Geneva: WHO; 2017.
10. WHO Reproductive Health Library. WHO recommendation on continuous positive airway pressure therapy for the treatment of preterm newborns with respiratory distress syndrome. 2015.
11. Newborn health in humanitarian settings: toolkit. 2019. Available from: https://www.healthynewbornnetwork.org/resource/toolkit/.
12. World Health Organization. Guideline: delayed umbilical cord clamping for improved maternal and infant health and nutrition outcomes. Geneva: WHO; 2014. Available from: http://www.ncbi.nlm.nih.gov/books/NBK310511/.
13. World Health Organization. WHO recommendations on interventions to improve preterm birth outcomes. Geneva: World Health Organization; 2015.
14. Kangaroo mother care: a practical guide. WHO; 2003.
15. AAP. Neonatal resuscitation program. Available from: https://www.aap.org/en-us/continuing-medical-education/life-support/NRP/Pages/NRP.aspx.

16. European Resuscitation Council. Available from: https://cprguidelines.eu/.
17. APLS: Advanced pediatric life support resources. Available from: https://apls.org.au/resources.
18. APLS Newborn life support. Available from: https://apls.org.au/sites/default/files/uploaded-files/Newborn%20life%20support.pdf.
19. WHO. Malaria in infants. 2018. Available from: https://www.who.int/malaria/areas/high_risk_groups/infants/en/.
20. UNICEF. Infant feeding in emergencies module 2. 2007. Available from: https://www.ennonline.net/ifemodule2.
21. Edmond K, Bahl R, Organisation mondiale de la santé. Optimal feeding of low-birth-weight infants: technical review. Geneva: World Health Organization; 2007.
22. Thwaites CL, Beeching NJ, Newton CR. Maternal and neonatal tetanus. Lancet. 2015;385(9965):362–70.
23. Slusher TM, Vreman HJ, Olusanya BO, Wong RJ, Brearley AM, Vaucher YE, et al. Safety and efficacy of filtered sunlight in treatment of jaundice in African neonates. Pediatrics. 2014;133(6):e1568–74.

Ante Wind, MD is a general pediatrician with an interest in global and immigrant health. She completed medical school at the University of Virginia and pediatric specialty training at Virginia Commonwealth University. Dr. Wind spent 6 years working for Médecins Sans Frontières in various roles including clinical pediatrician, deputy medical coordinator, and pediatric educator. She was based in Haiti, Honduras, Niger, South Sudan, the DRC, Tanzania, and Switzerland. She now lives in Washington, DC and works at the Upper Cardozo Clinic of Unity Health Care and at the National Institutes of Health.

Daniel Martinez Garcia, MD, MPH is a pediatrician and Pediatric Advisor in the Medical Department of Médecins Sans Frontières (MSF), GVA, Switzerland. He is clinical coordinator of MSF's Telemedicine platform and part of MSF's Paediatric Days organizing committee. He is an affiliate of the Johns Hopkins School of Public Health Centre for Humanitarian Medicine, as well as Chair of the Strategic Advisory Group for Children in Disasters for the International Paediatric Association (IPA). He has participated in the AAP Pediatrics in Disasters Course. He received his medical degree from UNAM, Mexico City, completed pediatric residency training at INP, Mexico City, and an MPH from Johns Hopkins Bloomberg School of Public Health, Baltimore, MD. His research focus is pediatric care in resource-limited, humanitarian and disaster settings, telemedicine in pediatrics, nutrition in critically ill children, and pediatric early warning systems. He has 15 years of experience in humanitarian and resource-limited settings. In 2016, he founded EveryWhereSchools, an NGO dedicated to Education in Emergencies & Humanitarian crisis.

Burns, Bites, and Stings

Ante Wind

General Overview

When providing care in humanitarian health settings you will likely have to manage various traumatic injuries such as burns, animal bites, and insect stings. Even if your familiarity with managing these conditions is minimal, diligent supportive care is often all that is needed to help your patient recover.

This chapter will cover practical information and technical guidance about burns, animal bites, and insect stings appropriate for a low resource pediatric setting.

Remember that the local community and staff will often be able to share valuable information with you. Most likely, they will be familiar with the regional venomous animals and insects. They may know the species names, or at least their descriptions, and their common medical sequelae (e.g., localized symptoms, coagulopathy, or neurotoxicity). They will also be familiar with local cooking and heating practices that may put children at risk for burns.

Take note of the supplies that are available to you. Advocate for your organization to have the minimum standard supplies for the management of burns, bites, and stings as these are common injuries in these contexts.

Burns

Overview

An estimated 180,000 people die from burn injuries annually. The vast majority of victims are from low- and middle-income countries. Children are particularly vulnerable, dying from burns seven times more frequently than in high-income countries [1]. Burns occur more often in low resource settings because there are fewer

A. Wind (✉)
Unity Health Care, Washington, DC, USA

© Springer Nature Switzerland AG 2021
C. Harkensee et al. (eds.), *Child Refugee and Migrant Health*,
https://doi.org/10.1007/978-3-030-74906-4_29

mandated electrical safety precautions, more primitive living conditions and heat sources, higher risk cooking conditions, and more frequent placement of young girls in household roles such as cooking and childcare [1, 2].

Prevention

Identify the main causes of burns in your community and include burn prevention and first aid treatment as part of a health promotion strategy. Providing safer stoves, fuels, and fire-retardant aprons can decrease the incidence of burns, as can advocating for safer shelters and fire safety measures within refugee camps or other resettlement locations [1]. Remember that burns can be intentional. Always consider the possibility of child abuse.

Management

Burns can result from direct flames, scalding with hot liquids, inhalation from smoke, or exposure to chemicals or electricity. While there are some differences in care per underlying cause, the general approach is similar. For most pediatric burns you will need soap, clean water, gauze, antibiotic ointment, petroleum jelly, tetanus vaccine, and possibly intravenous (IV) fluids. As a last case resort, if you do not have some of these supplies, be creative (see Figs. 29.1, 29.2, 29.3). Your diligent care is better than no care at all. You can use boiled clean cloths or clean cotton balls instead of gauze, and unscented petroleum jelly and povidone when you have no antibiotic ointment.

The fundamentals of initial care, whether inpatient or outpatient, include the following, all of which are explained in further detail below: safety and first aid, airway management, treatment of pain, wound irrigation and debridement, wound evaluation and dressing, fluid resuscitation, and appropriate disposition to the hospital,

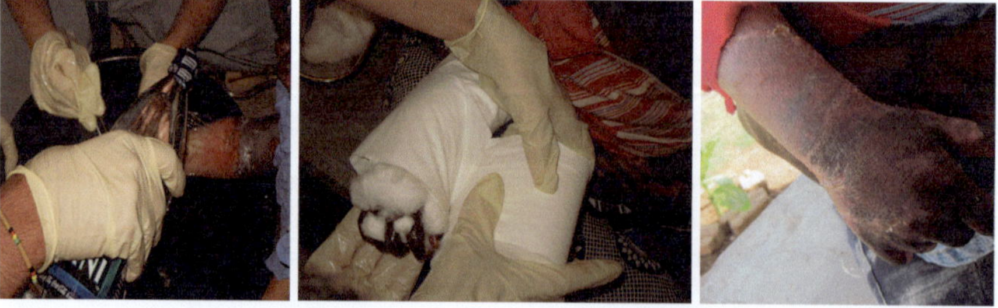

Figs. 29.1, 29.2, 29.3 Creative burn management with minimal supplies: Debridement of second-degree burns with tweezers and punctured water bottle, dressing with antibiotic cream, cotton wool, and toilet paper (later covered with cloth), healing injury several weeks later. (Photo credit Ante Wind)

home, or referral center. Most importantly, hygiene and diligence in treatment are critical.

Risk factors for mortality include larger total body surface area (%TBSA) involved, inhalation injury, multi-organ failure, age <4 years old, non-accidental burns, and infection [3].

Safety and First Aid

The first step in burn management is to ensure that both you and the patient are safe. In the case of chemical burns, ensure that medical personnel is wearing personal protective equipment if available. Make sure that the fire is contained and that there is no active electrical current. Remove any constricting jewelry or clothing. Remember to "cool the burns and warm the patient," by managing the wound while at the same time ensuring that the child does not become hypothermic [3]. If it is a chemical burn, submerge or soak the affected area in water to dilute the strength of the chemical. Do not apply ice to any burns as this can damage the tissue.

Airway Management

Next, evaluate the airway. Any soot around the nares, stridor, hoarseness, or tinged nasal hairs may indicate inhalation injury, which needs special attention to ensure that the patient maintains a patent airway. Because children have much smaller airways than adults, any degree of swelling can quickly lead to airway obstruction. In many refugee and migrant settings, oxygen and intubation are not available, but simple maneuvers like the jaw thrust and chin lift can help maintain an open airway [3].

Pain Management

Pain can be managed with acetaminophen (paracetamol), NSAIDS, ketorolac, opioids (if available), or non-pharmaceutical measures. Codeine is not indicated in children [3]. The itching that develops as the wound heals can be treated with petroleum jelly, diphenhydramine, or hydroxyzine [3]. Elevation of the wound will help prevent edema and improve pain control [2]. Consider how you can minimize discomfort, whether via medications or other techniques, prior to every dressing change. The chapter on non-pharmaceutical pain management can offer you further guidance.

Irrigation and Debridement

Irrigate the wound with copious amounts of lukewarm normal saline or clean water with soap. In case of a chemical burn, irrigate the wound as long as possible to stop any continued burning. Next, with clean dry gauze, or clean cloths if you do not have gauze, debride any dead tissue. The care of blisters is debatable: some advocate for removal of blisters and others advocate for leaving them intact. However, all agree that if the fluid is cloudy or if the blister limits mobility, the blister membrane should be removed [4]. Check the distal extremities for perfusion and capillary refill.

Wound Evaluation and Calculation of the %TBSA Burned

While you are irrigating and debriding, evaluate the wound to determine if it is superficial, partial thickness, or full thickness, and simultaneously make a rough estimate of the %TBSA burned.

Superficial wounds are dry and painful, partial thickness burns are wet and painful, and full thickness burns are dry and insensate or have visible bone and muscle [2]. Wounds may evolve over the first few days, and a wound that initially looks like a partial thickness burn may evolve into a full thickness burn [2].

While examining the burn, you should also calculate the %TBSA affected. This will help determine proper management and prognosis. The %TBSA constitutes the percent of the body covered by partial or full thickness burns only, not superficial burns [4]. For children, a quick and easy rule of thumb is that the child's palm will equal 1% of their TBSA. This can help you get a rough calculation of the %TBSA affected. If less than 15% of the TBSA is involved, the burn does not include the face, hands, or feet, the child is able to drink, and he/she has access to transportation for proper follow-up, then the burn can be managed in an outpatient setting [3]. If greater than 15% TBSA is affected, or when in doubt, refer the patient for hospitalization as quickly as possible. If there is no referral hospital, do the best you can with what you have. The care you provide in the most hygienic environment possible will be better than no care at all.

Dressing and Further Management

Once the burn is debrided, cover the freshly debrided burn with an antibiotic ointment. There is no added value of using povidone/iodine [3].

The dressing should have three layers. The first layer is a contact (or non-adherent) layer, like gauze (or cotton wool if no gauze available) covered in unscented petroleum jelly. If necessary, even cling wrap can suffice as a non-adherent dressing [3]. If the burns involve the fingers or toes, separate the digits with non-adherent dressing to prevent the digits from adhering to one another. The second layer should be an absorbent layer, for example, a clean, dry, fluffed gauze (or, if necessary, cotton wool or additional clean and dry boiled cloths). The third layer is a holding layer to ensure a clean and moist environment optimal for wound healing. For this layer you can use a mesh netting, a roll of gauze, or a clean tube sock with the end cut off [4]. Alternatively, in the inpatient setting, if hygienic conditions can be maintained, the burns can be covered only with a clean damp towel instead of gauze wraps. The child's bed should be covered with a mosquito net [4].

Initially, the dressing should be changed daily. You can decrease the frequency if the wound is healing well without signs of infection and as long as the absorbent dressing does not become soaked with exudate. The dressings should not dry out between dressing changes as this may cause freshly healing skin to tear, making wound care much more painful.

Once there is only healthy tissue and no signs of infection, antibacterial ointment is no longer needed, and you can proceed with simple wound care using non-adherent dressings and overlying dry gauze. Most burns will heal within 3 weeks.

For outpatient cases, remember to take the time to teach the parents about how to maintain a clean wound dressing plus how to recognize the signs of infection: fever, malaise, site erythema, swelling, and drainage [2].

Antibiotics and Tetanus

Prophylactic antibiotics are not indicated for burns. Fevers in the first 3 days are often due to inflammatory mediators rather than infections. After 3 days, fevers likely indicate infection [3]. Remember to provide a tetanus vaccine (±tetanus immunoglobulin) for anyone with less than three doses of tetanus vaccine or anyone vaccinated more than 5 years ago [3]. If there is no tetanus vaccine available in your clinic, work with the ministry of health or camp coordination to find out if other organizations have the tetanus vaccine and refer the patient.

Fluid Management

After a severe burn, there is a massive release of inflammatory mediators leading to capillary leak. This, in addition to evaporative loss from damaged skin, means that if there is greater than 15–20% of TBSA involved, the child should be managed in a hospital where intravenous (IV) fluids can be administered, and urine output can be monitored.

For children weighing less than 40 kg, to determine the volume of Lactated Ringers (LR) that should be administered over the first 24 hours after the burn, multiply 2–4 × %TBSA burned × weight (in kg) [4]. Half of that volume should be administered over the first 8 hours, and the remainder over the next 16 hours. Additionally, administer the regular D5LR maintenance fluids which can be calculated using the 4:2:1 rule outlined in the box below [5]. If IV access cannot be obtained, fluids via nasogastric (NG) tube can be given [2]. If you do not have LR, Normal Saline (NS) will suffice.

These formulas are a good starting point but ultimately fluids should be titrated up or down with the goal of having the child void 0.5–1 ml/kg/h [2].

The 4:2:1 Rule of Hourly Pediatric Maintenance Fluids [5]

Weight (kg)	Hourly
<10	4 ml/kg/kg
10–20	40 ml + 2 ml/kg for every kg >10 kg
>20	60 ml + 1 ml/kg for every kg >20 kg

Nutrition

The importance of nutrition cannot be overstated. In larger burns, the metabolic rate and cardiac output of the child increase substantially [2]. Providing good nutrition early will decrease the risk of gastrointestinal bleeding, treat unrecognized hypoglycemia, and improve wound healing [3]. The food should be high in protein content, and if available, supplementation with multivitamins, calcium, folic acid, and iron should be given if needed. Consider adding a proton pump inhibitor in higher risk children4].

Disposition

Whether or not you refer the patient to a higher level of care will depend on the capacity of your own health center and the availability of a referral surgical or burn center. Regardless of disposition, management of severe burns is resource intensive in any setting and requires diligent attention to hygiene, analgesia, and systemic support.

If you do not have access to a higher level of care and/or IV fluids, create a separate space to provide proper burn care and avoid cross-contamination. Focus on rehydrating and maintaining hydration via oral fluids, like ORS (oral rehydration solution). Monitor the heart rate and urine output to guide your fluid management. Collect urine in a soda bottle or any available vessel. Even if you can not measure the urine, the color can help you determine hydration status.

Bites and Stings

Overview

Animal bites and stings are a common occurrence in migrant and refugee settings. Crowded, unhygienic conditions, poor lighting, tasks such as searching for firewood and water, and location of camp setting are just some examples of the factors that may increase the risk of animal and insect bites and stings. Below we will discuss the prevention and management of animal-related injuries that you may encounter.

Prevention

Several strategies can be implemented to prevent animal and insect bites. If providing support to camps, consider preventative measures as part of camp set-up; ensure good lighting and clear spaces around toilets and kitchen areas. If possible, advise long sleeve shirts to minimize insect bites and advise/provide footwear to prevent snake and scorpion bites. Inexpensive footwear can even be made using old car tires. To prevent scorpion bites, shoes and clothing should be shaken out before being worn. Vibrations (feet stamping, hitting the ground with a stick) and noise disturb snakes, and often they will move away from oncoming humans. Debris on the floor should be minimized. Proper rubbish collection will prevent food scrap build-up and thus decrease insect infestations and help prevent mice, and subsequently snakes, from coming into homes or shelters.

If possible, provide and encourage the use of insect repellent and mosquito nets tucked underneath the mattress. Mosquito nets prevent not only insect bites but also bites from scorpions, snakes, and bats. Larger preventative interventions, that may not always be possible in migrant and refugee settings, include vector management such as insecticide spraying and optimizing housing conditions.

To ameliorate the impact of any traumatic injury, work with the local medical community to ensure that tetanus vaccinations are offered to all refugees and migrants. Ideally, local dogs should be vaccinated against rabies.

Management

Dogs, Cats, and Humans

Depending on the location, dog bites can be very common and pose a great risk for localized infections and more serious consequences such as rabies or tetanus. If there is a cluster of patients with dog bites, consider that there may be one rabid dog on the loose.

General care for any dog, cat, or human bite includes extensive and meticulous irrigation and debridement of the entire wound. There is no need to use alcohol or other disinfectants [5]. In general, avoid primary closure of an animal bite. If there is a very deep wound you can close the deeper tissues with stitches, leaving the remainder of the wound open for several days after which you can perform a secondary closure [5].

Always provide prophylactic antibiotics, such as amoxicillin clavulanate, that cover staphylococcus species and anaerobes. Most importantly, provide postexposure prophylaxis for tetanus and rabies. Refer to the tetanus guidelines for dirty wounds to determine whether or not to give the tetanus vaccine. Unless the victim is vaccinated against rabies you will need to provide both rabies vaccine and rabies immune globulin since it is unlikely that an animal in a refugee setting has been vaccinated. If there is no tetanus vaccine or rabies vaccine and immunoglobulin available in your clinic, work with the ministry of health or camp coordination to find out if other organizations have them and refer the patient.

Monkeys

Monkey bites are managed similarly to other animal and human bites with one exception. Macaques are known to carry Herpes B Virus, which can lead to fatal encephalomyelitis in humans. In case of monkey bite, scratch, or mucosal exposure to monkey secretions, treat as above and also consider prophylaxis with acyclovir [6].

Bats

Bats are ubiquitous, living in all continents except Antarctica. Bats are vectors for rabies along with other less common zoonotic diseases. Human bat bites occur at night and the person bitten may not even wake but simply find a bleeding wound with a double puncture site. Children are particularly vulnerable [7]. Upon presentation of a child with a bat bite, wash the wound thoroughly and if available, rabies vaccine and rabies immunoglobulin should be administered. Once a patient displays clinical symptoms of rabies, the disease is almost always fatal.

Snakes

The WHO estimates that there are 5 million snakebites annually resulting in 81,000–138,000 deaths, plus 400,000 amputations every year. Children disproportionately suffer from snakebites because of their small body mass. Although antivenom is part of the WHO Essential Medications list, due to limited global supply and prohibitive cost, it is difficult for many countries to obtain the appropriate antivenom for their region. For these reasons, since June of 2017, snakebites are now officially considered a neglected tropical disease in need of better treatment options including improved access to antivenom [8].

In regions where snakebites are a common occurrence, local staff should be able to provide insight into which species are common and their respective medical sequelae.

Depending on the species, snakebite envenomation may cause clotting problems, local swelling and pain, or neurotoxicity with paralysis of the respiratory muscles. Please refer to the Oxford Handbook of Humanitarian Medicine for a detailed outline of the different snake species and the typical presentation of their respective bites [9].

While management may differ slightly per species, in general, you can treat all bites using a similar approach. Start by removing any constricting jewelry or clothing. Then rinse the wound copiously with clean water. Do not cut or apply suction to the bite and do not use an artery constricting tourniquet. Immobilize the limb and if you are far from a health center, construct a simple stretcher to bring the patient to a health center. If it is a neurotoxic venomous snake, you can apply a pressure bandage to the limb to prevent systemic spread of the venom [9]. Create a pressure bandage by wrapping an ace bandage from the toes to the groin (or fingers to axilla). This has to be done carefully, it should be neither too tight nor too loose. A finger should easily slide under the bandage [10]. If it is not a neurotoxic venomous snake, then a simple pressure bandage can be placed [9].

In addition to wound care, pain should be managed with acetaminophen or even opioids. Avoid ibuprofen or other NSAIDS because they may exacerbate bleeding. If the snake has been killed, take a photo, or bring it with you, to help identify the species.

During transport, place the victim on his/her left side to prevent aspiration in case of vomiting [7].

Upon arrival to a medical center, once medically stabilized, or once the antivenom has been administered, the pressure bandage should be slowly and carefully removed [10]. All symptoms should be treated symptomatically. You may need to manage limb swelling, hypovolemia, kidney failure, respiratory failure, and/or localized infection. Anaphylactic symptoms can be treated with adrenaline and antihistamines [7].

In limb or life-threatening situations, antivenom should be administered if available [8]. General indications include spontaneous bleeding, prolonged clotting time, shock, paralysis, or swelling of over half of the bitten extremity. However, each antivenom will have its own specific indications for use [9]. Unfortunately, antivenom is prohibitively expensive, requires a working cold chain, and is limited in supply worldwide, especially for the types of snakes present in sub-Saharan Africa. If it is available to you and indicated, be prepared to treat anaphylaxis and note that you may need to give repeated doses [9]. Neurologic symptoms should start to subside within 30–60 min and bleeding disorders should start to improve after 6 h [7].

When feasible, all patients should be observed in a medical facility for 24 h because the presentation of symptoms may vary by species [7].

Scorpions

Scorpions are prevalent throughout tropical and subtropical regions. They are most active at night and tend to hide under rocks, branches, shoes, and anything on the floor during the day. Scorpions are not predatory towards humans and bites are usually accidental.

Different scorpion species will cause different constellations of symptoms. Because of children's smaller body mass, they are at higher risk for more severe symptoms. A bite can cause excruciating pain and swelling, severe abdominal pain, muscle twitching, tachycardia, dysrhythmias, pulmonary edema, and in certain cases neurologic manifestations such as slurred speech, eye deviation, seizures, and life-threatening paralysis of respiratory muscles [9]. You may not be able to see a sting mark. Symptoms usually resolve within 48 h.

Treatment starts with removing the stinger. The pain should then be treated. For minimal pain NSAIDS can be used, but in many cases local infiltration of lidocaine and possibly opioids are needed to dull the pain. For the remaining symptoms, provide wound care and supportive management. Antihistamines and steroids may be helpful. In some centers, you may have access to an antivenom [9].

Marine Animals

Depending on your location, you may need to treat injuries caused by venomous marine animals such as stonefish, jellyfish, man-o-war, and others. Symptoms of stings caused by these animals can range from an itchy rash to a sharp, agonizing pain with localized swelling, to severe systemic symptoms and even death. It is often difficult to be certain which type of animal has stung the patient, but management is similar. The venom can be neutralized by placing the stung body part in hot, not scalding water. Treat pain with pharmacologic and non-pharmacologic methods. For severe pain, you can consider injection of local anesthetic around the wound. All other symptoms should be treated with supportive care [7].

Mosquitos

Mosquitos not only transmit malaria but also dengue, chikungunya, zika virus, yellow fever, and other diseases. All refugee and migrant families and staff should have access to a mosquito net in areas where these diseases are endemic. Widespread insecticide spraying may also be available. For more detail, refer to the infectious disease chapter.

Wasps and Bees

Wasp and bee stings should be treated with ice and pain control using NSAIDs and acetaminophen (paracetamol). Remove the stinger by carefully scraping the skin with a nail or dry gauze. If there is constricting jewelry on the bitten limb it should be removed. Elevate the affected limb to prevent swelling. Scratching will aggravate symptoms and should be avoided as much as possible. If there is an anaphylactic reaction, treat with IM epinephrine. If no epinephrine is available, treat with diphenhydramine and provide supportive care.

Spider

Toxicity of a spider bite depends on the species and region. Management is supportive including analgesics and, if needed, muscle relaxants. Please refer to the Oxford Handbook of Humanitarian Medicine for further information on different spider bites and their respective management [9].

Ticks

Ticks are vectors for numerous diseases and should be removed as soon as possible. Remove with fine tipped tweezers by grasping the tick close to the skin, do not squeeze the body. Slowly and steadily pull upwards, do not twist as this can cause the mouthpiece to break off. If it does break off, leave it, do not dig into the skin to retrieve it. Once the tick is removed, clean the wound with soap and water and drown the tick in rubbing alcohol or throw it down a toilet or latrine [11].

Scabies and Bedbugs

Scabies is caused by the bite of the insect Sarcoptes scabiei. It presents as small, exquisitely pruritic papules, linearly arranged, typically in areas such as the webs of the fingers, wrists, the waistline, and the lateral and posterior aspects of the feet. In severe cases, children may present with diffuse crusted scabies. It is treated with agents such as topical permethrin, benzyl benzoate, or, in children weighing more than 15 kg, oral ivermectin. Make sure to provide specific instructions to the parents about how to apply the topical solutions and how quickly to wash it off as this varies by age. All affected family members should be treated at the same time. Bedding and clothes should be washed in hot water or sealed in a bag for at least 72 h. Scabies outbreaks are common in crowded conditions and, if needed, can be managed with mass drug administration of ivermectin.

Bedbug bites present as batches of erythematous pruritic papules. Some patients will develop large wheals around the individual bites. Treat with antipruritic agents and provide guidance to the family about eradication of the bedbugs. Bedbugs can spread rapidly in a crowded camp setting and all effort should be made to help the family eradicate these insects to prevent spread to other shelters and families.

Chagas Disease

Chagas disease, or American Trypanosomiasis, is a vector-borne disease caused by the parasite Trypanosoma cruzi which is spread by the triatomine insect or in rare cases by vertical transmission from mother to child or via blood transfusion. Only 5% of infected patients will present with acute symptoms but 30–40% will go on to develop chronic cardiac or gastrointestinal Chagas disease which may not present until 10–30 years after initial infection [12]. It is the most common cause of cardiomyopathy in Latin America [12].

Both diagnosis and treatment of Chagas disease are complicated. Antibody tests are the most accurate, but in resource limited settings these may not be available. The parasite can be visualized directly on a blood smear but only during the first 6 weeks after infection, while the parasite burden is high. All children with clinical suspicion of infection should be treated with either benznidazole or nifurtimox. Please note that these drugs have significant risks of side effects including skin manifestations [12].

Sleeping in insecticide impregnated bed nets, tucked under the mattress, plus vector control via insecticide spraying and better housing conditions are effective to minimize exposure to the triatomine insect and subsequent infection [12].

References

1. WHO. Burns. 2018. Available from: https://www.who.int/news-room/fact-sheets/detail/burns.
2. Sheridan R. Burn care for children. Pediatr Rev. 2018;39(6):273–86.
3. Strobel A, Fay R. Emergency care of pediatric burns. Emerg Med Clin N Am. 2018;36(2):441–58.
4. Beveridge M. Burns. In: Kravitz AS, van Tulleken X, editors. Oxford handbook of humanitarian medicine. 1st ed. Oxford, Oxford University Press; 2019. p. 921–48. (Oxford handbooks).
5. Harriet Lane Service (Johns Hopkins Hospital), Flerlage J, Engorn B, Johns Hopkins Hospital, Children's Medical and Surgical Center. The Harriet Lane handbook: a manual for pediatric house officers. 2015 [cited 2019 Nov 4]. Available from: https://www.clinicalkey.com/dura/browse/bookChapter/3-s2.0-C20110078213.
6. Cohen JI, Davenport DS, Stewart JA, Deitchman S, Hilliard JK, Chapman LE, et al. Recommendations for prevention of and therapy for exposure to B virus (Cercopithecine Herpesvirus). Clin Infect Dis. 2002;35(10):1191–203.
7. Warrell DA. Animals hazardous to humans. In: Hunter's tropical medicine and emerging infectious disease. Elsevier; 2013 [cited 2020 Apr 22]. p. 938–65. Available from: https://linkinghub.elsevier.com/retrieve/pii/B978141604390400134X.
8. World Health Organization. Snakebite envenoming. 2019. Available from: https://www.who.int/snakebites/disease/en/.
9. Warrell D. Venomous animal bites and stings and marine poisoning. In: Kravitz AS, van Tulleken X, editors. Oxford handbook of humanitarian medicine. 1st ed. Oxford: Oxford University Press; 2019. p. 555–68. (Oxford handbooks).
10. Parker-Cote J, Meggs W. First aid and pre-hospital management of venomous snakebites. Trop Med Infect Dis. 2018;3(2):45.
11. Tick removal. https://www.cdc.gov/ticks/removing_a_tick.html.
12. Franco-Paredes C. American trypanosomiasis. In: Manson's tropical infectious diseases. Elsevier; 2014 [cited 2020 Apr 22]. p. 622–30.e1. Available from: https://linkinghub.elsevier.com/retrieve/pii/B9780702051012000479.

Ante Wind, MD is a general pediatrician with an interest in global and immigrant health. She completed medical school at the University of Virginia and pediatric specialty training at Virginia Commonwealth University. Dr. Wind spent 6 years working for Médecins Sans Frontières in various roles including clinical pediatrician, deputy medical coordinator, and pediatric educator. She was based in Haiti, Honduras, Niger, South Sudan, the DRC, Tanzania, and Switzerland. She now lives in Washington, DC and works at the Upper Cardozo Clinic of Unity Health Care and at the National Institutes of Health.

Managing Epilepsy in Low Resource Settings

30

Venkateswaran Ramesh

Introduction

The management of epilepsy in resource-limited settings is particularly challenging due to often very limited diagnostic and treatment options. Because misdiagnosis or mismanagement may have severe detrimental effects, it is relevant to look at epilepsy management in more detail.

It is known that epilepsy affects far more people in low and middle income than in high-income countries, mainly due to a higher incidence of birth complications, infections, and head trauma; yet the "treatment gap"—the proportion of people with epilepsy who receive no treatment—is over 75% in most low-income countries as identified by the World Health Organization. There are likely to be added difficulties in epilepsy care in refugee and disaster settings, analogous to the challenges faced in low-income countries where many refugees will be from. There may be significant societal prejudice against epilepsy due to low levels of understanding among the general population and significant stigma, which leads to under reporting of symptoms and choosing to hide away people suffering from seizures, even when treatment costs are low or free. Beyond the cultural barriers are the logistic difficulties relating to the availability of trained personnel, diagnostic tests, and treatments; for example, personnel trained in managing childhood epilepsy, electroencephalography, and brain imaging, which are cornerstones in epilepsy diagnosis in western settings, may only be available in big city hospitals. Only a fraction of a large number of anti-epilepsy drugs (AEDs) may be available, and only in limited formulations for administration thus making treatment of seizure disorders more challenging—as well as giving emergency treatments where intravenous access and suitable preparations are often required.

V. Ramesh (✉)
King's College Hospital, London, UK
e-mail: venkateswaranramesh@nhs.net; venkateswaran.ramesh@icloud.net

© Springer Nature Switzerland AG 2021

C. Harkensee et al. (eds.), *Child Refugee and Migrant Health*,
https://doi.org/10.1007/978-3-030-74906-4_30

Despite these difficulties, the importance of appropriately managing seizures, epilepsy, and identifying non-epileptic phenomena (where unnecessary diagnostic investigations and treatments could be avoided) cannot be underestimated and should be emphasized to health care personnel and parents of children in refugee camps. This includes raising awareness of the risks of serious accidents during epileptic seizures like drowning, falls, and sustaining burns as well as sudden death with untreated epilepsy, developmental delay, and cognitive impairment in severe untreated epilepsy. It is also important to understand and recognize psychogenic non-epileptic seizures (sometimes called "pseudoseizures") in children who have had traumatic experiences which are very likely in this setting.

The information contained in this chapter was gleaned from the compilation of resources listed in the Further Reading section.

Epilepsy, or Not Epilepsy?

A **seizure** is any event which seizes the patient suddenly. It includes both epileptic and non-epileptic seizures. A **convulsion** refers to an attack of generalized shaking/jerking that involves the trunk and all four limbs. It is a nonspecific term and can refer to both epileptic and non-epileptic events. The terms seizure, convulsion, and fits are often synonymously used by the lay public in this context.

Epilepsy is a problem where the brain spontaneously produces sudden and recurrent bursts of abnormal electrical activity that result in recurrent seizures; in these, the brain and associated structures spontaneously generate them rather than being in response to an external trigger. Patients need to have had at least two similar or stereotyped attacks before they can be labeled epileptic. If a child has had only one epileptic seizure, he or she cannot be said to have epilepsy, as another attack may never occur. It is important to educate parents of children in refugee camps about this key difference between seizures and epilepsy, owing to the stigma and prejudice associated with the condition. It is also worth emphasizing that epilepsy is not due to a single cause; many different conditions affecting the brain can lead to epilepsy. The causes can be genetic or due to acquired brain injury.

In non-epileptic seizures, the primary event is not a spontaneously occurring abnormal electrical discharge originating in the brain. In infancy, childhood, and adolescence a wide variety of non-epileptic seizures occur commonly and form the majority compared with true epileptic seizures. There are a number of conditions that mimic (or look like) epilepsy and when an individual presents with such a seizure, they may be mistaken for epileptic seizures, through they are not associated with a spontaneous electrical discharge arising in the brain. They include the following:

- Febrile seizures
- Fainting/syncope
- Cardiac rhythm disturbances causing syncope
- Breath-holding attacks (blue and white/pallid) resulting in syncope
- Jitteriness in newborn babies, e.g., due to hypoglycemia, hypothermia, sepsis

- Benign sleep myoclonus
- Benign "tonic upgaze" of infancy
- Behavioral "stereotypies"
- Day dreaming
- Benign nervous tics
- Benign paroxysmal vertigo
- Migraine
- Altered/Dissociated mental states due to overwhelming psychological stress

Further details on distinguishing these different types of epileptic and non-epileptic seizures are provided in the Appendix, describing the observed symptoms and principles of medical management.

Clinical Assessment of Seizure Disorders

A careful history and witness account is the cornerstone of making a diagnosis of epilepsy or its many mimics. The history and examination may be all that is possible in resource poor settings. Hence, time spent in this exercise will be invaluable. The most important information that helps distinguishing these different types of seizures is an accurate account from an eyewitness, ideally accompanied by a video recording (e.g., mobile phone) of the event. Important features to ask for include:

- Was the seizure triggered by something?
- What were the symptoms at the start (e.g., losing consciousness, changing color, floppy/stiff)?
- Good description of the movements (which parts of the body, how did they move?) and how long they lasted.
- What did the eyes do?
- Was the face involved?
- Was there a head turn to one side or another?
- Was the child completely unconscious, semi-conscious, or awake? If consciousness was affected, for how long?
- Was the child incontinent?
- Was the patient drowsy/sleepy/non-rousable after movements stopped, if so for how long? Did they vomit afterwards?
- Is there a family history of seizures?
- Does the child have a history of developmental delay, past history of meningitis, head trauma? Any difficulties during pregnancy, delivery, or during the newborn period?

To make a confident *clinical diagnosis* of epilepsy, the patient must fulfill the following criteria

- Attacks are recurrent; should have had more than 1 or 2 seizure events

- Attacks are stereotyped
- Patient is rhythmically shaking or jerking with or without alteration of conscious level
- Attacks occur without fever

"A picture is worth a thousand words" as the old saying goes… Some parents even in refugee camps and war zones may possibly possess a smartphone or someone known to the patient may have a smartphone. If they are able to obtain a video of the child's attack and show it to a health care professional or a medical practitioner, it can be helpful in making a diagnosis of epilepsy without an EEG. Some humanitarian organizations run a telemedicine service with remote access to a specialist.

General examination looking for tell-tale birthmarks may indicate a neurocutaneous condition like Tuberous sclerosis or Neurofibromatosis and should be specifically looked for.

Many low resource settings may not have access to investigations, but if possible fasting blood sugar and calcium estimations as well as an ECG with a rhythm strip should be obtained in all patients who give a history of generalized convulsive seizures. The ECG helps the diagnosis of a cardiac rhythm disorder causing brain hypoperfusion and hypoxia leading to seizures. The commonest cardiac dysrhythmia misdiagnosed as epilepsy is the "Long QT" Syndrome which is estimated to occur in 1/2000 live births worldwide with no sex or ethnic predilection.

When the history and examination point to epilepsy as being probable, an EEG will be very helpful. It is extremely unlikely that one will have access to such tests in refugee camps or disaster areas, where the history, examination, and accompanying video is pivotal.

While the majority of typical presentations of epilepsy can be reasonably and reliably diagnosed on history and examination alone, the lack of access to further diagnostics by way of ECG, EEG, or brain scanning can lead to potential consequences in a small minority of cases. Firstly, there is the risk of missing a cardiac cause, e.g., dysrhythmia which could be potentially fatal and where anti-epilepsy drugs will not help. Secondly, there is a risk of misdiagnosing benign childhood movement disorders of non-epileptic origin, or psychological distress manifested as non-epileptic functional seizures, and consequent inappropriate administration of anti-epilepsy drugs which can have undesirable side effects, e.g., drowsiness, impaired mental functioning. Finally, though very unusual as a cause of seizures in children and people under the age of 40 years, tumors affecting the cerebral cortex can present as focal epilepsy and in their early stages there may be no focal neurological signs. In these cases, lack of access to brain imaging which is done more routinely in western settings could miss these.

One of the main advantages of modern telemedicine is the potential to share video clips easily by Whatsapp or similar software to consult with specialists in epilepsies of children and adults who are based remotely, and who would be more than happy to advise and offer diagnostic steer where there is uncertainty among health workers on the ground.

Management

Holistic management involves a confident diagnosis of epilepsy, exclusion of non-epileptic seizures, in particular, cardiac syncope and resulting anoxic seizures. Treatment is aimed at stopping the seizures and patient and parental education. Untreated and unmanaged epilepsy is a major cause for developmental delay, poor educational attainment, low quality of life, and stigmatization or exclusion.

Over 80% of children and adults diagnosed with epilepsy respond to an appropriately chosen anti-epilepsy drug (AED) to prevent further seizures. The drug regime should be kept simple and it is seldom necessary to use more than 2 AEDs. Ideally treatment with a single AED (monotherapy) is preferred. Optimal dosage and incidence of side effects vary between individuals.

It is important that you consider long-term availability and affordability in your setting of the medication you are intending to start. It may be better to start a medication that may be less effective but more easily available, than another that is more effective but runs out of supply or cannot be afforded by the patient long-term. Serum anticonvulsant levels are helpful and often necessary in assessing therapy with some but not all AEDs; e.g., Phenytoin, Phenobarbitone, Carbamazepine. However, this may not be available in many settings.

In the resource poor setting, you will be limited by anticonvulsant availability and formulations. Typically only the older broad spectrum AEDs are available, e.g., phenytoin, phenobarbitone, carbamazepine, valproate, and benzodiazepines. While they may be used less often in high resource settings due to their side effect profiles and having access to newer "cleaner" drugs, the older AEDs are highly effective and can be put to good use in the resource poor setting to treat most epilepsies and seizure types.

Phenobarbitone has been used as an AED from the early 1960s is very effective with a broad spectrum of action and can control almost all types of seizures including absence seizures. It is inexpensive and readily available. It is the drug of choice for neonates and infants. It can be given orally and intravenously as a loading dose of 20 mg/kg stat for rapid onset of action in status epilepticus. The recommended maintenance dose is 5–8 mg/kg/day split into 2 doses.

Carbamazepine is another excellent AED and superior to Phenobarbitone beyond infancy. It is very useful in generalized and focal convulsive seizures. The drug must also be started at a low dose and increased slowly each week until a target dose is achieved. The recommended dose is 15–30 mg/kg/day split into 2 doses and taken after food. It is contraindicated in absence seizures as it can make the seizures worse. It has few short- and long-term side effects, the important ones being double vision and tiredness some 30–40 min after administration. It can cause a maculo-papular skin rash in 3–4% of patients, which will worsen on continued use of the drug, in which case it has to be stopped.

Phenytoin is another broad spectrum AED, very useful in convulsive status epilepticus and for control of generalized and focal motor seizures. It has cosmetic side effects, in particular gum hypertrophy, as well as a narrow therapeutic window which requires regular blood monitoring facilities, all of which can limit its use as an AED in chronic epilepsy. It is absorbed well after oral administration and is often given intravenously in status epilepticus. If venous access is not possible 18 mg/kg can be given via nasogastric tube in convulsive status epilepticus. Maintenance dose is 4–6 mg/kg/day given in 2 doses. Its side effects include facial changes, gum hypertrophy, and cerebellar ataxia with toxic blood levels.

Sodium Valproate is another broad spectrum and highly effective AED with few side effects. It is non-sedating. Availability and cost may make it unsuitable in low resource settings. The dose range is 10–40 mg/kg/day split in 2 doses. It must be started at a low dose and titrated up each week to a target level. It takes approximately three months to achieve maximum effect. It is not recommended for children under 3 years in low resource settings as a regular AED.

Diazepam is only useful in convulsive status epilepticus. It is not effective as a regular, preventive medication for epilepsy.

Experience shows that certain types of epileptic seizures respond best to particular AEDs. If the setting allows, the choice can be rationally based on the type of seizures and the epilepsy syndrome.

Anti-epilepsy Drug Therapy

Type of epilepsy	Drug of first choice	Other drugs
Simple absences	Ethosuximide	Valproate, Phenobarbitone
Complex absences	Valproate	Phenobarbitone Lamotrigine, Topiramate, Clonazepam
Myoclonic	Sodium valproate	Benzodiazepines like Clonazepam
Infantile spasms	Vigabatrin or ACTH	Sodium Valproate, Clonazepam or Levetiracetam
Genetic generalized tonic clonic epilepsy	Levetiracetam	Lamotrigine, Topiramate, Valproate, Carbamazepine, Phenobarbitone
Simple partial seizures	Carbamazepine or Phenytoin	Phenytoin
Complex partial seizures	Carbamazepine	Lamotrigine, Topiramate, Levetiracetam, Phenytoin
Secondarily generalized tonic clonic seizures	Carbamazepine	Levetiracetam, Lamotrigine, Topiramate, Phenobarbitone. Phenytoin
Status epilepticus	Rectal Diazepam	Buccal Midazolam, Rectal Paraldehyde, intravenous Diazepam, Midazolam or Lorazepam

Further information on side effects can be found in the Appendix.

How to Start Anti-epilepsy Medication

Keep instructions simple. Dosing of AEDs in the refugee setting can be difficult. It may be difficult to get an accurate weight, patients may not understand or follow complex dose regimes, and time between reviews can be long.

Spend a few minutes educating the patient and his parent/carer regarding epilepsy and the drug you are planning to use. The dose needs to go up weekly and the drug has to be taken regularly and continued for up to 2 years. It should not be stopped suddenly as it can then lead to dangerous convulsive status epilepticus.

For children it is possible to estimate the weight of the child by using the formula:

$$\text{Weight}\left(\text{kg}\right) = \left(\text{Age} + 4\right) \times 2$$

So a 1 year old would normally weigh 10 kg and a 3 year old 14 kg. This formula becomes inaccurate in children who are malnourished. In this instance make an educated guess or reduce the dose for a normal child by 1/3.

For young adults or adolescents, a rough estimate would be 45 kg for a small adult and 60 kg for a taller man or woman. These weights are rough estimates.

An important consideration when prescribing anti-epileptic medication is the strength of tablets available. Check what strength the tablets or liquid formulations are.

Pregnant teenagers and women who are on epilepsy medication should be given folic acid 5 mg daily to prevent birth defects.

Education and Permitted Physical Activities

The majority of children with epilepsy have normal intelligence and have the potential to attend ordinary schools and progress well. However, learning disabilities are more common in children with epilepsy and should be looked for and addressed.

Epilepsy diagnoses often raise considerable fears in parents as well as among other adults who deal with the child. Children with epilepsy do not require much limitation of their activity. They should be advised not to swim unsupervised and should not ride a bicycle in traffic.

Young adults with epilepsy should be cautioned about swimming in open water, handling power tools or heavy machinery, and driving. If they suffer a seizure while being engaged in such activities it can be fatal.

Stopping Anti-epilepsy Drugs

This may be due to side effects, lack of efficacy, or when the patient has been seizure-free for 2 consecutive years when remission of epilepsy is assumed. It should be done slowly over 4–6 weeks. Sudden stopping can lead to convulsive status epilepticus and patients should be warned about this complication.

Prognosis

The overall prognosis for epilepsy is good with modern management. Over two-thirds of children diagnosed as having epilepsy in childhood grow out of their epilepsy in a time frame of 2–5 years. Anti-epilepsy drug therapy can be discontinued if they have been free from attacks for more than 2 years as they are then probably in remission. A minority continue to have epileptic attacks despite anticonvulsant therapy.

Death in Epilepsy

Untreated Epilepsy in resource poor settings carries a significant risk of death due to convulsive status epilepticus, accidents, and drowning. Further risk comes from a rare occurrence and entity called "sudden unexpected death in epilepsy (SUDEP)." Known risk factors for SUDEP include young males, living alone, generalized convulsive seizures, nocturnal seizures, and poor compliance with anti-epilepsy medication.

Status Epilepticus

This is defined as the occurrence of epileptic seizures continuously for a period of 20–30 min. It usually presents with generalized tonic clonic seizures though absence and focal motor and focal dyscognitive status can be seen in a small number of patients.

A convulsing child should be briefly assessed, then one must attempt to stop the convulsion as soon as possible. A child in convulsive status epilepticus (CSE) is in danger of death or other serious harm if the attacks are not stopped promptly. Healthcare professionals should be knowledgeable and skilled to stop CSE, and basic life support principles (Airway, Breathing, Circulation) should be employed regardless of the setting. Details about the management of CSE and status epilepticus are found in the Appendix.

Conclusion

Seizures and epilepsy remain a very common and important cause of morbidity in the developing world and are likely to occur in patients in refugee camps and disaster zones. There are additional challenges to be faced: the lack of access to trained personnel and diagnostics, unavailability of many drugs, coupled with beliefs about seizures and epilepsy that are difficult to change. The differential diagnosis will also be significantly different with more emphasis on tropical infections, birth complications, and trauma. However, a healthcare worker who can think calmly and carefully about the patient's history and examination findings can make a considerable difference to the patient.

The history and examination will be that much more important in this setting, with particular emphasis on birth history and childhood infections. Video evidence is tremendously helpful and parents and caregivers should be encouraged to try and capture this in some way even with a basic smartphone. Many of the common epilepsies and seizure types can be confidently diagnosed based on history and analysis of recorded footage without the need for further specialist tests. If there is doubt, a video can be easily shared with specialists working remotely who can provide expert advice and guidance.

Basic life support principles are the cornerstone of managing convulsive status epilepticus irrespective of location, and parents anywhere can be taught basic life support measures. The limited arsenal of drugs available will still treat and stabilize most seizure scenarios you are likely to encounter. The AEDs Phenobarbitone, Carbamazepine, Phenytoin, and Diazepam are all safe and highly effective and are more likely to be available in these settings.

As there may be superstition and stigma attached to the lay public's view of epilepsy, importantly parents should be educated about epilepsy and seizures. They should be counseled that it is not infectious and cannot be caught from another person, that it is not the fault of the patient or family, not due to supernatural forces, and can be treated and controlled to allow children to live normal lives.

Acknowledgments My thanks to Dr. Christopher Harris, Dr. Aravind Ramesh, and Dr. Anand Ramesh for helpful discussion and amendments.

Appendix: Epilepsy in Resource Poor Settings

Non-Epileptic Seizure Phenomena

The following are common occurrences that may be mistaken for seizures by parents and important to recognize and educate in the refugee setting.

Phenomena	Features
Febrile seizures	Caused by immaturity of the brain to cope with a sudden rise in body temperature. Most common type of non-epileptic seizure, affects 4% of children, mainly in second year of life, but can occur between age 6 months and 6 years. Usually short (<5 min) and self-limiting. Should be treated (e.g., rectal diazepam) if >5 min. Important to consider the presence of brain infection (e.g., meningitis, encephalitis, malaria)
Breath Holding Attacks	**Blue** breath-holding attacks: toddlers having a temper tantrum/crying—hold their breath—faint or have a brief motor generalized/focal seizure. Distraction may help to prevent these. **White/Pallid** breath-holding attacks: Painful stimulus causes a sudden low heart rate (vagocardiac reflex) with short loss of consciousness and seizure.

Phenomena	Features
Jitteriness	Exaggerated startling in awake newborn babies. Movement can be stopped by holding the jittering limb. Hypoglycemia, hypothermia, and infection should be excluded.
Benign sleep myoclonus	Jerky limb movements in healthy infants <4 months of age during sleep, not involving the face. Harmless and resolves over time.
Behavioral stereotypies	Infants in the second half of the first year of life, when restrained shows complex repetitive stereotyped movements of the head, trunk, and limbs
Syncope/fainting	School children and teenagers—triggered by postural change, standing for a long time, heat, dehydration, skipping meals. May have a brief seizure (reflex-anoxic seizure) without postictal confusion
Benign paroxysmal vertigo	Young children <4 years, episodes of sudden falling or swaying but remains conscious. Resolves within 6–12 months, often a forerunner of migraine
Daydreaming	Common in primary school children—often mistaken for absence seizures, child is staring but is distractable and responds to name or tactile stimulus
Dissociative state	Adolescents/adults, caused by panic or anxiety, triggered by emotionally charged situations when individual feels anxious, agitated, or overwhelmed.
Tic or habit spasm	Irregular contractions of muscle groups—face or limbs. Can be voluntarily controlled for a short period of time. Often runs in families.
Cardiac dysrhythmia	Some heart rhythm abnormalities (e.g., long QT syndrome) can result in sudden onset of extremely low or fast heart rates, leading to loss of consciousness and anoxic seizure. A 12 lead ECG with rhythm strip should be performed if this is suspected.

Different Types of Epilepsy

Tonic clonic or major or grandmal seizures consist of a sudden loss of consciousness with collapse or fall and initial stiffness (tensing) of the whole body followed by generalized convulsive movements. The attack involves the facial muscles, the trunk, and limb muscles. Urinary and fecal incontinence and tongue biting may occur. Most attacks are self-limiting and cease in a matter of minutes. Occasionally attacks go on for longer periods.

The EEG between attacks (interictal record) usually shows epileptic abnormalities in 50–80% of patients but in other 20% it may be normal.

The prognosis for major motor seizures is variable. In most children attacks cease with natural remission after 2 or 3 years.

Carbamazepine, Phenobarbitone, Phenytoin, and Valproate are useful drugs in epilepsy with generalized or focal tonic clonic seizures. Newer anti-epilepsy drugs (AEDs) are available in resource rich nations and those include Levetiracetam, Lamotrigine, and Topiramate being most commonly used.

Focal motor seizures are episodes of twitching and jerking involving one side of the body which can spread to become generalized. This epilepsy suggests structural pathology in both children and adults. However, in a significant proportion of children there may be no lesion. In fact, the commonest focal motor epilepsy occurring in older children is "benign centro-temporal/rolandic epilepsy" of childhood which is genetically determined and shows no structural brain lesion.

It is benign as the prognosis is very good for cessation of seizures after 2–3 years. The EEG shows sharp and spike wave focus in one and the other central and temporal regions. Carbamazepine is very effective and less desirable alternatives are Phenobarbitone and Phenytoin.

Myoclonic and drop attacks are sudden shock like jerks which are bilateral and symmetrical associated with sudden head flexion or extension. They can be violent as to make the child drop/collapse to the floor and the child may immediately get up. They are associated with generalized discharges of slow spike and wave on EEG.

Other types of drop attacks involve temporary loss of postural tone (atonic attacks) and cuse the child to collapse to the floor.

Such attacks may occur in genetic generalized epilepsy though more often they are seen in epilepsy due to an underlying cause or brain damage.

Absence/Petit Mal seizures are episodes of impaired consciousness without significant motor accompaniments. The child stops, ceases whatever activity he is engaged in ("motor arrest") and looks vacant for 5–20 s and then resumes normal activity as though nothing had happened.

The EEG shows burst of generalized and regular 3 per second spike and wave discharges and these can be precipitated by hyperventilation.

It is very age-related commencing usually between 5–10 years of age. Attacks usually remit after 2 or 3 years in the younger child or by early teenage years. In a small proportion of such children, estimated to be less than 10%, grand mal seizures can occur, particularly in the early hours of the morning.

This epilepsy is always genetic and there can be a helpful family history.

Ethosuximide is the drug of choice in typical absence epilepsy. Sodium Valproate is an excellent alternative.

It is important to remember that Carbamazepine and Phenytoin are specifically contraindicated in absence epilepsy and will make it worse.

Atypical absences are those which do not fit the description of the classic absence seizure—e.g., the seizures last for longer than 30 s or there may be associated complex motor symptoms like twitching of the eyelids (myoclonus) or automatisms.

The EEG does not show the regular 3 per second spike and waves of classic childhood absence; instead it may show generalized bursts of irregular polyspikes and wave or slow spike and wave pattern. Often these children have associated developmental delay. The prognosis is less favorable. Sodium Valproate is very useful. An alternative would be Phenobarbitone. Carbamazepine and Phenytoin are specifically contraindicated.

As mentioned earlier daydreaming can often be mistaken for absence epilepsy.

Temporal lobe epileptic attacks are focal and dyscognitive with altered or impaired consciousness associated with the patient experiencing strange, odd sensations while displaying complex semi-purposeful movements. The sensations patient experiences may be visual, auditory (sounds and voices may appear), sensations of vertigo may be experienced or gustatory/olfactory (peculiar tastes and sensations of smell) or emotional sensations, for example loss of reality, fear, laughter or excessive familiarity and so on. The child may talk nonsense during the episode and may display chewing or swallowing movements. Very often patients have an aura before the attack commences. The child may also display complicated movement during the attack such as aimless wandering. If fear is a significant accompaniment the child may look terrified and wide eyed. Such attacks commonly last a few minutes with significant postictal tiredness. It is quite conceivable that in developing countries or areas of the world that retain beliefs in possession and witchcraft, temporal lobe epilepsy may be mistaken for such supernatural phenomena with consequent mismanagement or failure to present.

The EEG often shows epileptic focus with spike and sharp waves in one or the other temporal region. Such attacks may progress to major motor seizures.

Behavioral disorders and specific learning disorders are often seen in children with temporal lobe epilepsy than among children with genetic generalized epilepsy. Drugs which are very helpful include Levetiracetam, Carbamazepine, and Phenytoin.

Epileptic spasms are seen in infancy when they are called "epileptic infantile spasms," commencing usually between 3–8 months of life. The majority show flexor spasms or Salaam attacks occurring in clusters of several seizures. The child may also show extension of the head and neck and limbs. Individual spasms last 1–3 s and occur in clusters lasting 10–20 min. In most instances epileptic spasms indicate an underlying serious brain disorder and no cause is found only in a small minority. Such children may have had normal development until the spasms commence although the majority have preexisting developmental delay before the onset of the infantile spasms.

Epileptic spasms can be caused by multiple causes, including perinatally acquired brain injury, post meningitic and posttraumatic brain injury, and genetic conditions like tuberous sclerosis.

The EEG in epileptic infantile spasms shows the pattern known as "hypsarrhythmia" which is a chaotic high voltage irregular EEG with superimposed multifocal spikes and spike wave bursts followed by periods of suppression.

Treatment is with either Vigabatrin or corticosteroids though the latter has a minor superiority.

Once again smartphone videos can be invaluable in the resource poor setting to help diagnose this condition in the absence of EEG, and steroids should be widely available (?)

Symptomatic epilepsies commonly associated with underlying structural brain injury or genetic or chromosomal conditions. Hence, it is commonly associated with cerebral palsy or severe learning disability and concurrent abnormal neurological findings.

The cause may be prenatal, perinatal, or acquired. Genetic conditions associated with brain malformations may be associated with epilepsy, for example, tuberous sclerosis, arteriovenous malformations, and hydrocephalus.

Epilepsy is an uncommon mode of presentation of brain tumors as most tumors of children are infratentorial affecting the brain stem and the cerebellum.

Many of the cerebral degenerative disorders associated with epilepsy are symptomatic. Most often tonic clonic, myoclonic, and complex absences may be the clinical seizure types seen in symptomatic epilepsy with the exception of true absence. Myoclonic seizures, drop attacks and infantile spasms are particularly associated with symptomatic epilepsy.

Anticonvulsants which are helpful include Levetiracetam, Lamotrigine, and Sodium Valproate.

The prognosis is generally poor for seizure control with AEDs.

Side Effects of AEDS

All anti-epileptic drugs (AEDs) can have side effects on chronic usage though only a small proportion of patients suffer them. All AEDs should be started at low dose and the dose increased every 4–7 days to avoid excessive tiredness and sleepiness.

Phenobarbitone can cause sedation at higher doses.

Phenytoin can produce cosmetic side effects including coarsening of facial features and gum hypertrophy and cerebellar ataxia with high blood levels.

Carbamazepine can cause double vision and tiredness 30–40 min after administration. For this reason, this medication is also available in slow release form. Carbamazepine can cause a skin rash in 3–4% of children and it may have to be stopped.

Valproate does not cause sedation. In children with undiagnosed mitochondrial metabolic disease, it can cause severe liver dysfunction and may be fatal. For this reason, this AED is best avoided in children under 3 years of age as a regular AED in refugee and disaster zone settings.

Common Anticonvulsants Dose and Side Effects

AED	Common	Rare
Ethosuximide	Nausea, Rash	Bone marrow depression
Carbamazepine	Rash, fatigue, dizziness	Bone marrow depression
Phenobarbitone	None with low doses	Sedation
Phenytoin	Ataxia, gum hyperplasia, hirsutism, rash	Facial coarsening
Levetiracetam	None	Behavior disturbance
Lamotrigine	Rash	Stevens Johnson's syndrome
Benzodiazepines	Drowsiness, salivation	

Treatment of Convulsive Status Epilepticus (CSE)

A convulsing child should be seen immediately and after a brief assessment, attempt to stop the convulsion as soon as possible. A child in CSE is in danger of death or other serious harm if the attacks are not stopped promptly. Healthcare professionals should be knowledgeable and skilled to stop CSE and there are basic life support principles (A,B,C) that can be employed regardless of the setting.

Make sure the Airway is clear, the child is breathing, and check the pulse (circulation)

First Aid

The individual should be placed in the safe semi-recumbent recovery position to ensure patency of the upper airway. The tongue remains on the side of the mouth with an opportunity for the saliva and secretions to flow out.

Insert an oral airway (Guedel) or a tracheal tube that can be passed as far as the back of the throat.

Anti-epilepsy Drug Treatment in Status Epilepticus

First line is Diazepam or Paraldehyde rectally.

Diazepam can be given rectally 0.5 mg/kg and it acts almost immediately to stop the seizure. This is very safe and is an excellent anti-epilepsy drug.

An alternative will be rectal Paraldehyde if available. This is given at a dose of 0.3 ml/kg mixed with an equal volume of Arachis or Olive oil. It is an excellent AED, which will almost always stop the seizures without respiratory depression.

In advanced countries, buccal Midazolam is used as first line and administered at a dose of 0.3 mg/kg, into the cheek pouch. It is dispensed in ready prefilled syringes for buccal administration. The doses are as follows:

- Infants <12 months 2.5 mg
- Children between 2– and 5 years, 5 mg
- Children between 5 and 8 years, 7.5 mg
- Children between >9 years, 10 mg

Parents of children with established epilepsy and prone to recurrent seizures in advanced countries are instructed in the use of these drugs and are provided with a supply to be kept at home.

What to Do If Rectal Medication Fails to Stop the Seizure

One of either Diazepam, Midazolam or Lorazepam if available can be given intravenously, but has to be injected slowly over 2–3 min. They will cause respiratory depression if given rapidly and there should be facilities for resuscitation.

Venous access and access to intravenous drugs are likely to be nonexistent in refugee camps and disaster zones; so it is likely that rectal diazepam will be the mainstay of initial stabilization and this is an excellent choice.

Second line AED for CSE is intravenous Phenytoin 18 mg/kg given over 10–15 min. Phenytoin ideally needs to be given with heart rate monitoring or by feeling the child's pulse continuously.

Third line AED if the first two drugs fail to stop the seizures, diverge depending on the resource setting the patient is in. In low resource settings intravenous Phenobarbitone 20 mg/kg injected over 10–15 min is very effective and helpful. An alternative would be intravenous Sodium Valproate 20 mg/kg given over 5–10 min.

In advanced countries, if second line Phenytoin fails after 30 min of the patient presenting to the Accident Emergency Department, rapid induction of anesthesia with Thiopentone and artificial ventilation is employed and the patient is transferred to an intensive care unit.

Management of Convulsive Status Epilepticus

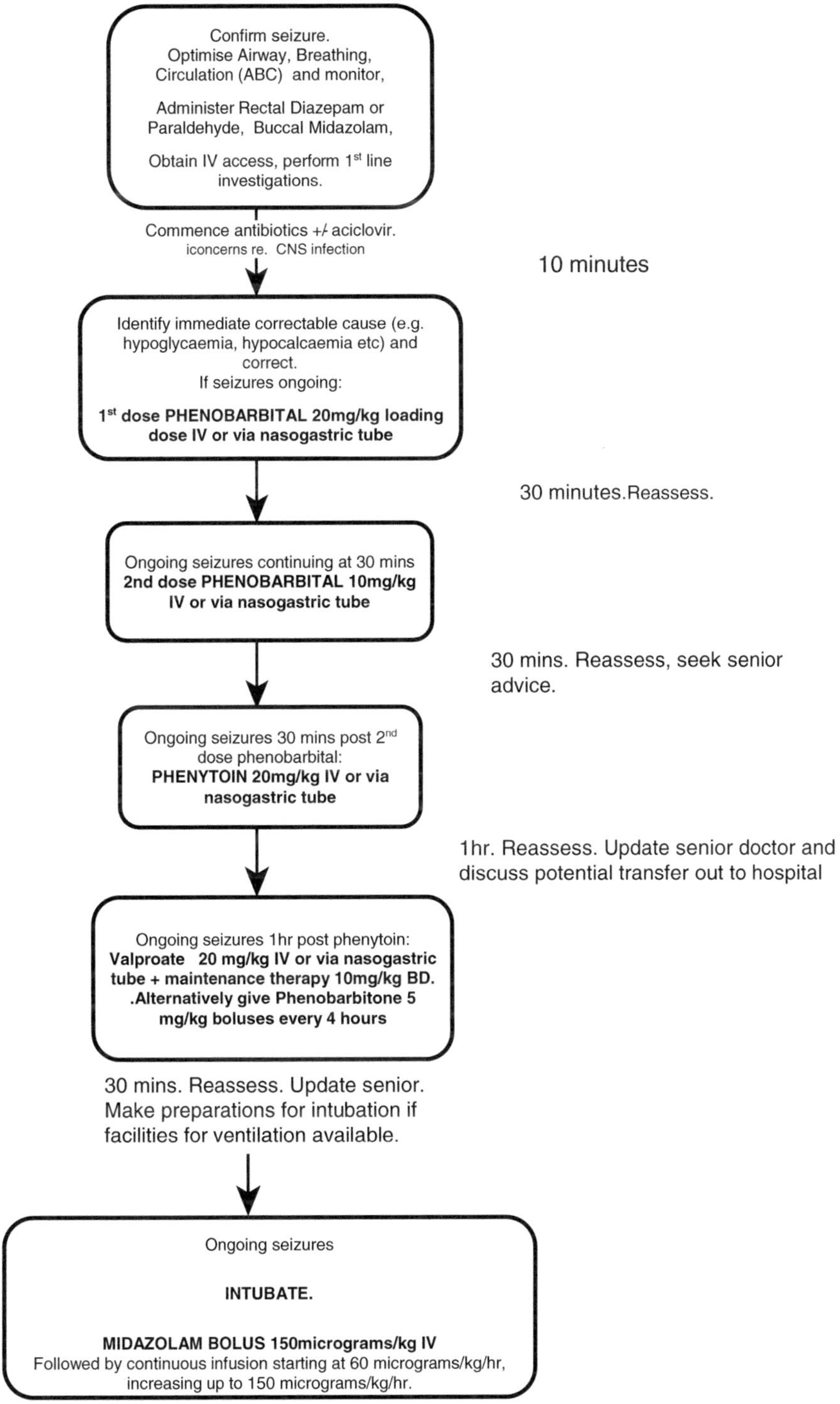

Confirm seizure.
Optimise Airway, Breathing, Circulation (ABC) and monitor,

Administer Rectal Diazepam or Paraldehyde, Buccal Midazolam,

Obtain IV access, perform 1st line investigations.

Commence antibiotics +/- aciclovir.
iconcerns re. CNS infection

10 minutes

Identify immediate correctable cause (e.g. hypoglycaemia, hypocalcaemia etc) and correct.
If seizures ongoing:

1st dose PHENOBARBITAL 20mg/kg loading dose IV or via nasogastric tube

30 minutes.Reassess.

Ongoing seizures continuing at 30 mins
2nd dose PHENOBARBITAL 10mg/kg IV or via nasogastric tube

30 mins. Reassess, seek senior advice.

Ongoing seizures 30 mins post 2nd dose phenobarbital:
PHENYTOIN 20mg/kg IV or via nasogastric tube

1hr. Reassess. Update senior doctor and discuss potential transfer out to hospital

Ongoing seizures 1hr post phenytoin:
Valproate   20 mg/kg IV or via nasogastric tube + maintenance therapy 10mg/kg BD. .Alternatively give Phenobarbitone 5 mg/kg boluses every 4 hours

30 mins. Reassess. Update senior. Make preparations for intubation if facilities for ventilation available.

Ongoing seizures

INTUBATE.

MIDAZOLAM BOLUS 150micrograms/kg IV
Followed by continuous infusion starting at 60 micrograms/kg/hr, increasing up to 150 micrograms/kg/hr.

Further Reading

Aicardi J. Textbook of epilepsy in children. New York: Raven Press; 1994.

Berhanu S, Alemu S, Prevett M, et al. Primary care treatment of epilepsy in rural Ethiopia: causes of default from follow-up. Seizure. 2009;18:100–3.

Chin JH. Epilepsy treatment in sub-Saharan Africa: closing the gap. Afr Health Sci. 2012;12:186–92.

Kale R. Bringing epilepsy out of the shadows. BMJ. 1997;315:2.

Meyer AC, Dua T, Ma J. Global disparities in the epilepsy treatment gap: a systematic review. Bull WHO. 2010;88:260–6.

World Health Organization. Epilepsy in the WHO African region: bridging the gap. The global campaign against epilepsy: "Out of the shadows". Geneva: WHO; 2004.

Online Resources

Online 'Paediatric Epilepsy Training level 1 (PET 1) is run by British Paediatric Neurology Association (BPNA), it is a low-cost course accessible from anywhere in the world. https://courses.bpna.org.uk/index.php?page=paediatric-epilepsy-training

Venkateswaran Ramesh, MBBS, DCH, FRCP graduated in medicine from Pondicherry, India. He trained in pediatrics in India and later in Birmingham and Glasgow, UK. He then specialized in pediatric neurology in Newcastle at Tyne and Manchester. He has worked as a consultant in pediatric neurology for the past 28 years currently at Kings College Hospital London, a major international hospital with clinical problems seen both in resource poor settings as well as in an advanced developed country. Its location is in a deprived part of London, meaning it has huge ethnic diversity and draws patients from over 40 different nations across five continents. The UK NHS has allowed him to provide comprehensive healthcare to patients, free at the point of delivery, and to practice ethical medicine delivering high quality, evidence-based care to children and young people, without monetary or external pressures.

Children with Chronic Diseases in Refugee and Disaster Settings

31

Eva Holsinger

Introduction

Worldwide, chronic diseases (noncommunicable diseases or NCDs) affect 10–30% of children and continue to rise. Duration and management (versus cure) of the condition are the main factors in defining chronic diseases well as their primarily noninfectious nature. Common chronic conditions include asthma, type 1 diabetes, leukemias and lymphomas, hemoglobinopathies, acquired and congenital heart disease, food and respiratory allergies, kidney disorders, epilepsy, and metabolic, genetic, and neurodevelopmental disorders. In addition, malnutrition and stunting, obesity, anemia, tooth decay, and psychiatric disorders and PTSD may be included. Some of these will be discussed in more detail in other chapters and are only briefly referenced here.

While some countries have fairly well-established systems to care for children with chronic diseases, low-and middle-income countries often have many competing priorities for health care. This reduced prioritization of NCDs often leads to crisis intervention as the primary treatment modality, rather than having a prevention and monitoring strategy for children with these diseases and their families. Even in higher income countries, access to appropriate care may be challenging for subsets of a country's population, including minority groups, immigrants, and refugees. Mental health concerns related to chronic diseases in children remain a challenge for families and health care systems even in optimal circumstances.

E. Holsinger (✉)
Liaoning International General Health Trainers, Shenyang, China

H'Image Doctor International Clinic, DeJi Hospital, Shenyang, China

© Springer Nature Switzerland AG 2021
C. Harkensee et al. (eds.), *Child Refugee and Migrant Health*,
https://doi.org/10.1007/978-3-030-74906-4_31

Practical Issues in Disaster Settings

The challenges facing children with NCDs in relatively stable settings become magnified exponentially in emergencies. As resources become even more scarce, the needs likewise grow. A study from Syria showed that 1 in 5 refugees had emotional, physical, or intellectual impairment [1]. As displaced children and their families leave their communities of origin in states of crisis and move unpredictably and often transiently from place to place, much attention to chronic conditions will fall by the wayside. Medical records, continuity of care, access to necessary supplies and long-term medications, as well as to laboratory and radiologic monitoring become inaccessible. Health care providers will likely be fewer than before, and the experience and knowledge base regarding chronic childhood diseases among health care providers encountered en route may be limited [2]. Language and cultural barriers as patients move away from their home communities form additional obstacles to providing even minimal care for many chronic diseases in children. In addition, if even available, the cost of obtaining necessary services and supplies (Table 31.1) may be insurmountable barriers for the family in a refugee or disaster setting. When medications are available, their potency is reduced in situations with increased heat and humidity. New onset diagnoses may present too late and result in otherwise preventable morbidity and mortality in unstable contexts.

Circumstances in the community of origin that lead to flight, or conflicts en route, may also create new conditions resulting in chronic disability—for example, exposure to products of chemical warfare in Syria has been shown to result in adverse pregnancy and birth outcomes in exposed women, including various congenital birth defects [3]. Bombs, guns, fires, and landmines can lead to permanent disability from injuries sustained, including traumatic brain injury, loss of vision, hearing, and limbs as well as disfiguring burns. Infectious diseases such as measles or malaria may result in permanent disabilities. Less conspicuously, multiple studies have demonstrated general immunosuppression in both children and adults during disasters, placing children at greater risk of acquiring infectious diseases and other secondary conditions. Physical symptoms such as chronic abdominal pain and chronic headaches may also result from ongoing stress and trauma, leading to increased distress in the child and caregivers.

Table 31.1 Supplies that may be difficult to procure in disaster settings

Insulin	Special foods and formula
Steroids	Devices to assist mobility
Inhalers	Physical therapy
Materials for kidney dialysis	Psychotherapy
Analgesics	Special education
Antibiotics	Anti-seizure medication
Epi-Pen	Supplemental oxygen

Social Barriers to Care

Children in disaster and refugee settings experience multiple obstacles to receiving appropriate care due to cultural views about the origin of diseases. For example, some cultures uphold that if a family has a disabled child, they must have done something to offend evil spirits, or made a serious mistake resulting in this punishment. Children with disabilities or chronic diseases may be hidden out of sight of the general public, whether due to cultural beliefs and fears or social stigma and ostracization by the community at large.

With the accessibility of social media in virtually every country in the world, rumors and misinformation often spread more rapidly than factual information, and can plant seeds of doubt about the role of health care professionals. While some myths are less destructive (such as eating raw onions or bathing in saltwater to prevent illness), efforts to control Ebola virus outbreaks in Guinea in 2014 were significantly hampered by the false belief that foreign health workers had brought the virus with them to the country [4, 5]. Local and foreign health care workers' attitudes, as well as discrepancies between international regulations and local laws and opinions, may further hinder treatment efforts. While health workers from outside the community may be viewed with suspicion and mistrust, reliance on traditional health providers within the community is often quite strong. Potential partnerships with key local persons of influence may significantly enhance building of trust. Furthermore, conflict may occur among health care workers about best approaches to diagnosis and treatment of chronic conditions, and acute illnesses are frequently prioritized for treatment. Resources for acute diseases may be more readily available.

Models of Care and Practical Solutions

Approaches to identifying and caring for children with chronic diseases in a disaster context must consider the location and context, balancing safety with access to services and distance to needed specialties. Local resources and appropriate alternatives should be identified, and an understanding of cultural preferences is essential. The skills of readily available health care workers and the knowledge base of parents and caregivers about the condition must be assessed. One must also ask whether the existing conditions can be prevented by certain changes in health behaviors and other mitigating factors.

Advocacy for children with chronic illnesses is a key aspect. General health surveys and community assessments should include ways to identify these children and learn which chronic diseases may be more prevalent in a particular setting. Sources of needed medications and supplies should be found, as well as acceptable alternatives in the community. A number of international associations focusing on specific chronic illnesses may have online consultation options with specialists if none are available in the local area (Table 31.2).

People with specific skills and backgrounds in the community should also be identified and given opportunities to get involved in caring for these children. For

Table 31.2 International networks with resources to help children with chronic illnesses

International Society for Developmental Pediatrics https://developmentalpediatrics.net/
Neph Cure Kidney International for children with nephrotic Syndrome https://nephcure.org/
International Society of Nephrology https://www.theisn.org/
International Society for Children with Cancer (ISCC) https://iscc-charity.org/
International Diabetes Federation https://idf.org/
The International League Against Epilepsy https://www.ilae.org/
Society for the study of Inborn Errors of Metabolism https://www.ssiem.org/
World Allergy Organization https://www.worldallergy.org/
World Asthma Foundation https://worldasthmafoundation.org/
International Children's Heart Foundation https://www.babyheart.org/
International Children's Palliative Care Network http://www.icpcn.org/
Meg Foundation for Pain www.megfoundationforpain.org
Hesperian Health Guides www.hesperian.org

instance, some people may help build mobility devices, administer physical therapy, and provide much-needed play therapy and mental health support for children and their caregivers. Community volunteers and caregivers should be trained as needed to ensure that minimum standards are maintained and that interventions are not inadvertently harmful to the child. Consider organizing respite care for families, if possible.

Nonpharmacological Pain Management

Pain can be a component of many chronic diseases of childhood, whether due to the disease process or due to the result of medical testing and interventions. Type 1 diabetes, for example, requires frequent blood glucose monitoring and multiple daily administrations of insulin in many situations. Although technology reducing the frequency of injections such as continuous glucose monitoring and insulin pumps may be available in a child's community of origin, these methods require an ongoing need for very specific supplies, which may not be accessible in refugee settings. This may necessitate changing treatment modalities for the child with Type 1 diabetes to multiple daily injections and glucose sampling. Other chronic diseases require intermittent painful procedures, such as blood draws, catheterization, or biopsies. Some children have experienced multiple surgeries and painful recoveries as a result of their chronic condition, including debridement of burns, setting fractures, suturing lacerations, lumbar punctures, blast injuries, arthritis, or juvenile migraines.

Different cultures have varying beliefs about pain, and it is important to recognize these deep-seated beliefs. For instance, pain may be seen as a punishment from God. It may be considered virtuous and honorable to suffer silently through pain. If pain is expressed, this can be seen as a sign of weakness in one's character. The presence of pain can be viewed as a reflection of disharmony and imbalance. While young children (and even many adults) may be unable to verbalize these thoughts, the expectation of what is deemed an acceptable response to pain is instilled from a young age.

Patients in a western context will often receive analgesics and/or benzodiazepines to assist with comfort during painful procedures, but these medications are used infrequently in some cultures even under typical conditions and often are in scarce supply in disaster settings. Hospitals and clinics in developing countries often lack pain medications as well as nonpharmacologic pain management programs, and families often cannot afford to purchase medications for pain. Children, adolescents, and adults suffer unnecessarily.

In approaching children who may be experiencing pain, it is important to understand that a child's reaction to pain relates to both tissue damage and emotional state. Health care providers can speak to children in a way that enhances their sense of mastery and implies that they will recover from this event. Basic cultural understanding about views on pain is crucial to help support both children and families. It is important to use a pain assessment method that takes into account both the child's culture and developmental age. The International Children's Palliative Care Network has developed an app that can be used in a variety of cultural and ethnic contexts to help individuals track pain type and levels over time [6]. Please refer to Chap. 32 for further resources on pain assessment and management.

Nonpharmacological Pain Management Tools

Guidelines for helping a child with pain include first assessing one's personal experiences about pain, assessing parental perceptions and expectations about pain management, and considering the impact of the treatment team on the child. With regards to the child, consider his/her age and developmental stage, learning styles, strengths and difficulties, as well as preferences and dislikes. The child's control and mastery should be emphasized. Caregivers and health care workers should avoid trying to control a child's perception or understanding of pain.

Children with a history of multiple painful procedures and/or recurrent pain may have severe behavioral responses to stimuli such as seeing a hospital, a uniformed staff, or an object associated with traumatic events. Even very young children may have nightmares, flashbacks, and other symptoms of PTSD. Whether or not pharmacologic treatments are used, children with recurrent pain may benefit greatly from learning self-regulation methods. These include comfort kits, simple biofeedback, self-hypnosis, and phone apps such as Healing Buddies, Bounceback, or Inner Balance. The care team can offer massage, music therapy, acupressure, distraction such as blowing bubbles or pinwheels, and even simply watching videos on a phone or computer. Children can participate in making suggestions for pain control. Positive feedback should be given. These skills help children acquire self-confidence and a sense of being in control, which helps them cope as adults as well as during childhood.

The Meg Foundation for Pain [7] has produced free high-quality videos directed at children and their caregivers, to empower children with nonpharmacological strategies to reduce pain. The videos have been translated into Arabic, Chinese, Spanish, and Thai languages.

Downloads in multiple languages are also available on www.hesperian.org for a number of resources for helping children with disabilities and chronic diseases.

References

1. Jabri S. The children with autism spectrum disorders in syrian crisis: challenges and recommendations. IJEMH. 2015;17(4):676–7.
2. Medecins Sans Frontieres. Children with chronic diseases need our attention. 9 Apr 2019 [cited 2020 Jun 18]. Available from: https://www.msf.org/children-chronic-diseases-need-our-attention-child-health
3. Omar H, Jabri S. Adverse birth outcomes in women exposed to Syrian chemical attack. Lancet Glob Health. 2015;3(4):e196. Available from: https://www.thelancet.com/action/showPdf?pii=S2214-109X%2815%2970077-X
4. World Health Organization. Busting the myths about Ebola is crucial to stop the transmission of the disease in Guinea. Apr 2014 [cited 2020 Jun 18]. Available from: https://www.who.int/features/2014/ebola-myths/en/
5. Buli BG, Mayigane LN, Oketta JF, Soumouk A, Sandouno TE, Camara B, et al. Misconceptions about Ebola seriously affect the prevention efforts: KAP related to Ebola prevention and treatment in Kouroussa Prefecture, Guinea. Pan Afr Med J. 2015;22(Suppl 1):11. https://doi.org/10.11694/pamj.supp.2015.22.1.6269. Available from: https://pubmed.ncbi.nlm.nih.gov/26740839/
6. International Child Palliative Care Network. ICPCN pain assessment tool for children. 2015 [cited 2020 Jun 18]. Available from: http://www.icpcn.org/icpcn-pain-assessment-tool-for-children/
7. Meg Foundation for Pain. Pain management and prevention resources to help you #beapainchampion [cited 2020 Jun 18]. Available from: www.megfoundationforpain.org

Eva Holsinger, MD completed her medical training at the University of Oklahoma College of Medicine, and her pediatric residency at Akron Children's Hospital in Ohio. She completed a fellowship in Global Child Health at Rainbow Babies and Children's Hospital in Cleveland, Ohio, and has lived and served in northeast China since 2009. Her focus has been vulnerable children in orphanages and in the community, focusing on children with special needs, and pediatric education of family medicine doctors. She is passionate about advocating for children and mothers. She is the happy wife of Brian and mother of five children as well.

Palliative Care

32

Megan Doherty, B. Emily Esmaili, and Farzana Khan

Introduction

This chapter addresses care for children with serious health-related suffering in the humanitarian context, focusing on the provision of palliative care. Palliative care for children aims to relieve pain and other physical symptoms while addressing the emotional, social, and spiritual needs of children and their families. Focusing on improving the quality of life both for the child and the family, palliative care promotes comfort and dignity for any child with a serious health problem, regardless of whether the illness is expected to be cured. Palliative care does not seek to hasten death and instead may prolong survival for those with serious illnesses [1].

In humanitarian crises and low-resource settings, there may be illnesses where potentially curative or disease-controlling treatments are not available and palliative care is provided. Palliative care should not be considered a substitute for illness prevention, diagnosis or treatment, and efforts to increase access to palliative care

M. Doherty (✉)
Program Director, Pediatric Palliative Care, Two Worlds Cancer Collaboration Foundation, Kelowna, BC, Canada

Children's Palliative Care Initiative in Bangladesh, World Child Cancer, Dhaka, Bangladesh

Pediatric Palliative Care, Children's Hospital of Eastern Ontario and Roger Neilson House, Ottawa, ON, Canada

University of Ottawa, Ottawa, ON, Canada
e-mail: mdoherty@cheo.on.ca

B. E. Esmaili
Duke Global Health Institute, Duke University, Durham, NC, USA

Lincoln Community Health Center, Durham, NC, USA
e-mail: bee6@duke.edu

F. Khan
Fasiuddin Khan Research Foundation (FKRF), Dhaka, Bangladesh

© Springer Nature Switzerland AG 2021
C. Harkensee et al. (eds.), *Child Refugee and Migrant Health*,
https://doi.org/10.1007/978-3-030-74906-4_32

"

should be accompanied by work strengthening access to medical care aimed at illness prevention, diagnosis, and treatment. It is never acceptable medically or morally to abandon a sick child. Palliative care should be universally accessible and is an essential component of humanitarian crisis response.

It is appropriate to start palliative care early in the course of a serious illness. Palliative care should not be reserved only for children reaching the end-of-life. Palliative care should be continued throughout the course of treatment for any serious illness, whether the outcome is cure or death [2]. When curative treatment for an illness is no longer possible, palliative care may then be the only beneficial type of care, and thus always should be accessible for children at the end-of-life.

Palliative care should be available and accessible in all settings, including children's homes or shelters, clinics, hospitals, refugee camps, and hospice facilities. The nature of palliative care provision will depend on the resources available, but there are common principles and treatment options that should be applied in all settings and resource levels.

Clinical Vignette

Mojibor is a 10-year old Rohingya boy with bone cancer living in a refugee camp in Bangladesh. When he was diagnosed at the refugee camp field hospital, Mojibor and his mother cried all night fearing he would soon die. Mojibor has two little sisters. His father is missing. We found Mojibor in a tent lying on a mat, unable to move or walk because of his pain. In the past, Mojibor was a typical football-loving boy. His nickname was 'bhuissya,' meaning 'buffalo'. We started pain treatment with paracetamol and then morphine, and soon Mojibor began to walk and even smile a little. Palliative care has improved the quality of Mojibor's life and has given much needed comfort to his family.

Which Children Should Receive Palliative Care?

Palliative care is appropriate for children with serious health-related suffering, including illnesses which are life-threatening (potentially curable) or life-limiting. Children with life-limiting illnesses have unique palliative care needs that are distinct from adults. Palliative care can help children with a range of illnesses, including neonatal conditions, congenital anomalies, cancers, as well as cardiac, respiratory, gastrointestinal, infectious, and neurological conditions in which the prognosis is difficult to predict. There are four broad groups of serious health conditions (Table 32.1) that can help professionals understand which children would benefit from palliative care. Additionally, in humanitarian crises and low-resource settings, palliative care clinicians should seek to address untreated acute suffering whenever it occurs [3].

Worldwide, children with neonatal conditions, such as prematurity, hypoxic ischemic encephalopathy, and those with congenital anomalies, constitute the largest groups requiring palliative care (Fig. 32.1).

Table 32.1 Categories of life-limiting and life-threatening conditions [4]

Category 1	*Life-threatening conditions for which curative treatment may be feasible but can fail* Access to palliative care services may be necessary when treatment fails or during an acute crisis, irrespective of the duration of threat to life. On reaching long-term remission or following successful curative treatment there is no longer a need for palliative care services. Examples: cancer, irreversible organ failures of heart, liver, kidney.
Category 2	*Conditions where premature death is inevitable* There may be long periods of intensive treatment aimed at prolonging life and allowing participation in normal activities. Examples: cystic fibrosis, Duchenne muscular dystrophy.
Category 3	*Progressive conditions without curative treatment options* Treatment is exclusively palliative and may commonly extend over many years. Examples: Batten disease, mucopolysaccharidoses.
Category 4	*Irreversible but nonprogressive conditions causing severe disability, leading to susceptibility to ill health* Children can have complex health care needs, a high risk of an unpredictable life-threatening event or episode, health complications, and an increased likelihood of premature death. Examples: severe cerebral palsy, multiple disabilities, such as following brain or spinal cord injury.

Reprinted with permission from Together for Short Lives (Bristol, UK)

Common Barriers to Palliative Care and Potential Solutions

Delays in Initiating Palliative Care for Children

Uncertainty about the likelihood of survival often causes clinicians to delay initiating palliative care, and while the trajectory for many serious pediatric illnesses can be uncertain and unpredictable, palliative care is recommended for all children with a serious condition starting at the time of diagnosis [2]. Many times, palliative care is only started once aggressive medical treatment or potentially curative therapies are stopped or are no longer effective; however, early palliative care is recommended, since it provides symptom management, psychological, social, and spiritual support for children and families facing the challenges of serious illness and its treatment.

Parents may be hesitant to accept palliative care, possibly believing that this means their child's condition is incurable. Clinicians should address this misconception, and it can be helpful for clinicians to specifically state that introducing palliative care does not necessarily mean that the child's condition is incurable. Clinicians should explain the role of palliative care, including focusing on ensuring comfort and providing additional support for the whole family, including parents, siblings, extended family, and the child's wider community (e.g., friends, neighbors, schoolmates, etc.)

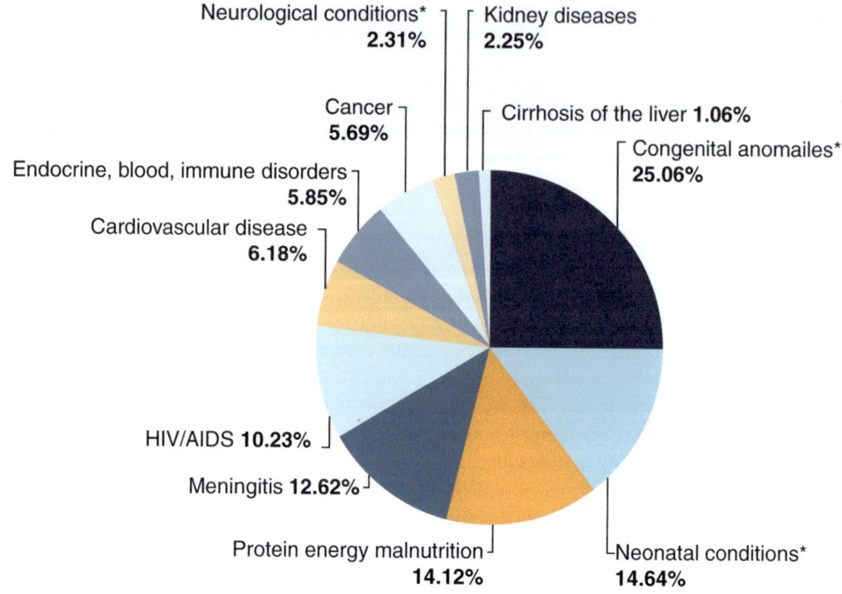

* see excluded conditions Appendix 6

N = 1,170,011

Fig. 32.1 Distribution of children in need of palliative care at the end-of-life by disease groups [5]. (Reprinted with permission from the Worldwide Hospice Palliative Care Alliance (London, UK))

Obtaining Essential Medicines for Children

Restricted access to opioids is another common challenge in palliative care, due to overly strict opioid regulations and lack of awareness about the safety and efficacy of these medicines for children. Clinicians should be aware of the important role of opioids in the relief of moderate to severe pain in children and should advocate for appropriate access to opioids in all settings where children receive health care.

Principles of Symptom Assessment and Relief

Adequate and appropriate symptom management and relief of physical suffering should be viewed as a human right and should be available to all children irrespective of the probability of survival. Children's physical symptoms are frequently under-recognized by health care providers due to limited knowledge of appropriate assessment tools for children and limited skill in assessing or communicating directly with children. Adults may wrongly assume that children are not experiencing pain or other symptoms if they are quiet or do not voice any complaints. However, children may not express due to fear of receiving painful treatment or out of a desire to please the adults around them. Developing a trusting relationship with the child is the foundation of effective symptom assessment and should be a priority for health care professionals providing symptom relief for children.

Most symptoms can be addressed following a stepwise approach (discussed in further detail below):

1. Assessment (rapid assessment if the symptom is severe)
2. Treatment of the symptom
3. Treatment of the underlying cause, if possible
4. Regular reevaluation and modifications to the treatment as needed

A complete symptom history may include:

- Location (especially relevant for pain)
- Onset
- Duration
- Severity (see below for suggested pain severity scales)
- Quality—which words are used by the child to describe the symptom (e.g., burning or stabbing for pain)
- Aggravating or relieving factors
- Effects on the child's sleep, daily activity, appetite, and mood

Detailed guidance for relief of all symptoms in children with serious illnesses is beyond the scope of this chapter and can be found in other resources, such as Basic Symptom Control in Pediatric Palliative Care [6].

Pain Relief

Palliative care extends well beyond pain relief, but effective analgesia is a critical component of palliative care. Opioids can be safely and effectively used in children of all ages who have moderate or severe pain. For clinicians who have limited experience in the use of opioids, we recommend connecting with colleagues in pain medicine or anesthesia for guidance and support, if available. Although confusion is common, providing adequate pain relief with opioids is very different from euthanasia or medical assistance in dying. When used appropriately, by following dosing and titration guidelines, opioids do not hasten death.

Pain Assessment

There are validated tools for assessing pain severity in children of any age and any ability to communicate:

- FLACC scales (Table 32.2) may be used for **infants, toddlers, and older non-verbal children**
- Faces Pain Scale-Revised (Fig. 32.2) can be used for **children 4 years and older**
- Numerical Rating Scale (where the child is asked to rate their pain from 0 to 10, with 10 representing the worse pain) can be used for **children 8 years and older**

Table 32.2 Revised FLACC scale [7]

	0	1	2
Face	No particular expression or smile	Occasional grimace/frown; withdrawn or disinterested; appears sad or worried	Consistent grimace or frown; frequent/constant quivering chin, clenched jaw; distressed-looking face; expression of fright or panic
Legs	Normal position or relaxed; usual tone and motion to limbs	Uneasy, restless, tense; occasional tremors	Kicking, or legs drawn up, marked increase in spasticity, constant tremors, or jerking
Activity	Lying quietly, normal position, moves easily; Regular, rhythmic respirations	Squirming, shifting back and forth, tense, or guarded movements; mildly agitated (e.g., head back and forth, aggression); shallow, splinting respirations, intermittent sighs.	Arched, rigid, or jerking; severe agitation; head banging; shivering (not rigors); breath holding, gasping or sharp intake of breaths, severe splinting
Cry	No cry/ verbalization	Moans or whimpers; occasional complaint; occasional verbal outburst or grunt	Crying steadily, screams, or sobs, frequent complaints; repeated outbursts, constant grunting
Consolability	Content and relaxed	Reassured by occasional touching, hugging, or being talked to. Distractible.	Difficult to console or comfort; pushing away caregiver, resisting care, or comfort measures

Instructions: Each of the five categories is scored from 0 to 2, giving a total score of 0–10
Source: From Malviya, Voepel-Lewis, Burke, Merkel, and Tait (2006)

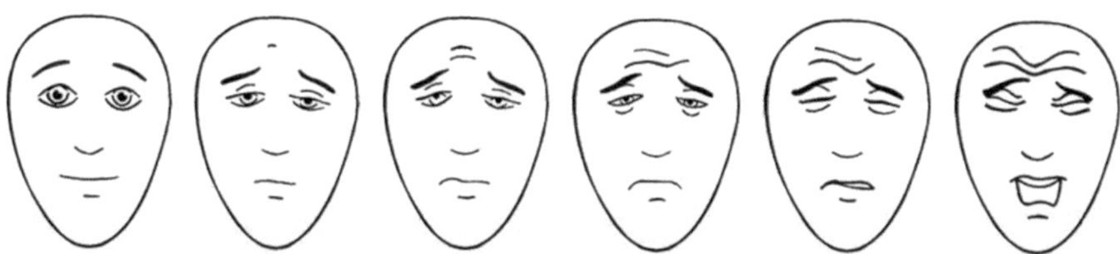

Fig. 32.2 Faces Pain Scale—Revised (FPS-R) for children 4 years and older. Translations and instructions available at: https://www.iasp-pain.org/Education/Content.aspx?ItemNumber=1823& navItemNumber=1119. (Reprinted with permission from Mapi Research Trust)
*These faces show how much something can hurt. This face [point to left-most face] shows **no pain**. The faces show more and more pain [point to each from left to right] **up to this one** [point to right-most face]—it shows **very much pain**. Point to the face that shows how much you hurt [right now].*

General measures, including keeping the child comfortable (warm or cool, depending on conditions) and providing regular human contact (being held by parents or trusted adults), should always be provided. Providing opportunities to play is particularly important for distraction and as a support for psychosocial aspects of a child's pain. Additional non-pharmacological techniques, such as music, massage, relaxation and breathing techniques, and hypnosis, should be considered; however, such non-pharmacologic treatments alone are not first line for severe pain. Several resources describing these treatments in more detail can be found at the end of this chapter.

When pharmacological treatment is needed for severe pain, the following four principles should guide treatment [8]:

- **By the ladder—If pain occurs drugs should be administered following a two-step ladder as follows.**
- **By mouth**—the oral route of administration is simplest and safest, and thus preferable if the child can swallow medicines.
- **By the clock**—pain medicines should be given at fixed intervals for pain, which is constant or persistent, with the next dose given before the previous dose has worn off. This will improve pain control and reduce the amount of medicine needed for adequate analgesia.
- **For the individual**—pain treatment is tailored to the child's unique needs and response to treatment, relieving the child's pain to a level which is acceptable for the child and caregivers. Generally, the dose of pain medicine should be titrated by 25–50% when pain control is inadequate.
- **With attention to detail**—the pain relief regimen should be clearly explained and written out for the patient and their family. The possible adverse effects of each medicine should be explained.

Initiation of Pain Relief

- Children should be started on analgesics which are appropriate to their type and severity of pain
    - Step 1: Mild analgesics (e.g., paracetamol, NSAIDs) should not be given alone for moderate or severe pain
    - Step 2: Strong opioids (e.g., oral morphine) should be started for moderate or severe pain (generally 4–10/10 on pain severity scales)
    - Dosing guidelines for morphine or other strong opioids are shown in Table 32.3

Codeine should not be used in children due to the significant risks of respiratory depression and toxicity due to indivdual variation in the rate of drug metabolism. Tramadol also should be avoided in children due to concerns about safety and variation in drug metabolism with age and nutritional status. However, the choice of opioid may be determined by availability, and if tramadol is the only strong analgesic available, it may be used with caution. Acceptable PO tramadol dosing is 1–2 mg/kg every 4–6 h (maximum initial single dose of 50 mg; maximum of 4 doses in 24 h) [6].

Clinicians should be aware of common opioid side effects of constipation, nausea, and drowsiness (generally resolves after several days and often represents children catching up on sleep now that their pain is adequately managed).

Table 32.3 Strong opioid dosing guidelines [4, 6]. (Disclaimer: Medication and doses are provided here for general guidance only. Prescription requires a qualified medical professional and appropriate individual medical assessment)

Drug	Route	Usual Starting Dose		Dosing Interval	Maximum Starting Dose
Morphine	PO (immediate release)	0.2-0.3mg/kg/dose		4 hrs	10mg
	IV, SC	0.05-0.1mg/kg/dose		2-4 hrs	5mg
	IV/SC Infusion	0-6 mon	10-20mcg/kg/hr	Continuous	
		>6 mon	10-40mcg/kg/hr		
		Breakthrough	20-50mcg/kg/dose	2 hrs	
Hydromor phone	PO	30-80 mcg/kg/dose		3 hrs	2mg
	IV, SC	10-20 mcg/kg/dose			0.6mg
	IV/SC Infusion	4-6 mcg/kg/hr		Continuous	
		Breakthrough	10-20mcg/kg/dose	2 hrs	
Fentanyl	Trans-dermal	Do not use for opioid naïve patients, convert from rapid acting opioids once pain is controlled with stable dose of opioid		48 or 72 hrs	25mcg/hr
	IV	0.5-1mcg/kg/dose		1 hr	Dose limit of 4 mcg/kg/dose
	IV Infusion	1-3mcg/kg/hr		Continuous	3mcg/kg/hr
		Breakthrough	0.5-1mcg/kg/dose	1 hr	

Discussing Goals of Care and Advance Care Planning

To minimize confusion and encourage trusting therapeutic relationships, it is crucial to clarify the goals of care for a seriously ill child with all stakeholders, which may include the child, their caregivers or other family members, and clinicians. For such meetings, clinicians should begin by clarifying the child and/or family's understanding of the illness, with gentle correction of any misunderstandings, which may entail giving bad news (see section on "Communication"). If possible, bad news should be communicated in a quiet, private location, and clinicians should prepare by turning off mobile phones and pagers, requesting not to be disturbed during the encounter, and considering in advance what they will say and what next steps to suggest. Clinicians should be prepared for strong emotional responses, including anger and grief, and should always listen patiently. Sometimes, bad news can be communicated gradually over several hours or days.

To reach agreement about goals of care, clinicians also should explore the family's values and perspectives regarding health, disability, and suffering. Treatment options should be reviewed, and the potential benefits and harms of each treatment should be described.

Families have multiple goals. For example, for a child with leukemia and a serious infection, the goals may be to treat the infection and to prepare the child for treatment of leukemia, but also to maximize comfort. This is a typical situation in which disease treatment and palliative care should be simultaneous and complimentary. However, in different situations where further disease-specific or life-sustaining treatment is not available, would provide no benefit, or would be more harmful than beneficial, the only goal of care may be comfort. In this situation, focussing exclusively on palliative care may be appropriate.

Symptom Control in the Last Hours and Days of Life

If symptoms are not well managed, not only the child will suffer, but this suffering may be the family's final memory of their child's life. Anticipate and plan for how to manage physical symptoms, by following guidelines and standardized protocols.

For a dying child admitted to the hospital, clinicians often recognize that certain assessments (e.g., routine vital signs) and treatments are not clinically indicated. However, it may be difficult for some families to accept discontinuation of these treatments, which they may perceive as an indication that the medical team is "giving up" on their child.

Thus, a flexible approach, such as intermittent monitoring of vital signs, may be considered. It is important to recognize that in resource-limited settings, monitoring and intravenous fluids administration ensure that nurses provide regular bedside visits. If these are discontinued, then it is important to ensure that there will be regular visits, which can often be done by initiating regular pain and symptom assessments and treatments.

Rapid titration of symptom control medicines is often necessary for the last days and hours of life and providing adequate appropriate symptom relief is not the same as euthanasia or medical assistance in dying. If dosing and titration guidelines are followed, these medicines will not hasten death.

Pain, Dyspnea, and Agitation

Pain, dyspnea, and agitation are common symptoms requiring intensive treatment near the end-of-life. To facilitate rapid titration (over minutes to a few hours), ensure that all medicines, including opioids, are available at the bedside. There is no ceiling dose of opioids for symptom management in the last hours or days of life, as the correct dose is that which relieves the symptoms. Do not be afraid to increase the dose of morphine and other medicines to ensure pain and other symptoms are well controlled. See Box 32.1 for a suggested symptom management protocol.

The subcutaneous (SC) route is particularly useful in this phase of illness, to avoid needing to maintain IV access. A SC butterfly needle can be kept in place for up to 7 days provided the SC site does not have any significant redness or tenderness. SC doses are the same as the IV dose with maximum volume per SC injection of 1.5–2 ml. Pediatric dosing information can be found in the references listed at the end of the chapter [6].

Medicines which can be given SC include:

- *Opioids*: Morphine, hydromorphone, fentanyl, methadone, oxycodone, diamorphine
- *Sedative-hypnotics*: Midazolam, clonazepam, phenobarbital
- *Antiemetics*: Haloperidol, metoclopramide, levomepromazine (methotrimeprazine)

> **Box 32.1: Suggested Guidelines for Management of Escalating Pain, Dyspnea, and Agitation in Children (Adapted from Interdisciplinary Textbook of Pediatric Palliative Care [4]).**
> **(Disclaimer: Prescribing requires an individual assessment of the patient by a qualified medical practitioner. Doses provided may not be suitable for all ages.)**
> **Loading dose:**
>
> - *For patients already on opioids*: administer loading dose of opioid equal to 10% of total dose in past 24 h
> - *For patients not already on opioids*: administer IV or SC loading dose as follows:
> - *Less than 12 years*: 0.1 mg/kg
> - *12 year or older*: IV/SC morphine 5 mg
> - (Note: this same dose of morphine can be started for opioid naïve patients with moderate to severe pain)
>
> **Subsequent dosing:** doses may be given every 10 min PRN for end-of-life symptoms
> Escalate dose as follows: (Note: 5 mg is given as an example, actual dose may vary)
>
> - First dose: 5 mg, if ineffective after 10 min, then give
> - Second dose: 5 mg, if ineffective after 10 min, notify prescriber then give
> - Third dose: 7.5 mg (1.5× starting dose), if ineffective, after 10 min then give
> - Fourth dose: 7.5 mg (1.5× starting dose), if ineffective, after 10 min then give
> - Fifth dose: 10 mg (2× starting dose)
>
> Once good pain relief is achieved, provide the total dose administered during the rapid titration phase regularly every 4 h and as a PRN (as needed dose for breakthrough symptoms). Do not use only as needed doses as this will allow the symptoms to return and will lead to more distress. Pain assessment may be by pain scale or observations of verbal and nonverbal behavior (crying, grimacing, and moaning either at rest or when moved).
> **Adjuvant therapy for symptoms which may accompany pain or dyspnea:**
> **For agitation:** (recommended starting dose)
>
> - PO/IV/SL/PR Lorazepam 50 mcg/kg/dose or PO/SC/IV Midazolam 100 mcg/kg/dose: PRN for anxiety/agitation
> - SC/IV/PO Haloperidol 12–25 mcg/kg/dose: PRN for hallucinations/agitation

- *Anti-secretory agents*: Hyoscine butyl bromide, hyoscine hydrobromide, glycopyrrolate, octreotide
- *Antihistamines (which have antiemetic properties)*: Cyclizine, promethazine
- *Miscellaneous*: Dexamethasone, Methylnaltrexone, Naloxone, Furosemide

Seizures/Convulsions

Seizures may be uncomfortable and disturbing, so anticonvulsant therapy should be continued even when the goal of care is comfort only. Generally, in end-of-life situations, a full investigative workup is not necessary. If the child has a known seizure disorder and can no longer swallow medicines, SC medicines should be used.

For acute treatment of status epilepticus, give Diazepam, Lorazepam, or Midazolam. Repeat after 15 or 30 min if needed. If ineffective, consider doubling the dose of Midazolam or Diazepam, or give Phenobarbital. This should be followed with regular doses of Phenobarbital to prevent further seizures. The starting doses for medicines to treat status epilepticus are shown in Table 32.4.

If a child is likely to have prolonged seizures at home, parents should be trained in the use of sublingual lorazepam (if available) or rectal diazepam as abortive medicines. Rectal administration can be by syringe through a small feeding tube cut at 5 cm, inserted up to 4–5 cm beyond the anal margin for an older child and 1–2 cm for an infant [10].

Anorexia or Loss of Appetite

Reduced oral intake is a normal part of the dying process and children who are close to death typically do not feel hunger or thirst. Parenteral fluids should be avoided as these do not improve symptoms or quality or duration of life for patients who cannot drink, and instead may cause distress from edema or dyspnea [11, 12]. Swabbing the child's mouth with water and applying petroleum jelly or lip balm to the lips will provide comfort by preventing dry mouth.

Table 32.4 Seizure treatment dosing guidelines [6, 9]

Drug	Route	Pediatric dose		Dosing interval	Maximum dose
Midazolam	Buccal or IM	IM: 0.3 mg/kg/dose		5 min	10 mg
		Buccal: 0.5 mg/kg/dose		5 min	
	Intranasal	0.2 mg/kg/dose		5 min	5 mg per nostril
Diazepam	IV	0.3 mg/kg/dose		5 min	5 mg (<5 years) I 10 mg (>5 years)
	PR	0.5 mg/kg/dose		5 min	20 mg
Lorazepam	Buccal/SL, PR, IV	0.1 mg/kg/dose		5 min	4 mg
Phenobarbital (loading dose)	PO, IV/SC	Neonate	10–20 mg/kg	Once, see below	Maximum cumulative loading dose: 40 mg/kg Given over 20 min
		>1 month	20 mg/kg	Once, see below	Given over 20 min
Phenobarbital (maintenance)	PO, IV/SC	Neonate	3–5 mg/kg/day	12–24 h	5 mg/kg/day
		Infants	5–6 mg/kg/day	12–24 h	200 mg/day

Respiratory Secretions

Children often have impaired ability to swallow at the end-of-life and difficulty clearing secretions and this can result in gurgling or rattling sounds, aspiration, coughing, choking, and dyspnea. If there is respiratory congestion (e.g., gurgling or rattling sounds), but no evidence of discomfort, the family should be reassured that the child is comfortable, while if there is evidence of discomfort (e.g., crying, panicked look) then treatment should be provided.

Positioning the child on his/her side with the upper body elevated will allow secretions to passively drain out of the mouth. Medicines such as **Atropine 1%** (eye drop solution—apply 1–2 drops to oral mucosa q1h as needed), **Glycopyrrolate** (PO 40 mcg/kg q6–8h, can titrate up to 100 mcg/kg/dose), **Hyoscine butyl bromide** (PO or IV 0.3–0.5 mg/kg q6–8h), or **Hyoscine hydrobromide** (PO or SL 10 mcg/kg/dose q6–8h) can also be used to reduce oral and respiratory secretions [6]. Glycopyrrolate and hyoscine butyl bromide may be preferable as they do not cross the blood-brain barrier and thus do not cause sedation.

Communication and Psychosocial Support

Refugee and migrant children frequently experience significant psychological and emotional trauma resulting from loss of family members or friends, forced displacement, witnessed violence, and living in unpredictable contexts. Among children with serious illnesses, such trauma increases the risk of long-term morbidity and mortality. Careful planning and communication are needed to ensure the continuum of care. It is important to make available multidisciplinary support from social workers, psychologists, chaplains, teachers, art therapists, play therapists, or child life specialists, whenever possible. Spiritual support should be available to children and can be facilitated by linking with chaplains and religious leaders in the community.

The role of play as a means of expression and emotional support is particularly important for children and should be considered integral to the provision of palliative care for children, particularly since ill children are made more vulnerable due to their illness or disability. It is important to consider how to provide appropriate toys as well as sufficient play opportunities even in places where resources are limited [13].

A child's age and developmental stage should be taken into consideration when communicating with them about their health and prognosis. Table 32.5 outlines general conceptions of and reactions to death at different ages. In addition, Boxes 32.2 and 32.3 provide communication strategies.

Care of the Dying Child (Last Days and Hours)

It can be challenging to identify when death is imminent. Observations which can help identify when children are in the final stages of life include:

- Very tired and weak, majority of time spent sleeping or lying down
- Little or no oral intake and difficulty swallowing
- Decreased urine and stool output
- Altered level of consciousness—confused, agitated, restless, or drowsy
- Changes in pulse, blood pressure, and breathing
- Cool and mottled extremities

Table 32.5 Conceptions and reactions to death by age

Age	Common conceptions and reactions to death, and expressions of grief
Infants (0–2 years)	• Nonverbal communication • Tone, volume of speech, gestures, and facial expressions are particularly important at this stage • Physical contact such as hugging and rocking may be effective and soothing • No concept of death, but aware of separation, which may be disturbing
2–4 Years	• Verbal, prefer concrete questions • Conceive of death as something reversible (e.g., may still expect deceased family members to return)
4–8 Years	• Still prefer concrete questions, more ability to respond to open-ended questions • Later in age range idea of death as permanent develops • Some magical thinking about causes of death (may include assigning blame, e.g., "if I hadn't done that, this wouldn't have happened.")
8–12 Years	• May be more demanding of answers, more able to start engaging in developed conversations • Concept of personal mortality emerges • More interest in what happens after death, recognizing its permanence
12 Years and older	• Ability to understand abstract ideas (including abstract and philosophical ideas around death) • Able to express full range of emotions

---

Box 32.2: Tips for Communicating with Caregivers and Family Members of Seriously Ill Children

- Sit down and give the family your undivided attention for 5–10 min, in the most quiet and private location possible
- Involve additional health care team members such as the child's nurse and a psychosocial counselor in the meeting if possible
- Be gentle but honest. Honesty does not lead to a loss of hope for caregivers, but instead demonstrates truthfulness and transparency, which is valued by families and it allows them to plan for their child's future
- Avoid saying "there is nothing more that can be done," since there are always things that can be done, such as treating pain and other symptoms
- Use the checklist in Box 32.3 to guide the conversation when you expect that death is expected soon. This sequence follows evidence about the best structure for delivering difficult news and discussing goals of care, based on language which has been developed and tested with parents and families

> **Box 32.3: Key Steps for a Conversation to Inform a Family That Death is Expected (Adapted from Serious Illness Conversation Guide-Pediatric Adaptation [12])**
>
> - Set up the conversation by introducing yourself and asking permission to proceed: "Can I talk to you about what is happening to your child?"
> - Assess their understanding of the illness: "What is your understanding of where your child is with regard to his/her illness?"
> - Ask about how much information they would like: "How much are you willing to hear about your child's present condition and what is likely to come?"
> - Share prognosis: "I wish it were different, but I am worried that your child is very sick and will not be able to recover from this illness. We do not have any treatments which can cure this problem and I am worried that he/she is not going to live for very long."
> - Assess goals: "What are your goals or desires, given the information I have shared with you?"
> - Establish plan: "I recommend that we focus on providing care which ensures that he/she is comfortable and can be with those he/she loves."
> - Close the conversation: "We will be here to treat and support your child and your family." Share a telephone number so that they can reach a health care provider anytime they are needed.

When asked about how long the child is expected to live, it is best to acknowledge uncertainty while providing a general time range if possible. For example: "It can be difficult to predict, but I worry that because her condition is very unstable and we are seeing changes every few hours, she may live for hours to a few days." Changes in the child's condition are the best guide for prognostication. If changes are hourly, death is generally expected in hours to several days. If daily, death is expected in days to several weeks. If a change happens every week or every few weeks, death may be expected in weeks to months.

After a child dies, it is important to respect cultural values related to care of the body and burial and funeral rites. Engaging with local spiritual and religious leaders to better understand the community's cultural practices can assist health care providers who may be unfamiliar with these specific issues.

Home-Based Palliative Care

Many families will wish to provide end-of-life care for their children at home, and this can be facilitated in most settings, including refugee camps or temporary dwellings. Always ensure that the caregivers have a 24-h contact number for support if needed. Trained family members may be able to provide symptom management as outlined above, with appropriate support as needed. Remind them to keep the child clean and dry using cloths or pads for urinary incontinence. Do not force the child to eat or drink. Remind them to give the medicines to control symptoms at prescribed times; do not wait for the symptoms are severe as this will make them more difficult to control. Connect caregivers with spiritual or religious leaders for support if requested and emphasize the importance of self-care.

Memory Making

Parents should be encouraged to keep tangible objects (e.g., clothing, blankets, toys, photographs) to remember their child, as this helps support them in their grief. This is especially important in a pregnancy loss or infant loss, where the child's life was short and few people aside from the parents may have known or met the child. Do not encourage the parents to quickly forget the child, "move on" or have another child as this can lead to more complicated and prolonged grief [14].

Supporting Staff Who Provide Palliative Care

Staff who witness death and suffering in children may experience moral distress, compassion fatigue, and burnout. Staff support meetings can be used to create a safe space for staff to reflect and express their emotions. Commemorating patients through annual hospital memorial services, attending funeral services, or having follow-up contact with families is important for health care providers. Letters, phone calls, or text messages from staff are deeply valued by families who often treasure the memories of these small acts of kindness by staff [15].

Special Situations

Unsuccessful Resuscitation

During resuscitation, allowing the family to be present may lead to less anxiety, depression, and second-guessing about staff competence. A member of the health care team should update the family frequently about what is happening and provide emotional support.

In resource-limited settings, a clear policy should establish under what circumstances resuscitation should be initiated, continued, terminated, and withheld. Ideally, this policy should be written with involvement of both clinicians and the population being served. This can help to avoid accusations of discrimination or unjust use of resources. Resuscitation that continues longer than clinically indicated should be avoided as this may lead to unnecessary distress both for staff and for the family [16].

Discontinuing Ventilatory Support

It may be ethically appropriate to discontinue mechanical ventilation in certain circumstances. For example, it may become clear that the underlying cause of ventilator dependence is irreversible and that continued respiratory support will prolong or exacerbate suffering. It is essential to involve the family in the decision to discontinue ventilatory support. Involving religious or cultural leaders is also advised, if possible.

After discontinuing ventilation, most patients live only minutes or hours; however, there are some children who live for a few days or longer. Clinicians must prepare the family for the possibility that the child may continue to breathe on his or her own for some time, especially neonates and young children. Further guidance on the process of ventilator withdrawal is available [10].

Outbreaks, Epidemics, and Pandemics

Large-scale outbreaks of infectious diseases can be particularly devastating for vulnerable populations such as children with palliative care needs living in refugee camps or other similar settings. These children often have complex medical needs requiring significant care in an already resource-limited setting and may suffer significantly when resources are further depleted in an outbreak situation. Moreover, when demand for advanced medical equipment, such as ventilators, exceeds the capacity of the health system, children with preexisting serious health conditions may be subject to difficult rationing decisions. It is advisable for health care organizations and facilities to establish fair resource allocation guidelines prior to an outbreak to ensure that decisions follow ethical principles [17, 18]. During public health crises, it is particularly important to advocate for the needs of those who are the most vulnerable, including children with palliative care needs.

References

1. Hoerger M, Wayser GR, Schwing G, Suzuki A, Perry LM. Impact of interdisciplinary outpatient specialty palliative care on survival and quality of life in adults with advanced cancer: a meta-analysis of randomized controlled trials. Ann Behav Med Publ Soc Behav Med. 2019;53(7):674–85.
2. Palliative care for children. Pediatrics. 2000;106(2):351.
3. World Health Organization. Integrating palliative care and symptom relief into paediatrics: a WHO guide for health-care planners, implementers and managers. Geneva: World Health Organization; 2018. p. 66. Available from: http://apps.who.int/medicinedocs/en/m/abstract/Js23559en/.
4. Wolfe J, Hinds PS, Sourkes BM. Textbook of interdisciplinary pediatric palliative care. Philadelphia: Elsevier Health Sciences; 2011. 514 p.
5. Worldwide Palliative Care Alliance. Global atlas of palliative care at the end of life. London; 2014. p. 111. Available from: http://www.who.int/nmh/Global_Atlas_of_Palliative_Care.pdf.
6. Basic symptom control in paediatric palliative care: the rainbows children's hospice guidelines. 9.5. Bristol: Together for Short Lives; 2016. 356 p.

7. Malviya S, Voepel-Lewis T, Burke C, Merkel S, Tait AR. The revised FLACC observational pain tool: improved reliability and validity for pain assessment in children with cognitive impairment. Paediatr Anaesth. 2006;16(3):258–65.
8. World Health Organization. WHO guidelines for the pharmacological and radiotherapeutic management of cancer pain in adults and adolescents. WHO; 2018 [cited 2019 Apr 18]. p. 144. Report No.: 1. Available from: https://www.ncbi.nlm.nih.gov/books/NBK537492/pdf/Bookshelf_NBK537492.pdf.
9. Lexicomp, Inc. Lexicomp online database. Lexicomp, Inc. [cited 2020 Jan 10]. Available from: http://online.lexi.com.
10. A field manual for palliative care in humanitarian crises. Oxford, New York: Oxford University Press; 2019. 160 p.
11. Bruera E, Hui D, Dalal S, Torres-Vigil I, Trumble J, Roosth J, et al. Parenteral hydration in patients with advanced cancer: a multicenter, double-blind, placebo-controlled randomized trial. J Clin Oncol. 2013;31(1):111–8.
12. Tsai E. Withholding and withdrawing artificial nutrition and hydration. Paediatr Child Health. 2011;16(4):241–2.
13. Boucher S, Downing J, Shemilt R. The role of play in children's palliative care. Children. 2014;1(3):302–17.
14. Cortezzo DE, Sanders MR, Brownell EA, Moss K. End-of-life care in the neonatal intensive care unit: experiences of staff and parents. Am J Perinatol. 2015;32(8):713–24.
15. Macdonald ME. Parental perspectives on hospital staff members' acts of kindness and commemoration after a child's death. Pediatrics. 2005;116(4):884–90.
16. Jabre P, Belpomme V, Azoulay E, Jacob L, Bertrand L, Lapostolle F, et al. Family presence during cardiopulmonary resuscitation. N Engl J Med. 2013;368(11):1008–18.
17. Scheunemann LP, White DB. The ethics and reality of rationing in medicine. Chest. 2011;140(6):1625–32.
18. Emanuel EJ, Persad G, Upshur R, Thome B, Parker M, Glickman A, et al. Fair allocation of scarce medical resources in the time of Covid-19. N Engl J Med. 2020;382:2049–55.

Additional Resources

Basic symptom control in pediatric palliative care. https://www.togetherforshortlives.org.uk/resource/basic-symptom-control-paediatric-palliative-care/ (provides treatment recommendations for common symptoms and dosing recommendations for palliative care medicines).

Healing buddies comfort kit. http://www.healingbuddiescomfort.org/ (free app applying integrative medicine techniques for pain and symptom management).

Integrating palliative care and symptom relief into paediatrics: a WHO guide for health-care planners, implementers and managers. https://apps.who.int/iris/handle/10665/274565. Geneva: World Health Organization; 2018.

Integrating palliative care and symptom relief into responses to humanitarian emergencies and crises A WHO guide. https://apps.who.int/iris/handle/10665/274565. Geneva: World Health Organization; 2018.

Meg Foundation. https://www.megfoundationforpain.org/resources-home (age-appropriate videos and tutorials on pain management using various non-pharmacological techniques).

Megan Doherty, MD, FRCPC a specialist in pediatric palliative care at the Children's Hospital of Eastern Ontario and Roger Neilson House (pediatric hospice) in Ottawa, Canada. Dr. Doherty has experience in the development of palliative care programs for children in humanitarian crises and other resource-limited settings, while leading the Children's Palliative Care Initiative in Bangladesh and the Pediatric Palliative Care Program of Two Worlds Cancer Collaboration in Hyderabad, India, as well as in her role as a telemedicine consultant for Médecins Sans Frontières. She has also been instrumental in the development of palliative care programs for children in humanitarian crises situations, focusing on capacity building and training for health care workers and innovative models of community-based palliative care programs.

Emily Esmaili, DO, MA, FAAP is a pediatrician with global health experience both locally and internationally. After residency at Wake Forest Medical Center, she worked in Laos for 2 years as country coordinator and pediatric faculty for the NGO Health Frontiers. She then moved to Rwanda to serve as visiting pediatric faculty through Yale University and the Human Resources for Health program. While there, she helped start a "farm-to-bedside" nutrition program for food-insecure hospitalized children, which she later established as a 501c3, Growing Health, Inc. She then returned to the US to earn her Masters in Global Bioethics and Science Policy from Duke University, followed by a fellowship in refugee child health also from Duke. Dr. Esmaili now works for Lincoln Community Health Center in Durham, NC, which serves primarily low-income, immigrant, and refugee children in the local community, where she also leads a grant-funded outreach program for refugee and immigrant families post-COVID. She has volunteered with humanitarian organizations in Greece, India, Nepal, Rwanda, and along the Thai-Burma border.

Farzana Khan, MA, MPH, MBBS is a palliative care physician and researcher. She is the founder, president, and executive director of Fasiuddin Khan Research Foundation (FKRF), a local nonprofit organization based in Dhaka, which provides palliative care in vulnerable contexts like urban slums, refugee camps, etc. She is IAHPC appointed Advocacy Ambassador of Palliative Care for Bangladesh. She is an affiliated member of RESPIRE, University of Edinburgh. Graduating from Chittagong Medical College in 1994 with an MBBS, she went on to complete an MPH in Public Health at the Independent University, Bangladesh in 2006 and an MA in Palliative Care at the Lancaster University, UK in 2014. She is a fellow of International Pain Policy Fellowship (IPPF) at the Wisconsin University, USA. She has also completed a fellowship in Palliative Medicine from the Institute of Palliative Medicine, Kerala, India in 2011. Currently, she is doing a PhD in Global Health at the University of Edinburgh, UK.

Index

© Springer Nature Switzerland AG 2021

C. Harkensee et al. (eds.), *Child Refugee and Migrant Health*,

https://doi.org/10.1007/978-3-030-74906-4

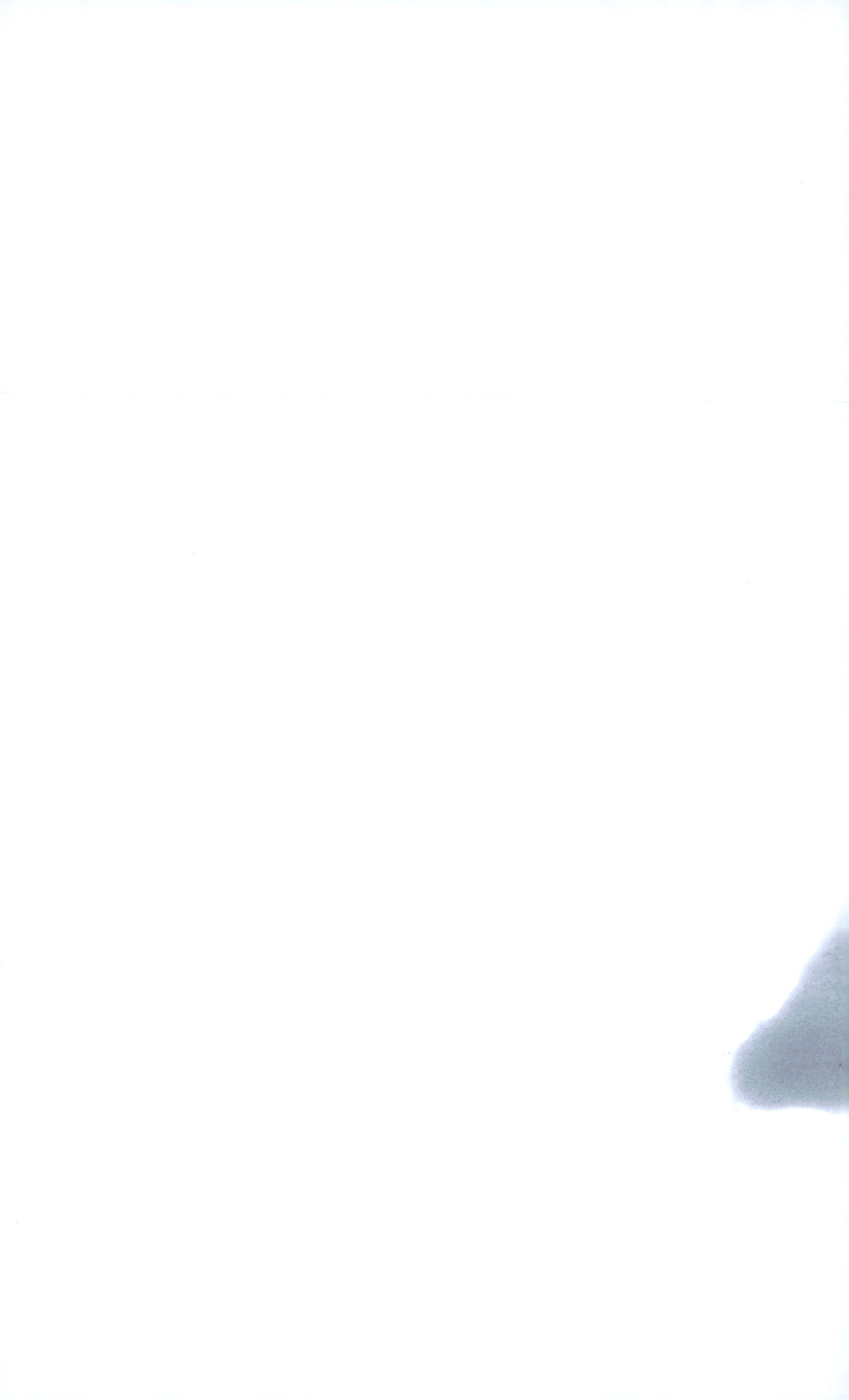